Praise for *Nourishing Menopause*

"Andrea Donsky's *Nourishing Menopause* is a gift to women everywhere. Andrea marries heart with hard data, exploding myths like 'hot flashes are the whole story' and revealing the real, nuanced spectrum of symptoms women live with. . . . If you want compassionate guidance backed by evidence and real-world wisdom, start here."

ANNA CABECA, DO, OB-GYN, FACOG, and the Girlfriend Doctor

"Andrea Donsky reframes menopause from something to endure into an opportunity to truly nourish yourself, connecting symptoms to evidence-based nutrition and lifestyle solutions. This book helps women feel seen, understood, and empowered with tools that make a real difference, physically, mentally, and emotionally."

SARAH WILSON, ND and founder of Canada's largest network of integrative women's health clinics, Advanced Women's Health

"Andrea's book is a gift to women in the menopause transition. . . . *Nourishing Menopause* gives us the knowledge and the tools to successfully make our way through the most significant physical, mental, and psychological transitions of a woman's life. . . Buy an extra copy to share with your bestie, your boss, and your doctor."

DR. FIONA LOVELY, creator of the *Not Your Mother's Menopause* podcast and clinician of twenty-plus years

"*Nourishing Menopause* is the book I wish existed years ago. One that's evidence-based, practical, compassionate, and written in a voice every woman can understand. Andrea blends science, personal experience, and expert insight so beautifully that this has officially become my new menopause bible."

ZORA BENHAMOU, gerontologist, menopause specialist, and host of the *Hack My Age* podcast

"Andrea Donsky is one of my most trusted voices on the relationship between food and health, and a respected advocate for perimenopausal and menopausal women. . . . This book is an invaluable resource for both women and the practitioners who support them."

LAKEISCHA WEBB McMILLAN, MD, integrative OB-GYN, and International Menopause Whisperer™

"Andrea Donsky's *Nourishing Menopause* is THE book I wish every woman had. It meets you with compassion and a clear 'you are not alone' message, while offering practical, science-informed, balanced nutrition and lifestyle support for women forty-plus. What sets this book apart is Andrea's original published research, her deep understanding of nutrition, and most importantly, her lived experience of going through perimenopause and menopause herself."

DANIELLE MEITIV, MS, PHC, thyroid coach,
and founder of ThyroidHealingSolutions.com

"What makes this book so impactful is the way Andrea blends her own lived experience with extensive research and a deep understanding of nutrition. This is powerful knowledge that can truly change how women care for themselves. This book gives women confidence, clarity, and practical tools to nourish their bodies during this important life stage. It is a must-read!"

ANGELA MACGREGOR, founder of the National Menopause Show

"*Nourishing Menopause* offers evidence-based fixes that start on the plate, balanced with movement and recovery tools that fit real life. . . . Whether you're forty-two and cycling irregularly or fifty-eight and years past your last period, this guide meets you where you are. I would place this book in the hands of every forty-plus patient, and every clinician who needs this education."

ASHLEY ALEXIS, ND, and licensed naturopathic medical doctor

"Andrea Donsky has achieved no mean feat: writing the most well-rounded book on how to handle perimenopause and menopause to hit the market. I love how deeply this book dives into symptoms, as Andrea is a leader in this area of research after all . . . I had a much better understanding of how my own body works after reading it!"

ANN MARIE McQUEEN, journalist and founder of Hotflash inc

"*Nourishing Menopause* fills a critical gap with clear, compassionate, evidence-based guidance. It is a modern road map for women and for the partners and clinicians who want to support them better."

Bryce Wylde, BSc, DHMHS, and founder of Husband™

"A thoughtful, evidence-based guide that cuts through confusion and gives women the tools they need to support their health during perimenopause and menopause. It's a resource you need on your bookshelf!"

Nicole Avena, PhD, associate professor of Neuroscience
and author of *Sugarless: A 7 Step Plan to Uncover Hidden Sugars, Curb Your Cravings, and Conquer Your Addiction*

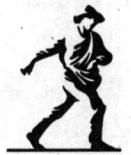

ALSO BY ANDREA DONSKY

Unjunk Your Junk Food: Healthy Alternatives to Conventional Snacks
(with Randy Boyer and Lisa Tsakos)

nourishing meno pause

Powerful Nutrition
and Lifestyle Strategies
to Feel Your Best

andrea donsky

registered holistic nutritionist (R.H.N.)

PUBLISHED BY SIMON & SCHUSTER

New York • Amsterdam/Antwerp • London • Toronto • Sydney/Melbourne • New Delhi

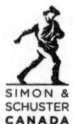

SIMON &
SCHUSTER
CANADA

A Division of Simon & Schuster, LLC
166 King Street East, Suite 300
Toronto, Ontario M5A 1J3

For more than 100 years, Simon & Schuster has championed authors and the stories they create. By respecting the copyright of an author's intellectual property, you enable Simon & Schuster and the author to continue publishing exceptional books for years to come. We thank you for supporting the author's copyright by purchasing an authorized edition of this book.

No amount of this book may be reproduced or stored in any format, nor may it be uploaded to any website, database, large language model, or other repository, retrieval, or artificial intelligence system without express permission. All rights reserved. Inquiries may be directed to Simon & Schuster, 1230 Avenue of the Americas, New York, NY 10020 or permissions@simonandschuster.com.

This publication contains the opinions and ideas of its author. It is intended to provide helpful and informative material on the subjects addressed in the publication. It is sold with the understanding that the author and publisher are not engaged in rendering medical, health, or any other kind of personal professional services in the book. The reader should consult a medical, health, or other competent professional before adopting any of the suggestions in this book or drawing inferences from it.

The author and publisher specifically disclaim all responsibility for any liability, loss, or risk, personal or otherwise, which is incurred as a consequence, directly or indirectly, of the use and application of any of the contents of this book.

Websites referenced in this book are provided for informational purposes only and are not intended as an endorsement or promotion of any website or its contents. Website addresses were accurate at the time the book went to press. The publisher is not responsible for the functionality, content, or legal compliance of any external website and expressly disclaims all responsibility and liability in connection therewith.

I dedicate this book to women in perimenopause and menopause. May you feel seen, heard, and validated. I encourage you to empower yourself with information, a support team you trust, and the treatment options you deserve.

contents

Full references for *Nourishing Menopause* are available online at www.nourishingmenopausebook.com.

FOREWORD

It started with a brain lapse. I had a brilliant idea, and by the time I opened my computer, it was gone. Then came the 4 a.m. wake-ups and itchy ears. I was asked, "Have you had phantom smells yet?" Not at the time . . . but then I did. A lovely sewer smell that only *I* could perceive, despite asking my husband to sniff harder.

My cycles got shorter for a few years. Now they're stretching out again, which, lucky me, cues up ocular migraines. Awesome.

When Andrea told me there are over 103 signs and symptoms of perimenopause, I believed her, but it still blew my mind. So many women are told their symptoms are just *stress*, *aging*, or *normal*, when in reality, it's so much bigger than that.

You might feel completely unprepared, and with good reason. Nobody talked about this for generations. My own mom suffered terrible hot flashes and heavy periods but wasn't offered any solution other than to "chin up." Because this is what women go through.

That narrative is finally changing, thanks to you. You're demanding better healthcare, better answers, and better options for yourself and for the women coming after you.

The perimenopause transition can last six to ten years, or longer, if you still have your ovaries. That's a long time! If you've had them removed, you're considered postmenopausal no matter your age. Either way, the decline in hormones affects *all twelve systems* of your body. That's why there are over 100 possible symptoms. Thankfully, you won't get them all (thank gawd), but you might notice some come and go while others hang out—like that extra belly weight you swear wasn't there last summer.

So does anything good come out of this transition? Oh yes.

I started off telling you about the symptoms I'm experiencing in my own perimenopause journey. But the best part is who I'm becoming. What I stand for. The things I no longer tolerate. The confidence

I've gained. The firmer boundaries. And the unexpected joy of stepping into the next phenomenal era of my life.

In *The Wizard of Oz*, Glinda the Good Witch tells Dorothy that she's always had the power, that she just had to learn it for herself. That applies to perimenopause too.

Because while you might be feeling lost, overwhelmed, anxious, or downright pissed about what's happening, there is *so much* you can do. You truly have the power—once you have the tools.

That's the beauty of this book.

It's your guide for when you're cursing hot flashes, hair changes, or the dryness down there. It answers the questions you didn't even know to ask because, let's be real, they didn't teach *this* in health class.

Why does digestion suddenly feel different—and what can you do about it? Why do you feel like a stressed-out mess whose nervous system is fried? (And WTF *is* a nervous system, anyway?) The internet has you tracking protein grams and scoops of creatine like it's your full-time job . . . except you already *have* a full-time job and don't have time for all this.

You have the power, and by reading this book, you'll learn exactly how to use it. Chapter by chapter, Andrea walks you through the who, what, where, when, why, and how of it all. Whether you're brand new to this phase or have been navigating it for a minute, she's got you.

Andrea is a nutritionist, educator, and published researcher, and she's one of the few voices making perimenopause and menopause feel understandable, hopeful, and even a little bit funny.

So grab your coffee (or your fan), take a deep breath, and get ready. This book is about to change how you think about your body, your hormones, and this wild, wonderful chapter of womanhood.

In joy,

Carrie Jones, ND, FABNE, MPH, MSCP

FOREWORD

Menopause is not an ending but rather a powerful new beginning. Few voices have championed this truth as passionately and effectively as Andrea Donsky has. For decades, Andrea has transformed the conversation around health and nutrition and, more recently, the often-overlooked realities of midlife. Her work is more than research; it is a movement, a call to action for women everywhere to reclaim vitality, confidence, and joy during one of life's most profound transitions.

As a nutritionist, educator, and menopause researcher, Andrea has dismantled myths and built bridges between science and empathy. Through her platform, WeAreMorphus.com, and her far-reaching media presence, she has become a trusted guide for millions. Her ability to blend evidence with actionable strategies makes her work groundbreaking and deeply personal. Andrea reminds women that menopause is not something to fear but something to embrace, a time to rediscover themselves and live fully, vibrantly, and unapologetically.

This book reflects Andrea's unwavering commitment to women's health. Every page is infused with her passion for education and her belief that knowledge is the ultimate tool for transformation. She has created a resource that empowers women to thrive, not just survive, through menopause and beyond.

As someone who has spent a lifetime advancing women's health, I am honored to write this foreword. My own journey as a board-certified ob-gyn, reproductive endocrinologist, and clinical professor at George Washington University School of Medicine has been dedicated to improving healthcare for women at every stage of life. Through more than 450 clinical research trials, 800 publications, and leadership roles as former president of both The Menopause Society and the International Society for the Study of Women's Sexual Health (ISSWSH), I have witnessed firsthand the urgent need for voices like Andrea's. Her work complements decades of medical research with practical, compassionate guidance that women can trust.

Andrea's vision aligns with my own mission: to ensure that every woman has access to accurate information and expert care, and the confidence to navigate midlife with strength and grace. She speaks not only as an expert but as an advocate, a champion for every woman who has ever wondered, *Why didn't anyone tell me this?*

To the reader: As you turn these pages, know that you are not alone. You are part of a powerful community rewriting the narrative of midlife. Let this book be your companion, your guide, and your reminder that you are strong, beautiful, and capable of extraordinary things.

Andrea, thank you for your courage, your wisdom, and your relentless pursuit of truth. This book is a testament to your vision, a vision where every woman thrives in body, mind, and spirit.

With admiration and gratitude,

James A. Simon, MD, CCD, MSCP, IF

CLINICAL PROFESSOR, GEORGE WASHINGTON UNIVERSITY SCHOOL OF MEDICINE

FORMER PRESIDENT, THE MENOPAUSE SOCIETY

FORMER PRESIDENT, INTERNATIONAL SOCIETY FOR THE STUDY OF WOMEN'S SEXUAL HEALTH

1.

Welcome
to the Change

How are you feeling? I mean, *really* feeling?

If I had to guess, I'd say you've had better days.

You're probably exhausted and struggling with brain fog, you've gained weight, your anxiety is out of control, your ears are itchy, you have joint pain, you forgot what you had for breakfast, you have a hard time putting together a sentence, you sweat (a lot), your sex drive is gone, or maybe you're experiencing vaginal dryness, which is making sex uncomfortable, and you're lucky if you get a few straight hours of zzz's a night.

How do I know? Because I've been there myself.

If you feel like someone or something has taken over your body, or you're wondering what happened to your old self, or you wake up every day with another ache, pain, or symptom you didn't have the day before, this book is for you. It's also for you if you want to take charge of your health as you enter into this new chapter of your life. And if you're younger, perhaps in your twenties or thirties, and you've had your ovaries removed and are in surgical menopause, this book is for you too.

I wrote this book with you in mind because, while you may feel like you're the *only one* experiencing what you're going through, I can assure you, you're not.

It's estimated that one billion of us are in menopause right now. That's 1,000,000,000 women around the world who understand you, including me. And this number is expected to increase to 1.2 billion by 2030, with 47 million women entering menopause every year.

Welcome to a New Phase of Your Life

Menopause is a natural biological process that marks the end of a woman's reproductive years, and it's as old as womankind itself.

Despite its long history and commonality, there are myths, misconceptions, prejudices, fears, shame, and misinformation about it that continue to persist, keeping us in a never-ending loop of confusion.

Some of the most common myths and dismissive comments I hear from women in our community are as follows: "You're too young to be in perimenopause or menopause in your forties and fifties," "Nothing can be done to ease your symptoms," "It's a natural part of life, so deal with it," and "You can't be in perimenopause if your periods are still regular." None of this is true. And unfortunately, oftentimes when women share what they're experiencing, they're dismissed.

Whether you've felt dismissed or gaslit or overwhelmed by the sheer volume of information available about menopause these days, this book offers a safe space for insight, compassion, and nourishment, which is exactly why I called it *Nourishing Menopause*.

The word *nourish* comes from the Latin word *nutrire*, meaning to feed, to foster, and to support growth.

I wanted to expand this concept beyond what we put on our plates, because perimenopause and menopause are times in our lives when we need continuous nourishment in every area—mental, physical, and spiritual—so we feel supported, comforted, and cared for as we enter the next chapter of our lives. I know how tough it is and how overwhelming, lonely, and frustrating it can feel when your symptoms take over and it's hard to find the answers you're looking for. I want you to know this: You're not alone.

Your body is asking for a different kind of nourishment now, one that honors the wisdom of slowing down, the power of saying no, and the practice of prioritizing self-care. It also means giving your body the nutrients it needs to thrive, learning how to move in ways that protect your joints and keep your muscles and bones strong as your body changes, saying yes to what helps you feel better without guilt or apology, and releasing what no longer serves you. It's also inviting you to be gentle with yourself as you get to know this new version of who you are, one that will flourish beyond what you can imagine once you move through the rough patches.

With the right nourishment in every area of your life, you can feel cared for, confident, and prepared for the years ahead.

Every part of you matters during perimenopause and menopause, and every part of you deserves attention. Think of this book as the kind of care that wraps around you like a warm hug and says, "You're going to be okay, and you deserve to feel amazing."

I'll help you to reimagine menopause, from how you think about it to how you navigate it. My mission is to help you understand the root causes of your perimenopause and menopause symptoms and provide nutritional and lifestyle guidance and solutions to support your hormones so you can feel like yourself again. Together, we'll look at the physical, emotional, mental, and spiritual changes this stage of life brings.

Before we dive in, let me introduce myself. I'm Andrea, a nutritionist for more than twenty years, a seven-time published menopause researcher, and, like many of you, a menopausal woman myself. Prior to dedicating my career to menopause education and research, I spent over twenty years in the health and wellness industry (starting in my late twenties) and won multiple awards for my work helping people understand what they were putting in and on their bodies.

I graduated from nutrition school in 2005, and my passion for health eventually led me to become the cofounder and CEO of Naturally Savvy, a digital marketing company that focuses on wellness education.

I've appeared in over 450 TV segments across major North American networks, and my work has been featured in national newspapers, magazines, radio shows, podcasts, and online platforms.

In 2011, I coauthored *Unjunk Your Junk Food*, one of the first books to call out questionable ingredients in ultra-processed foods and offer healthier alternatives.

I loved my work, but when I got my first hot flash in my late forties, everything changed. At first my hot flashes and night sweats were sporadic. They'd come and go for months at a time, and because they weren't consistent, I thought they couldn't be related to menopause (I didn't even know perimenopause existed at that point). It was such a confusing time, and even when I tried, I couldn't find the answers I was looking for from my doctor or other healthcare providers. Nobody, not even my mother, brought up the conversation about menopause. Then one day my hot flashes returned for good, and that was when I realized it was definitely menopause.

I went into menopause at either forty-nine or fifty. I'm not exactly sure because the first time I went twelve months without a period, it came back a month later. I also felt like I had a yeast infection, which went away after about a week. Then another year went by without getting my period, and the same thing happened. This time I was in excruciating pain. It felt like glass was cutting my insides. Like last time, I thought it was a yeast infection, only more severe, and the bleeding lasted two weeks, which was unusual for me, so I went to my gynecologist to have it checked out. She told me I didn't have my period, rather, I had severe vaginal dryness. She ran blood work and confirmed I was in menopause. All this to say, I'm not sure if vaginal dryness was the same issue I had the first time around, so that's why I'm not exactly sure when I went into menopause. I'll share more of my story later in this chapter.

I suffered for years with debilitating symptoms, including hot flashes and night sweats, anxiety, weight gain, sleepless nights, and mood swings. I felt helpless and frustrated.

I tried everything I could to relieve my symptoms, from therapies to wearables and hacks I read about online. I was so desperate for relief that I was willing to do anything, even if it meant chugging apple cider vinegar on an empty stomach right before bed while standing on my head because I heard it helps to relieve hot flashes (okay, I'm exaggerating, but you get the point).

I was especially hard on myself because, as a nutritionist and healthy-living expert, I felt I should have known better. I was supposed to understand what was happening to my body and be able to fix it. But I didn't, and I couldn't, because I didn't realize I was in perimenopause. I didn't have the awareness to recognize that my body was changing, that what had always worked for me before was no longer effective, and that I needed to adapt my nutrition and lifestyle to this new phase of life.

Then one day, when I had what seemed like my fiftieth hot flash of the day, I was at my wit's end and just couldn't cope anymore. I told my husband I was going to find answers about what was happening to my body and solutions on how to fix it, and I wouldn't stop until I found a formula that worked. Thankfully, I did. I spent years relearning how to eat, move, manage stress, sleep, take supplements, and adjust my mindset. As a result, my symptoms improved, I had more energy and focus, and I felt like myself again. That's what inspired me and my business partner, Randy, to start Morphus, the company we launched in 2021. Our goal is to teach and empower women in perimenopause and menopause about what's going on with their bodies and help them find their own winning formula to take control of their health and symptoms with nutrition, lifestyle, mindset, and science-backed supplements. With our background in health and wellness, launching Morphus felt like the perfect next step, and writing this book was a natural progression.

Now that I've learned how to truly nourish the body through perimenopause and menopause, I'm excited to share what I learned, so you can feel supported on your own journey.

I'll cover everything from how many symptoms there *really* are to the top forty-five most common ones, including fatigue and brain fog, along with lesser-known symptoms like itchy ears, tinnitus, vertigo, and phantom smells. I'll also share stress management strategies, sleep protocols, relationship insights, my published research, and the reasons we gain weight. We'll look at the foods and supplements that can support your hormones and how mindset affects your overall experience. Then, we'll tie everything together into a clear, actionable plan that shows you how to optimize nutrition and exercise now that you're in perimenopause and menopause.

I've also included quotations from experts I trust. I encourage you to check them out and follow them on social media. Buy their books, read their articles, and listen to their interviews on my podcast, *Menopause Reimagined*.

Let's get started!

Changing Attitudes

In Western societies, menopause is often seen as a negative experience. Zora Benhamou, a gerontologist and the host of the *Hack My Age* podcast, interviewed more than three hundred women in perimenopause and menopause around the world and asked them to share their experiences. She found that while symptoms such as hot flashes and mood swings are universal, attitudes toward menopause aren't. She says, "In Western countries in North America and Europe, menopause has traditionally been medicalized and often associated with negative stereotypes such as a loss of fertility, vitality, and attractiveness, aging, suffering, and a condition that needs to be 'cured' or 'fixed.' This line of thinking unfortunately creates a negative perception about menopause and often leads to fear and stigma, causing many women to feel anxious and stressed compared to women in other regions, such as Asia." I highly recommend listening to my interview with Zora on my podcast, *Menopause Reimagined*, episode #125, where we talked about her work in more detail.

What's encouraging is that I already see a shift in attitudes in the Western world. People like me, Zora, and many others are reframing menopause and aging as a time of empowerment, strength, experience, freedom, vitality, wisdom, confidence, radiance, and vibrance. It's also important to recognize that for decades, our medical system and research have largely overlooked women once they passed their reproductive years. Now female doctors and scientists are openly addressing these gaps and working together to champion change through education, research, and collaboration with others in this space.

That's why I'm so passionate about arming you with knowledge so you can step into perimenopause and then menopause feeling prepared, empowered, and fully aware about what's ahead and how to support yourself for the rest of your life. It's my hope that Gen X (people born between 1965 and 1981, myself included) will be the last generation caught off guard by perimenopause and menopause. Just like millennials destigmatized periods, Gen Xers are now leading the way to destigmatize menopause. And by the time Gen Z and future generations reach this stage, it won't be a taboo topic. Rather, menopause will be treated as another natural phase of life, just like puberty. We can help future generations by teaching them healthier eating and lifestyle choices in their teens, twenties, and thirties to support their future transition into perimenopause, then menopause.

It's time to end the silence. The shame. The stigma. And shout it from the rooftops. Are you with me?

History and Hormone Hoopla

The earliest references to menopause are believed to be around the time of Aristotle, but they didn't call it that. It wasn't until 1821 that a French doctor named Charles-Pierre-Louis de Gardanne gave it the name "menopause." Before that, it was just called the "climacteric," which covers perimenopause, menopause, and postmenopause.

Fast-forward one hundred years, and menopause was increasingly framed as a deficiency condition. In 1938, synthetic estrogen was introduced, and by the mid-twentieth century women going through menopause were commonly offered hormone replacement therapy (HRT) as a treatment option.

In 1991, the Women's Health Initiative (WHI), the largest study of its kind, was officially launched to look into strategies, including hormone replacement therapy, that might help prevent chronic diseases in postmenopausal women such as heart disease, osteoporosis, and breast and colorectal cancers. In July 2002, the estrogen-plus-progestin portion of the study was stopped early (after about five years) because of an increased risk of breast cancer, heart attacks, stroke, and blood clots. And in 2004, the estrogen-only trial was stopped early because of an increased risk of stroke. After the results were released, many women discontinued their HRT. More recent analyses, however, have questioned and reevaluated

> While hormone replacement therapy is a well-known and commonly used term to describe taking hormones that naturally decline as we go into perimenopause and menopause, many organizations now prefer the term *menopause hormone therapy* (MHT). This newer term better reflects the purpose of the treatment: to manage symptoms and support overall health rather than imply that menopause is a hormone deficiency.

the original results, and researchers now understand that age and timing matter. For most healthy women who start menopause hormone therapy before sixty or within ten years of going into menopause, and who have no contraindications, the positives outweigh the risks. Therefore, the pendulum has swung back to recognizing the benefits of hormone therapy, especially for hot flashes and night sweats, and for preventing bone loss and fractures, as well as vaginal estrogen for genitourinary symptoms that affect the vulva, vagina, urinary tract, and surrounding tissues.

It's important to note that the findings of the WHI study took place decades ago. Since then, many other big studies have been done, like the ESTHER study (2007), the E3N-EPIC cohort observational study with eighty thousand women (2008), and the Timing Hypothesis (2011). These newer studies, along with other research, have shown that hormone therapy can have real benefits, especially if it's started around the time we go into menopause. Even recent follow-up studies from the WHI in 2024 support a more balanced and positive view on hormone therapy. So, while the original study gave us important information, newer research has helped doctors better understand *when* and *how* hormone therapy can be helpful and safe for women in perimenopause and menopause. And in November 2025, after reviewing decades of research since the WHI study, the U.S. Food and Drug Administration (FDA) announced plans to update hormone therapy labels and asked manufacturers to remove parts of the "black box" warning on many systemic and topical hormone therapy products.

If you'd like to hear more about the WHI study, check out episode #77 of *Menopause Reimagined*. I spoke with Dr. JoAnn Manson, MD, DrPH, professor of medicine at Harvard Medical School, and chief of preventive medicine at Brigham and Women's Hospital, one of the leading researchers of the original study. And if you'd like to hear more about how things have changed since the WHI study, check out episode #175 with Dr. Tara Scott, FACOG, FAAFM, ABOIM, NCMP, a certified menopause practitioner with The Menopause Society and a fellow of the American College of Obstetrics and Gynecology.

The Change

Before we dive into the fun stuff, let's review the terminology that applies to each unique stage of a woman's life. This section is important because, according to my research, one in five of us don't know which stage we're in . . . and I was one of them until I started researching the topic of perimenopause and menopause.

Premenopause

Premenopause is the time between your very first menstrual cycle and the start of perimenopause. It's the stage of life when women are in their prime reproductive years. During this time, your monthly periods are generally regular, and estrogen and progesterone levels follow a predictable monthly pattern. You may still experience hormonal fluctuations, but most women don't experience the hallmark symptoms associated with perimenopause or menopause.

Perimenopause

Perimenopause (*peri* means "around"), also known as the menopausal transition, is when you start to notice changes in your body. It typically begins eight to ten years before menopause. This stage can start anytime after age thirty-five (and sometimes earlier), but most women will be in perimenopause between the ages of forty and fifty.

Perimenopause can last anywhere from a couple of months to ten-plus years. On average, it lasts three to four years. I was in perimenopause for a total of fourteen years. Research published in

2017 in the journal *Menopause* looked at 1,145 women from four ethnic groups (African American, White, Chinese, and Japanese) and found that perimenopause lasted longer for African American women than for White women. It also lasted longer for women who started the transition younger.

Perimenopause is typically broken down into two main stages, but because hormones gradually change and symptoms can worsen as time goes on, it's easier to think of it as three stages. For this, I turned to Dr. Tara Scott, MD. Here's how Dr. Scott identifies each stage:

Phase 1: The Launch Phase

This is when subtle hormonal shifts start. Testosterone levels have been decreasing since your mid-twenties, and now progesterone is dropping too. Your estrogen levels, however, are still stable and holding their own at normal levels. You may start to notice subtle body changes, like you can't lose weight as easily as you could before, you're more tired at the end of the day, your sleep may be off, you might feel more anxious or stressed, you have more intense PMS symptoms, like bloating and headaches, your cycle may change somewhat, you're hungrier, and you may be more irritable or moody.

Phase 2: The Roller Coaster or Turbulence Phase

This is when you notice major hormonal shifts. Estrogen levels start to fluctuate, and progesterone levels continue to fall. In this phase, estrogen becomes increasingly erratic and can spike to higher levels than when you were younger, and it may be high relative to progesterone levels. This is when many typical symptoms of perimenopause and menopause can start to manifest, such as irregular, lighter, or heavier cycles, hot flashes, night sweats, digestive issues, lack of concentration, lack of focus, anxiety, brain fog, memory problems, weight fluctuations, changes in body shape, and an increase in inflammation. Check out the full list of symptoms in Chapter 2.

Phase 3: The Transition Phase

This is the phase when your body goes through major hormonal shifts as it gears up for menopause and symptoms often peak. Your estrogen, testosterone, and progesterone levels are significantly lower, and your ovaries are preparing for their much-deserved rest.

Unfortunately, as of the time of writing this book, there's no single test to determine whether you're in perimenopause. However, according to LaKeischa Webb McMillan, MD, an OB-GYN, integrative gynecologist, and hormone specialist, there are certain markers your doctor can look at collectively, such as your age, when your mother went into menopause, changes in your menstrual cycle, and whether you're experiencing symptoms like hot flashes, night sweats, and sleep disturbances. Some doctors will also check a specific panel of sex hormones, which may include estrogen, progesterone, testosterone, follicle-stimulating hormone (FSH), and luteinizing hormone (LH). Oftentimes, the results will come back in the "normal" range, leading your healthcare provider to say you're not in perimenopause. However, that may not be the case, since your hormones can fluctuate so quickly that they may be in range one day and out of range the next. If you're in perimenopause and considering menopause hormone therapy (MHT), Dr. LaKeischa recommends having that conversation with your doctor sooner rather than later. For many women, starting hormones in perimenopause, instead of waiting until after menopause, can help ease symptoms such as hot flashes, night sweats, sleep disruptions, and mood changes. With the right treatment, early intervention may not only bring you relief more quickly but could also reduce other health costs in the future.

Yes, You Can Get Pregnant in Perimenopause. I Did.

During perimenopause, your ovaries function less consistently, so ovulation is more irregular, and its timing can change from one cycle to the next. Hormone levels rise and fall unpredictably, which makes cycles even harder to track. Even with all the irregularities, it's still possible to get pregnant until you reach menopause and your ovaries stop releasing eggs. If you're not planning on having children at this stage, keep using birth control until you've gone at least a full year without a period, including spotting, or your doctor confirms you're in menopause.

PERIMENOPAUSE PREGNANCY: MY STORY

I had my first child at thirty-three, my second at thirty-five, and my third at forty-one. Before my third was born, I got pregnant at thirty-nine, only to have a miscarriage in my first trimester. Unfortunately, I lost the baby right around my fortieth birthday.

When I went for a checkup right after, my doctor explained how there's a higher rate of complications and miscarriage for a pregnancy "of advanced maternal age" (formerly referred to as a geriatric pregnancy), which is the term used when you're thirty-five years old or older at the anticipated time of delivery.

I understood age was a factor, but I didn't really understand *why*.

When I was ready and recovered from the loss, my husband and I decided to try to conceive one more time. I told myself that if I lost this baby, too, it just wasn't meant to be.

Fortunately, we were successful, and I was blessed with a third pregnancy at the age of forty.

I had been seeing a fertility doctor (OB-GYN) since before I got pregnant with my oldest child because I have polycystic ovary syndrome (PCOS) and had trouble getting pregnant. As soon as I found out we were expecting again, I called my doctor, and she put me on progesterone suppositories.

When I was ten weeks pregnant, I started bleeding while I was at a friend's cottage for the weekend. Not just spotting but heavy bleeding. I thought for sure I had lost this baby, too, and mentally prepared myself for the news. When I went for an ultrasound the next day, I was shocked to hear a heartbeat. The baby was fine, but I had what was called a subchorionic hematoma. My doctor told me I had a 50 percent chance of losing the baby, so she put me on bed rest for the remainder of my first trimester. Thankfully, it healed with time, and I now have a healthy fifteen-year-old daughter.

About a year after giving birth, I started to notice subtle changes in my body. My sleep was different (I had a hard time falling asleep, and when I finally did, I woke up a few hours later and couldn't fall back to sleep). My anxiety worsened, I had pains in my body, my moods were all over the place, and I snapped at anyone and everyone around me (I had to apologize to my kids and husband on countless occasions!). As time went on, I couldn't deal with stress the same way I could before. I was easily overwhelmed and distracted, I lacked focus and concentration, and I smelled awful (the body odor was brutal, especially in my left armpit). My hair changed and started breaking, my appetite was voracious, and my weight fluctuated for years until I finally put on twenty pounds and it wouldn't come off. I couldn't fit into my clothes (even though I never changed what I ate or how I exercised), and I could no longer wear the cute tank tops I lived in because my boobs were huge and sore (I couldn't even get them over my chest). My stomach was constantly bloated, and the gas situation was out of control. I had phantom smells, vertigo, tinnitus, and honestly, I could keep going.

I was a mess!

Whenever I asked my colleagues and friends if they were feeling the same way, or if they knew *why* I was feeling the way I did, they always responded with a "No" or "I don't know."

I couldn't find any answers to why my body and mind were changing. I felt alone, sad, and ashamed.

I often asked myself, "Am I the only one feeling this way? What's wrong with me?"

It was as if someone, or something, had taken over my body.

This went on for five years.

Until . . .

Two months after my forty-seventh birthday, while I was working in my office, I got my first hot flash.

That's when I connected the dots and thought, *Wait a minute . . . aren't hot flashes associated with menopause? Am I in menopause? Aren't I too young to be in menopause? Isn't menopause for older women like my mother and grandmother? I'm not even fifty yet!*

I had absolutely no knowledge about this pivotal time in a woman's life, and I was ashamed to admit it because I had worked in the health and wellness industry for seventeen years at that point, and it was my job to educate others about their bodies. I thought I knew a lot about myself, but when it came to menopause . . . I knew nothing.

Nada.

Zilch.

Zero.

Looking back, I now realize that I got pregnant twice while I was in perimenopause, and I had no idea until years later.

Menopause

You're in menopause once you've gone 12 consecutive months, or 365 days, without a period and there's no other biological or medical cause. When menopause happens naturally, meaning you haven't had your ovaries surgically removed (bilateral oophorectomy) or undergone medical treatments that induce it, it's called natural menopause.

The average age of menopause in the United States and Canada is fifty-one or fifty-two, depending on the source, with most women going into menopause between forty-five and fifty-five.

When you're in menopause, hormones like estrogen and progesterone drop to low, more stable levels. Testosterone generally declines with age, and the change is slower and not as abrupt as it is with estrogen. Other hormones like follicle-stimulating hormone (FSH) and luteinizing hormone (LH) increase, and anti-Müllerian hormone (AMH), which reflects ovarian reserve, or the number of eggs you have left, falls and reaches undetectable levels. These changes can affect everything from your menstrual cycles and fertility to heart health, mood, and libido.

Menopause is technically just one day. It's the one-year anniversary of the last day of your final period. Every day after that is referred to as postmenopause (a term I dislike, as you'll see in a moment).

Postmenopause

I find the term *postmenopause* misleading.

Here's why: Oftentimes, when I'm asked what I do for a living, and I say I'm a published menopause researcher and educator, in many cases, they'll respond by saying, "Oh, I'm way past that!"

But the thing is, they're not. Once we're in menopause, we're *always* in menopause, so we're never past it; in fact, we're in it for the rest of our lives.

Considering we face an increased risk for health issues like osteoporosis, heart disease, and dementia once we're in menopause, and that many of us will live anywhere from a third to half of our lives in this phase of life, it's more important now than ever to pay attention to our nutrition, exercise, and other lifestyle choices that support our overall health. When we dismiss menopause by saying we're *way past it*, we risk ignoring important lifestyle factors that can affect not only our lifespan, how long we live, but also our healthspan, the years we can live in good health and enjoy a high quality of life, without any serious diseases or disabilities.

So if it were up to me, I'd do away with the term *postmenopause* completely and just use *perimenopause* and *menopause*.

For this reason, I'll refer to *menopause* as an umbrella term that includes both menopause and postmenopause throughout the book. As you'll notice, I put parentheses around *post* to reflect my thinking, and they're intentional.

Early or Premature Menopause

Some women go into menopause years, even decades, before the average age of fifty-one or fifty-two. It's considered "normal" (I don't like using this term, but that's how it's often defined) to go into menopause between forty-five and fifty-five.

If a woman goes into menopause before the age of forty-five, it's called "early" menopause, and if it happens before age forty, it's called "premature" menopause.

We're in This Together

I want to remind you that you're not alone. Every woman will go into menopause if she's blessed to live long enough.

A common question I hear is "How long does menopause last?" But I think what they're really asking is "How long will my symptoms last?" This distinction is important because many women, including myself when I was in perimenopause, can feel overwhelmed by our symptoms, leading us to worry that this is how we'll feel for the rest of our lives. That's why finding ways to manage them early is so important.

While managing symptoms is one aspect of menopause, and a *huge* one, implementing the nutrition, lifestyle, mindset, and supplement recommendations in this book can make a real difference and help you feel like yourself again. This book isn't just about getting you through perimenopause and menopause; it's about thriving during the transition and the years after.

You might find your body and mind changing in ways you didn't expect. Think of perimenopause as an upgrade to your current operating system and menopause as your 2.0 version: You're stronger, wiser, and fully in your knowing. Your body is figuring out how to work differently now. See it as stepping into your *queenager* era, a term I first heard on social media and love.

Be kind to yourself while you adjust, give yourself grace, and try to ease up on the self-criticism. These are all things I've been working on getting better at, too, along with self-compassion and self-forgiveness. Listening to what your body needs while you move through these changes can make a big difference in how you feel.

Also, take the time to learn and relearn what works for you, because what worked before may not work anymore. This might mean rethinking your diet and supplements, changing up your exercise routine, making lifestyle changes, and even shifting your mindset. This doesn't mean you have to do it all at once. Start slowly. Even small tweaks can make a difference in how you feel, how you move through your day, and how you show up for yourself.

I'm here to guide and cheer you on every step of the way.

2

The Signs and Symptoms of Perimenopause and Menopause

What's the first symptom that comes to mind when you hear the word *menopause*?

Whenever I speak in front of a live audience, I start by asking this question, and the answer is always the same: hot flashes!

And that makes sense because hot flashes are synonymous with the word *menopause*. It's the symptom we associate with it whenever we mention the word or search for it online.

Hot flashes are what made me think I was in menopause when I got my first one at forty-seven.

But what if I told you it's not the most common symptom? In fact, it's not even in the top five, according to research I conducted and published through my company, Morphus. Would that surprise you?

It surprised me.

I'm obsessed with data and have been for as long as I can remember. Many years ago, before I started Morphus, I bumped into an old friend who mentioned she was creating an app for menopause symptoms. I was intrigued and frankly a little shocked. I asked her if there were really enough symptoms to dedicate an entire app to them. She said yes, there were about thirty-four to forty of them. That stuck with me, so I created a document and started tracking every symptom I came across from friends, studies, social media, etc. I quickly discovered that women reported more than eighty-five symptoms, far more than the thirty-four

We collected survey responses through a variety of sources: the research page on our website (wearemorphus.com /pages/research-surveys); our social media pages including TikTok, Instagram, YouTube, and LinkedIn, and our Facebook group (wearemorphus); partners and healthcare practitioners we collaborated with, such as Dr. James Simon, MD, Dr. Carrie Jones, ND, Dr. Anna Cabeca, DO, Dr. Sarah Wilson, ND, Danielle Meitiv, MS, and Marcella Hill, who also shared the surveys with their patients, customers, and communities; and our weekly newsletter.

to forty recognized ones that my friend had mentioned. When I tried to confirm a specific number of symptoms in the medical research, I hit a wall. There wasn't much data, and every search led me back to the same thirty-four symptoms that were commonly cited: hot flashes, night sweats, mood swings, sleep issues, and so on.

Other than my own work and one study from the 1970s, there's been no research quantifying the number of perimenopause and menopause symptoms, so I turned to the women in our Morphus online and social media communities to ask them about their symptoms.

This inspired me to create the very first Morphus survey, called "The Signs and Symptoms of Perimenopause and Menopause," or "Signs and Symptoms" for short. I wanted to understand what women in this phase of life were experiencing and why, so they could get the answers and support they needed.

Since then, my team at Morphus and I have created several more surveys covering perimenopause and menopause topics including sleep issues, anxiety and stress, libido/sex drive, pelvic health, doctor's visits, healthcare practitioner insights, and women in the workplace. We even have a survey looking at men's perspectives of perimenopause and menopause, and we're always adding new ones.

I'm extremely proud of this research. I'm honored to have been published seven times in this area,* and I'm committed to continuing and expanding this work. You can find all seven abstracts in the journal *Menopause*.

I'm sharing some of my published research so you know you're not alone. Thousands of women are living with the same symptoms you have right now.

According to the Menopause Foundation of Canada, 75 percent of women experience menopausal symptoms that interfere with their daily lives, and 25 percent suffer from severe symptoms. Knowing the full range of possible symptoms helps you make sense of what you're experiencing and gives you the vocabulary to communicate how you're feeling with your partner, family, friends, coworkers, and healthcare providers. It also equips you with research-backed information to validate your experience.

Our published data shows that there are more than 103 reported signs and symptoms of perimenopause and menopause. You heard me right: 103, and counting! That number confirms our lived experiences and updates the commonly referenced thirty-four to forty recognized ones. In my opinion, the word *recognized* in this context can feel dismissive, as if the rest of our symptoms don't count. Given the high percentage of women in perimenopause and menopause who feel dismissed by their doctors and healthcare providers, acknowledging *all* the possible symptoms we may experience helps us feel seen, supported, and validated. It also empowers us to speak up for ourselves, look for the right help, and get the treatments we need.

If you've ever been dismissed or gaslit, remember this: Your symptoms are real. Don't let anyone tell you otherwise.

---

* These studies include: "The Wide Range of Symptoms of Perimenopause and Menopause and the Means by Which Women Seek Support" with Danielle Meitiv; "The High Prevalence of Sleep Disturbances in Perimenopause and Menopause" with Danielle Meitiv; "Beyond the Physical: The Psychological Toll of Perimenopause and Menopause" with Danielle Meitiv; "Women's Experiences with Healthcare Providers During Perimenopause and Menopause" with Danielle Meitiv; "Women's Sexual Health: Understanding Libido Changes During Perimenopause and Menopause" with James A. Simon, MD, Marcella Hill, and Danielle Meitiv; "Perimenopause and Menopause in the Workplace" with Danielle Meitiv; and "Understanding Men's Perspectives of Perimenopause and Menopause" with Marcella Hill and Danielle Meitiv.

Signs and Symptoms Survey*

Since our surveys are ongoing, here's the most current list of the signs and symptoms at the time of writing this book, based on more than 5,200 responses. The symptoms are ranked from most to least common based on the number of women experiencing them.

At least 60 percent of the respondents said they were experiencing the following:

1. Fatigue, lack of energy, exhaustion, tired all the time

2. Brain fog

3. Sleep issues or problems

4. Memory lapses or loss, or forgetfulness

5. Anxiety

At least 50 percent of the respondents said they were experiencing the following:

6. Loss of/low libido

7. Lack of concentration

8. Joint pain

9. Lack of focus

10. Hot flashes

11. Lack of patience

12. Night sweats

13. Slower metabolism/weight gain

---

* The official name of this research as published in the journal *Menopause* is "The Wide Range of Symptoms of Perimenopause and Menopause and the Means by Which Women Seek Support."

Forty percent or more of the respondents said they were experiencing the following:

14. Changes in body shape

15. Digestive problems

16. Dry, itchy skin

17. Itchy ears

18. Headaches/migraines

19. Emotional/weepiness

20. Lack of/low self-esteem

21. Pain (body)

22. Social anxiety

23. Depression

24. Hair loss

25. Inflammation

26. Tingling extremities

And 30 percent or more of the respondents said they were experiencing the following:

27. Vaginal dryness

28. Dry eyes

29. Weight fluctuations

30. Early waking

31. Dry hair

32. Flatulence

33. Wrinkles

34. Frequent urination

35. Dizziness

36. Shoulder pain

37. Clumsiness

38. Food cravings

39. Acid reflux/indigestion

40. Adrenal exhaustion

41. Brittle nails

42. Unwanted hair growth

43. Health anxiety

44. Increased hunger

45. Breast pain, soreness, tenderness

Page 26 includes a complete list of all 103+ symptoms for your reference. You can also find it on www.wearemorphus.com under the Signs & Symptoms tab. If you want a printable version to bring to your doctor or healthcare provider, go to: www.nourishingmeno pausebook.com under the Resources tab.

Lesser-Known Symptoms

Although hot flashes, night sweats, and mood swings are commonly associated with menopause, there are also lesser-known symptoms that may surprise you, such as itchy ears, bruising, body odor (in one or both armpits), social anxiety, impending doom, digestive issues (gas, bloating, indigestion, loose stools, and constipation), phantom smells (when you smell something that doesn't actually exist), internal tremors or vibrations, cold flashes, hot or burning feet, runny nose, pins and needles, the sensation of bugs crawling on your skin, electric shocks, dizziness, frequent urination, vertigo, tinnitus, loss of appetite, and nausea.

Other Key Findings from Our Published Research

In addition to discovering there are more than 103 symptoms related to perimenopause and menopause, we also learned the following:

- Nearly 20 percent of women were unsure what stage they were in, meaning whether they were in perimenopause or menopause.

- On average, respondents experienced thirty-one different symptoms.

- The nervous system is the most affected body system, followed by the endocrine system. This makes sense because while hormones may be the root cause of many of our symptoms, the nervous system is where many of the effects are *felt*. Hormones guide the messages that run through the nervous system, so when our hormone levels change, the messages they send can change too, and our nervous system reacts. That's why we can experience symptoms everywhere in our body, but feel the most effects in the nervous and endocrine systems.

- Weight gain is either directly or indirectly associated with eleven out of the top fifteen most common symptoms. I mention this because more than 50 percent of women experience this symptom, and it's a major concern for many women in our community. In Chapter 5, I explore all the reasons we gain weight in perimenopause and menopause (hint: there are seventeen of them!).

- Brain health, mental health, and cognition account for at least 50 percent of the top ten most common symptoms, but one could argue that this figure is closer to 90 percent. And at least 70 percent of the top twenty-five most common symptoms can fall into these categories as well.

103+ Signs and Symptoms of

Body

Acidosis
Adrenal exhaustion
Allergies
Bad breath
Bleeding gums
Blind spots
Blood pressure (high and low)
Blood sugar dysregulation
Body odor
Breast pain or tenderness
Breast size change
Bruising
Burning scalp
Burning tongue and mouth
Carpal tunnel syndrome
Changes in body shape
Changes in sense of smell
Chills
Clumsiness
Cold flashes
Crawling sensations
Dizziness
Double vision
Dry eyes
Dry mouth and tongue
Early waking
Electric shock
Fatigue/low energy
Fatty liver
Frequent urination
Frozen shoulder
Hard bloated stomach
Headaches or migraines
Hearing problems
Heart palpitations

High cholesterol
High or low cortisol
Hot feet
Hot flashes
Inflammation
Insomnia
Internal tremors/vibrations
Irregular heartbeat
Itchy ears
Joint pain (arthralgia)
Lightheadedness
Meibomian gland
    dysfunction
Metabolic syndrome
Muscle atrophy (sarcopenia)
Muscle cramps
Night sweats
Ocular migraine
Osteoporosis
Pain
Pelvic and rectal pain
Phantom smells
Restless legs syndrome
Runny nose
Shortness of breath
Shoulder pain
Sleep apnea
Slower metabolism
Sore nipples
Tingling extremities
Tinnitus
TMJ
Vertigo
Water retention
Weight fluctuations
Weight gain

Perimenopause and Menopause

Digestive Health

Abdominal pain
Acid reflux (indigestion)
Bloating
Burping
Constipation/gas/bloating
Difficulty swallowing
Flatulence (gas)
Food allergies and sensitivities
Food aversions
Food cravings
Heartburn
High liver enzymes
Increased hunger
Irritable bowel syndrome (IBS)
Lack of appetite
Loose stools
Metallic taste in mouth
Nausea

Mind

ADHD
A feeling of doom
Anxiety
Brain fog
Depression
Difficulty concentrating
Feeling emotional and crying
Health anxiety
Lack of focus
Lack of motivation
Lack of patience
Lack of self-esteem
Memory lapse/loss
Moodiness and mood swings
Nightmares

Panic attacks
Rage
Sleep problems
Social anxiety
Stress

Sexual Health

Bacterial vaginosis (bv)
Bladder spasms
Heavier periods
Increased libido
Irregular periods
Lighter periods
Loss/low libido
PMS
Prolapse (vagina, uterus, rectum)
Shorter periods
Urinary incontinence
Urinary tract infections
Vaginal dryness

Skin and Beauty

Acne
Brittle nails
Dry hair
Dry, itchy skin
Dull skin
Eczema, psoriasis, and rosacea
Frizzy hair
Hair loss
Hives
Itching
Melasma
Unwanted hair growth
Wrinkles

According to Dr. Fiona Lovely, host of the *Not Your Mother's Menopause* podcast, "Most of the symptoms we know about perimenopause and menopause are actually related to brain function, according to the latest research. Common symptoms like depression, anxiety, memory issues, mood swings, and trouble sleeping happen because hormone levels in the brain are dropping. To properly treat these symptoms, we need to better understand how the brain works, looking at hormone levels and assessing related systems." She adds, "As new research emerges, we're starting to see just how important the brain and brain health are during menopause. It's the part of us most affected during midlife, yet the least understood. People often think menopause is just about changes in the reproductive system, but that's only a small part of it, as Andrea's research and that of Dr. Lisa Mosconi and others are showing us. The brain is impacted by declining hormones, which influence multiple systems, and modern menopause care needs to consider brain health to better manage symptoms, promote healthy aging, and lower chronic health risks for women."

No Symptoms at All

My friend's mom, who is now in her late seventies, told me she didn't experience any symptoms when she transitioned into menopause. She said she remembers having just one hot flash, and that was it!

While she was fortunate to have gone through perimenopause and menopause without symptoms, this is not the norm for most women.

It's estimated that 8–20 percent of women in perimenopause and menopause don't notice or report having any symptoms. However, I question this number because there are so many symptoms on the list of 103+ that aren't typically linked to perimenopause or menopause. Therefore, in my opinion, it's highly likely that the true number is closer to the lower end of that range.

Research on Specific Symptoms

Since I can't go into depth about all the research I've done, I do want to call out two more of my published studies that I feel are important to mention since they're both in the top ten most common symptoms: sleep, and stress and anxiety.

Sleep Issues Survey*

When I realized how common sleep problems are for women in perimenopause and menopause, I wanted to better understand what's keeping us awake at night. So I created a sleep survey to find out.

The most up-to-date results, with 3,500 responses, show that the four leading causes of sleep disturbance for women in this phase of life are:

1. Waking up between 2 a.m. and 4 a.m.,

2. Frequent bathroom visits,

3. Night sweats, and

4. Anxiety, racing heart, adrenaline rushes, and stress.

My first thought when I saw these results was that stress is probably the main reason women are waking up between 2 a.m. and 4 a.m., but I couldn't confirm it from this survey alone. While I did ask what might be disrupting their sleep in general, I didn't ask specifically about the 2 a.m. to 4 a.m. time slot. I also didn't ask whether women had trouble falling back to sleep or what might be keeping them awake at that time, so I made sure to ask those specific questions in my stress and anxiety survey, which gave us a much clearer picture.

There can be several reasons for waking up between 2 a.m. and 4 a.m., some of which include high cortisol levels due to chronic stress, blood sugar fluctuations, sleep apnea, and emotional processing. For

---

* The official name of this research as published in the journal *Menopause* is "The High Prevalence of Sleep Disturbances in Perimenopause and Menopause."

many women, it's likely a combination of factors, but stress often plays a major role.

When it comes to frequent overnight bathroom visits, I've had women tell me they wake up every hour to use the bathroom. Age, urinary tract infections (UTIs), a prolapsed bladder, anxiety, alcohol, caffeine, drinking too much liquid before bed, and certain medications can all contribute to having to pee during the night. Also, high blood sugar levels can make us urinate more (it's our body's way of getting rid of the excess sugar), and low blood sugar levels can disrupt sleep and cause night sweats. Since we're more prone to blood sugar issues in perimenopause and menopause, managing it as best we can is really important, which I talk about quite a bit throughout the book.

Keep in mind that waking up more than twice a night on a consistent basis can be a sign that something else is going on, so speak to your doctor if you're concerned.

Stress and Anxiety Survey*

I created this survey for two reasons. First, because of my own experience with anxiety (which I talk about in Chapter 6), and second, because of how prevalent it is in perimenopause and menopause (it's the fifth-most-common symptom overall). This survey, which currently has more than 1,500 responses, shows that 66 percent of women in this stage of life are more stressed and anxious now than before.

Building on the data from the sleep survey, the majority of the women reported waking up between 2 a.m. and 4 a.m. When asked what prevents them from falling back to sleep, nearly 70 percent said anxiety, a racing mind or thoughts, overthinking, and other stress-related factors. This, combined with the sleep survey results showing anxiety is the fourth-most-common cause of sleeplessness, confirms that for many of us, stress is the main reason we're waking up during the night.

---

* The official name of this research as published in the journal *Menopause* is "Beyond the Physical: Shedding Light on the Psychological Toll of Perimenopause and Menopause."

Since our research is ongoing, I'd love for you to take a few minutes to fill out our surveys because your voice matters! By collecting more data, we can push for better services, policies, treatments, and resources.

You can find all our surveys on www.wearemorphus.com under the Research tab. By filling them out, you're helping to reshape the future of women's health and creating the change we deserve.

In the next chapter, I'll dive deeper into many of the symptoms I mentioned here and explain what they are and why they happen, so you can better understand how they're linked to perimenopause and menopause.

3.

Understanding Your Symptoms

"I don't feel like myself anymore!"
"I feel like someone else is living inside me!"
"OMG! What is happening to my body?"

These are some of the responses we received from women who completed our surveys.

Many of us feel lost and alone with our symptoms because we weren't prepared or properly educated about this stage of life. It isn't our fault. What matters now is that we're rewriting the story by learning, speaking up, and empowering ourselves to take control of our health and our symptoms. This chapter is one of the tools that will help you do exactly that. In the last chapter I shared the full list of 103+ symptoms. While I can't cover all 103+ symptoms in depth here, this chapter will walk you through many of the more common ones, what they mean, and their possible causes, and throughout the book I'll share practical tools to help you manage them.

The main driver behind the changes we experience is fluctuating and declining hormone levels and their interactions, kind of like a busy intersection when the traffic lights aren't working.

Although the hormonal swings level off over time, these changes can bring on physical and emotional symptoms. Lower estrogen affects the heart, bones, brain, and more, making us more susceptible to longer-term health issues like heart disease, osteoporosis, and cognitive decline.

But don't be discouraged. Every change your body and mind go through during this time is impacted, either directly or indirectly,

IMPORTANT: If any of your symptoms are severe, persistent, or interfere with your daily life, please speak to your doctor or healthcare provider so they can look for potential underlying causes. It's important to rule out any serious conditions first. Once you get a clean bill of health, you can consider connecting your symptoms to perimenopause and menopause.

by what you eat and drink, how much you move, how you sleep, your environment, how you think, and how you care for your body. In addition to the option of hormone therapy, there are many nutrition, lifestyle, and mindset approaches you can introduce right away to help manage your symptoms and reduce the risk of the potential concerns that come with this stage of life.

The Hormones at Play

The most well-known hormones affected during perimenopause and menopause are estrogen and progesterone, but there are other hormones involved as well.

Let's start with *estrogen*. Estrogen helps to regulate your menstrual cycle, keeps your bones strong, supports memory and brain sharpness, and helps maintain your skin's hydration and suppleness, among many other important functions.

During perimenopause, estrogen levels fluctuate. That's why one single blood test isn't a reliable predictor of whether you're in perimenopause. Your ovaries, which have been producing estrogen for years, start to wind down. A helpful way to think of how they function in perimenopause is like this: One day they're hard at work making estrogen, and the next they decide to take a vacation day. This on-again, off-again pattern is why symptoms and cycles feel so unpredictable: Sometimes they're heavy, sometimes they're light, sometimes they're early, sometimes they're late, and sometimes they don't come at all.

You'll notice a pattern in this chapter of how estrogen is linked to a majority of the 103+ symptoms.

Next is *progesterone*, estrogen's calmer, quieter partner. This hormone is typically made during the second half of your monthly cycle, after ovulation (called the luteal phase). As you get closer to menopause, ovulation becomes less dependable, and progesterone levels start to drop. Progesterone has a calming effect on the brain and helps regulate sleep, so when levels are lower, you might have sleep issues, feel more anxious, and experience mood swings. Progesterone also helps balance the effects of estrogen, and when progesterone levels drop too low relative to estrogen, it can lead to hormonal imbalance or dysregulation. If estrogen is on the higher side and progesterone is low, or even if estrogen is in a normal range but progesterone is low, it doesn't necessarily mean your body has "too much" estrogen. It's more about the ratio and how estrogen no longer has its usual partner keeping things in check. That's when you might notice breast tenderness, heavier periods, or stronger PMS symptoms.

Androgens are a family of hormones that include testosterone, dihydrotestosterone (DHT), and the precursor dehydroepiandrosterone (DHEA) and its sulfate form, DHEA-S. Androgens are produced in the ovaries and adrenal glands, and fat cells can convert some of them to estrogen. They help maintain muscle mass, bone density, mood, cognition, and sex drive. Over time, starting in your mid-thirties and continuing into perimenopause and menopause, androgen levels start to fall, which can contribute to less muscle tone, a drop in libido, less motivation, and noticeable physical changes like more belly fat. Menopause itself doesn't cause a sudden drop in androgens. Your ovaries and adrenal glands will continue to produce them even once you're fully menopausal, but your levels generally continue to taper off with age.

Another hormone you'll hear about is *follicle-stimulating hormone* (FSH). Produced by the pituitary gland, FSH tells the ovaries to grow follicles and prepare eggs for ovulation. As your ovaries wind down, your body compensates by making more FSH. Although it fluctuates in perimenopause, a consistent FSH level higher than about 30 IU/L can suggest you're in menopause. However, FSH alone doesn't give the full picture, so your doctor or healthcare provider will look at it alongside your symptoms and menstrual cycle history.

Luteinizing hormone (LH) plays an important role in the changes that happen during perimenopause and menopause. As the ovaries become less responsive during perimenopause, LH levels may fluctuate, contributing to the irregular menstrual cycles commonly seen at this stage.

Once you're in menopause when ovulation has stopped, LH levels tend to rise because the body is still trying to stimulate the ovaries, even though they no longer respond. According to the Cleveland Clinic, in menopause, LH can range between nineteen and one hundred, but can vary depending on the lab.

There's also *cortisol*, a major stress hormone. As you enter perimenopause and menopause, *how* your body handles stress can change. You might find yourself getting worked up quickly over things that never used to bother you or feeling like your stress levels are at an eleven for no reason. Cortisol affects several systems in your body, including digestion, appetite, sleep, energy levels, memory and focus, and your immune system. It can also affect your weight. Over time, chronic stress can disrupt your hormones and either bring on or worsen your symptoms. I talk about stress in Chapter 6.

And the last one I'll mention is *insulin*, the hormone that helps keep your blood sugar steady. When estrogen levels drop, we can become more prone to blood sugar issues and a condition called insulin resistance (which is often the step before type 2 diabetes). I talk much more about this hormone in Chapter 5 and throughout the book.

All these hormone changes, some gradual, others more abrupt, interact in complicated ways and can affect nearly every aspect of your physical and emotional health. Plus, other organs and systems jump in to help your body adjust, which is why there's such a wide range of symptoms and health quirks.

Understanding what's happening to your body prepares you to tackle perimenopause and menopause head-on, whether that's with lifestyle tweaks, dietary changes, or medical treatments and support. The more we know about what's happening, the better we can handle this stage of life with confidence.

Now that you recognize the hormones involved, let's review several of the symptoms they may either trigger or exacerbate.

Symptom: Fatigue

As you saw in Chapter 2, fatigue is the most common and, for many, the most draining symptom of perimenopause and menopause. That's why I'm starting here. Fatigue in menopause is more than feeling tired. It's a deep exhaustion that seeps into your mind, mood, and body. Every task you do demands effort, planning, and willpower. It's frustrating because you remember how much energy and focus you once had, yet no matter what you do, you can't seem to snap out of it. Unfortunately, it's so common during menopause that it's often considered "normal."

But *why* are we sooooo tired?

There are many possible reasons, including:

a. Hormones: Fluctuating and changing hormones can affect our energy levels. Lower estrogen can trigger hot flashes and night sweats, making it harder to fall asleep, and less progesterone makes it harder to stay asleep. Mood swings, anxiety, and depression can drain both our physical and mental energy (the mental fatigue is real!). And lower testosterone levels can zap our energy and motivation, making it harder to do physical activities.

b. Lack of sleep: Waking up between 2 a.m. and 4 a.m., bathroom visits, and night sweats are the top reasons we're not getting enough sleep. Less sleep equals more fatigue.

c. Sleep apnea: If you wake up dragging your feet and feel tired during the day, ask your doctor for a sleep test to see if you have sleep apnea since we become significantly more prone to it once we're in this stage of life.

d. Hypothyroidism: A symptom of a low, or underactive, thyroid is fatigue. Hypothyroidism can show up or worsen during peri-menopause and menopause due to hormonal shifts that impact thyroid function. For a list of blood work, including thyroid tests, you can ask your healthcare provider for, visit www.nour ishingmenopausebook.com and click on the Resources tab.

e. Stress: Chronic stress wears us down mentally and physically. It also affects our sleep.

f. Dehydration: Every system (digestive, circulatory, muscular, nervous, etc.) in our body needs water to function properly. Without enough of it, we can feel mentally and physically depleted.

g. Nutrient deficiencies: Fatigue is a symptom of low vitamin D, ferritin (iron), and B12 levels. Ask your doctor to check all three.

h. Emotional exhaustion: Mood swings, depression, and anxiety can take an emotional toll on our energy levels.

i. Physical discomfort: If you're dealing with pain and inflammation, you may feel more run-down and drained than usual.

Symptoms: Brain Fog, Memory Problems, Lack of Concentration and/or Focus

Menopause is a full-body experience, so your brain is intimately involved in the changes you're experiencing. Hormonal fluctuations can impact your mental health along with your physical health. You might feel like you're going crazy at times, but I assure you that what you're feeling mentally and emotionally is as real as any of your physical symptoms.

As we learned in Chapter 2, brain health, mental well-being, and cognitive function play a role in at least half of the top ten most common symptoms, and likely closer to 90 percent. Imagine these all-too-familiar scenarios: You go to get something from another room, and when you get there, you forget what you came for. You're in a meeting presenting a report or in the middle of a conversation and suddenly lose your train of thought. Or you're searching everywhere for your glasses while they're on top of your head, or your phone, which is in your hand (been there, done that!). And then there's the fun game of "Name That Person, Place, or Thing," where you can't remember what you had for lunch or your best friend's name but can recall every word from a song you listened to at a social in fifth grade (I'm talking about you, "Tainted Love").

I know it all too well.

In fact, I dealt with quite a bit of brain fog during perimenopause, but the memory loss, well, that was next level. On one very specific occasion I was driving in my neighborhood, on a route I must have driven no less than one hundred times, and I completely blanked on where I was. I mean, zero recognition of the streets, the intersection, and my surroundings. I thought I was losing my mind, and I was only in my late forties!

If you feel like your brain is on hiatus, you're not alone. Women in perimenopause and menopause are more likely to report memory problems than premenopausal women.

Estrogen, progesterone, testosterone, cortisol, and thyroid hormones all have an effect on your brain, and can impact areas tied to memory, focus, and mood. When these hormones shift, you may experience brain fog and forgetfulness, have trouble remembering words, lose your train of thought, need more time to understand and process something you're reading, or find it more challenging to learn new things. The good news is the brain often adapts over time. Implementing the nutrition and lifestyle strategies mentioned throughout this book can help.

Estrogen influences important brain chemicals like serotonin and dopamine, which affect mood and concentration. When those are out of balance, you might feel more scattered or mentally sluggish, anxious, moody, or irritable.

Interrupted sleep also affects your memory. When you don't get enough rest, you feel like you're in a mental fog, and it's harder to focus.

Stress can interfere with your ability to concentrate. Stress triggers the release of cortisol, and in perimenopause and menopause, fluctuating and lower estrogen and progesterone levels make it harder for the body to regulate it. These changes can lead to higher levels of cortisol, which can cause brain fog. Chronic stress can also affect the hippocampus, the part of the brain tied to memory and learning. High cortisol also affects sleep, which is critical for brain health.

The brain and gut (see Chapter 4 about the gut-brain connection) are closely linked through the vagus nerve and have a big impact on how we think and feel. Like any relationship, this "gut-brain romance," a term coined by Dr. Uma Naidoo, MD, a nutritional psychiatrist and the best-selling author of *Calm Your Mind with Food*, needs to be nourished to fend off symptoms such as depression, anxiety, and mood swings.

Menopausal women are more at risk of being deficient in choline (an essential nutrient) than premenopausal women because as estrogen levels fall, we become less efficient at making it. Choline has been shown to improve brain function, reduce inflammation in the brain, and protect brain cells. Low levels have been linked to brain fog, low mood, and memory issues. We need to get choline from our diet in order to have enough. Eggs with the yolk, chicken, turkey, salmon, cod, shrimp, soybeans, quinoa, broccoli, Brussels sprouts, and kidney beans are all good sources, so adding one or more choline-rich foods to your diet a day is beneficial. Aim for 425 mg a day. There's also the option of supplements, which have been shown to be beneficial for menopausal women.

Another contributing factor is oxidative stress, which increases in menopause (meaning we have more free radicals than antioxidants). Antioxidants, whose job is to neutralize free radicals, help to reduce inflammation and protect brain cells. I talk about antioxidants in Chapter 10.

If you're thinking, *This is f'ing scary*, it is, but don't panic! Research from neuroscientist Lisa Mosconi, PhD, shows that while gray matter (the area that helps you think, feel, and process information) dips in some parts of the brain during perimenopause, many of those areas stabilize or partially recover once you go into menopause. And research in *Neurology* suggests that memory and learning problems often seen in perimenopause tend to bounce back toward premeno-pausal levels in (post)menopause.

One thing to note: Brain fog and memory changes during peri-menopause or menopause can sometimes feel like mild cognitive impairment or even dementia. The key difference is that menopausal symptoms typically improve over time, especially as other symptoms (like hot flashes and sleep issues) are treated, while dementia symp-toms progress and worsen over time.

Symptoms: Anxiety, Stress, Mood, Mental Health

Many women experience feelings of depression, impending doom, anger, mood swings, rage, weepiness, anxiety, increased stress, sudden bouts of crying for no reason, social anxiety, detachment, newly onset phobias, low self-esteem, or other changes in their mental health. Several women in my social media community have said they feel dead inside. Some feel detached from everything and everyone. Others have said they feel "dissociated." Many feel their personalities have completely changed, and they went from being social beings to wanting to be left alone all the time. As one woman put it, "I don't have the battery life to keep it up. I can only manage small interactions with anyone."

Research from 2023 estimates that up to 70 percent of women in perimenopause and menopause experience emotional or mood-related symptoms such as irritability, anger, anxiety, depression, trouble concentrating, and lower confidence or self-esteem. Estro-gen plays a major role when it comes to mood changes because it affects the production of serotonin (the "feel-good" neurotransmit-ter). When estrogen levels fluctuate in perimenopause and drop in menopause, it affects how the brain makes, uses, and responds to serotonin. You might feel sadder or more emotional than usual. Fluctuating progesterone levels during perimenopause can also dis-rupt serotonin, leading to more mood swings. On top of it all, sleep disruptions and increased anxiety can influence our moods, so it can become a vicious cycle. Factors such as blood sugar fluctua-tions, stress and less ability to cope with stress, everyday responsibilities (such as taking care of aging parents, kids, work, etc.), or other health issues can also contribute to mood-related symptoms.

Our Morphus published research showed that 66 percent of women in perimenopause and menopause are more stressed now than they were before; 60 percent of women have anxiety; nearly 60 percent have trouble focusing and/or concentrating; more than 40 percent are emotional/weepy, have social anxiety, and/or are depressed; and nearly 30 percent experience rage and panic attacks.

Stress and anxiety aren't the same thing. Stress is usually a reaction or response to something specific, like an argument with a friend or a deadline you need to meet, and it disappears once the triggering event is over. Anxiety is different. It's more of a constant internal feeling of worry or fear that doesn't go away, even when there's no underlying reason or rationale for it. It can last long after a stressful event is over or show up out of nowhere and without a specific cause.

According to the Mayo Clinic, while occasional anxiety is normal, anxiety disorders involve constant, intense worrying that can trigger panic attacks and interfere with everyday situations. Many women in our community have shared that their anxiety is so debilitating, they'd rather stay home than go out and socialize with other people.

Other factors that can lead to mental health symptoms include hot flashes and night sweats, heart palpitations, restless legs, and health anxiety, all of which can make you cranky and irritable, especially if they're disrupting your sleep.

Women in perimenopause and the early stages of menopause are two to four times more likely to experience a major depressive event than they are at any other point in their lives. Perimenopause and menopause can also worsen existing conditions and symptoms, such as bipolar disorder and schizophrenia. Some women notice Attention-Deficit Hyperactivity Disorder (ADHD) symptoms for the first time, or experience worsening symptoms. This is likely because fluctuating and lower estrogen levels also affect brain chemicals, like dopamine and serotonin, both of which play a role in attention, mood, and ADHD-related symptoms.

Approximately 20 percent of women going through perimenopause and menopause experience feelings of impending doom. The best way to describe it is that a feeling of dread takes over, and your brain is convinced something catastrophic will happen and that the worst possible outcome of whatever situation you're in will come to fruition. It's different from a "gut feeling." It's more like an uncontrollable, deep sense of fear that manifests physically and emotionally and for no apparent reason because you're not in any immediate danger.

Symptom: Lack of Sleep

Sleep disturbances are the third-most-common symptom of perimenopause and menopause overall, and they affect 66 percent of women in this phase of life. Our research also shows it's more common in menopause than in perimenopause, and a lack of good-quality, restful sleep makes everything else feel harder to handle. As a result of sleep deprivation, you may wake up feeling tired, groggy, and unrefreshed, even if you went to bed early. Poor sleep disrupts the body's natural sleep cycle, leading to fatigue, irritability, increased hunger, and difficulty concentrating during the day. I go into detail about sleep in Chapter 7.

Symptoms: Joint and Muscle Pain and Stiffness, Bone Loss, Mobility Changes, Frozen Shoulder

When I was in perimenopause (before I knew I was), there was a period of about a year where I couldn't lift my left arm higher than my shoulder. It seemed to appear out of nowhere, and I had no idea why. Nothing seemed to help, not even massages. After doing a ton of research, I realized I had something called frozen shoulder. Years later, in 2022, research from Duke University found a possible link between frozen shoulder and lower estrogen levels in menopausal women, and women who were on hormone therapy had a slightly lower chance of developing it.

Recently, a good friend of mine shared that she's been dealing with terrible back pain that also appeared out of nowhere. She also finds it harder to recover after being active, like when she plays pickleball. She's fifty-five and in perimenopause.

If you start to notice aches, pain, stiffness, swelling, or burning or warming sensations in your hands, wrists, fingers, knees, elbows, neck, back, shoulders, or other joints, especially first thing in the morning or after sitting for long periods, you may be experiencing what's referred to as the musculoskeletal syndrome of menopause (MSM), a term coined by Dr. Vonda Wright, a double board-certified orthopedic surgeon with a subspecialty certification in sports medicine, and the author of *Unbreakable: A Woman's Guide to Aging with Power*.

More than 70 percent of women in this stage of life experience musculoskeletal symptoms as they move from perimenopause into menopause. Roughly a quarter report severe symptoms, and about 40 percent have pain and stiffness even though nothing shows up structurally on scans or tests. Women in menopause have a greater chance of experiencing moderate or severe pain than women in perimenopause.

According to Dr. Wright's research, musculoskeletal symptoms don't only include joint pain; they also involve changes in the tendons, ligaments, and cartilage, along with muscle and bone loss. Loss of bone density increases the risk of osteoporosis and fractures, changes in tendons and ligaments increase the chance of injury, and when the cushioning in your joints weakens, it can trigger or worsen osteoarthritis. And as I mentioned earlier, musculoskeletal symptoms in menopause can also include adhesive capsulitis, or frozen shoulder, which affects the shoulder capsule.

Estrogen helps keep your joints, connective tissues, muscles, and bones healthy by keeping inflammation in check, protecting collagen, and supporting the turnover of tissue. When estrogen levels decrease, inflammation can increase, and connective tissues can feel stiff and less flexible over time.

Also, extra weight gained as a result of hormonal changes adds pressure on the joints, especially in the knees, hips, and lower back.

On top of that, muscle loss, poor sleep, stress, and less physical activity can make symptoms worse.

When it comes to bone loss, early prevention matters. According to Dr. Doug Lucas, a double board-certified orthopedic surgeon and osteoporosis specialist, and founder of The OsteoCollective, "Many women don't start thinking about their bones until their sixties or beyond. What most women don't realize is that bone loss can start with hormone fluctuations even before menopause. The time to screen for bone loss and act on bone preservation is now. Start thinking of bone health as a biomarker of healthspan and longevity instead of an afterthought of aging."

Symptoms: Hot Flashes, Cold Flashes, Night Sweats

If you've never experienced a hot flash or night sweat, I'll try and explain what it feels like: One minute you're perfectly fine, then out of nowhere, an intense wave of heat, which feels like an inferno, takes over your body, and you start sweating profusely. Then, just as quickly, the feeling passes, and you're freezing. Then the cycle repeats itself. This was my own personal experience, and each episode would last for at least thirty seconds, and they'd come and go many times a day. Eventually, I stopped counting because they happened so often.

Some women don't have hot flashes during the day but rather at night. These are called night sweats, and they're similar to hot flashes as far as the body's physiological response, but they tend to show up while you're sleeping (or trying to!). You may wake up drenched in sweat or feeling overheated, even when the temperature in your room is comfortable or cool. And similar to hot flashes, you may cycle between extreme heat and extreme cold. However, we're all different. Some women experience flushing (face, chest, upper back, and neck), and for many women, hot flashes and night sweats can be accompanied by an increased heart rate, nausea, or anxious feelings. How intense they are and how often they happen is different for everyone.

Hot flashes, cold flashes, and night sweats are known as "vaso-motor symptoms," which can happen when changes in the brain's temperature control system make blood vessels widen (dilate) and narrow (constrict), leading to sudden feelings of heat, sweating, or cold. Some researchers also include palpitations, changes in blood pressure, and migraines in this group. It's estimated that 75–80 per-cent of women in perimenopause and menopause suffer from vaso-motor symptoms.

Our research shows that 56 percent of women in perimeno-pause and menopause get hot flashes, and they're more common in menopause than perimenopause.

On average, hot flashes last about 7.4 years.

Our research also shows that 53 percent of women have night sweats. They're disruptive because they interfere with sleep, often waking us up multiple times a night, leading to exhaustion, mood changes, mental health struggles, and an overall lower quality of life because of the sleep deprivation.

While hot flashes and night sweats aren't exclusive to perimeno-pause and menopause, they can also happen during pregnancy, as side effects of medications, and as a result of thyroid issues, infec-tions, and stress and anxiety. However, when they happen around perimenopause and menopause, there's a good chance they're likely due to hormonal changes.

Here's what's happening: Body temperature is regulated by the hypothalamus (a part of the brain and central nervous system). Think of it as the body's thermostat, and estrogen, among other things, helps to fine-tune its controls. According to Dr. Lisa Mosconi, author of *The Menopause Brain*, "When estrogen doesn't activate the hypo-thalamus correctly, the brain cannot regulate body temperature cor-rectly. So those hot flashes that women get, that's the hypothalamus."

Factors that may affect how severe and long vasomotor symp-toms can last include genetics, lifestyle, obesity, race, and ethnicity. For example, smoking can influence blood vessels and hormone metabolism, interfering with your body's ability to control body tem-perature. Black women, on average, experience hot flashes and night sweats for much longer than White women (about ten years compared to approximately six and a half years), and their symptoms tend to be more severe. The Study of Women's Health Across the Nation (SWAN) suggests that these differences tend to be due to a combination of factors, including hormonal differences, increased chronic stress, limited access to care and treatment options such as menopause hormone therapy (MHT), going into menopause earlier (on average), socioeconomic factors, and systemic healthcare biases that can lead to Black women's concerns being dismissed or overlooked by healthcare providers. Other factors that affect the severity and duration of hot flashes and night sweats across all racial and ethnic groups include psychological and social factors, including a history of trauma or adversity (for example, child abuse or neglect), and anxiety.

Anxiety often comes before hot flashes and is strongly linked to how often and how severe they are, even after accounting for other factors. One possible reason for this may be that anxiety sets off the body's fight-or-flight system, which may make the brain's thermostat more sensitive. This, combined with lower estrogen levels, can make the body more reactive to stress and hot flashes.

One promising treatment to explore is clinical hypnosis, as it has been shown to decrease hot flashes by about 70 percent, performing better than cognitive behavioral therapy (CBT), and in some trials, the relief can be similar to what some women see from hormone therapy. Beyond hot flashes, hypnosis can improve sleep and reduce anxiety. Ann Marie McQueen, a journalist and founder of Hotflash inc, wishes more people knew how powerful and underused hypnosis is for perimenopause and menopause symptoms. She pointed out: "All of the major research in this field traces back to Dr. Gary Elkins, professor of psychology and neuroscience at Baylor University. He originally developed his hypnosis protocol more than twenty years ago to help breast cancer survivors who could not take hormones, and the improvements were immediate and powerful. He views hypnosis as a way of helping the brain return to balance, a different mechanism from hormones yet often producing a similar outcome."

It's accessible, evidence based, and can now be used in self-guided formats through apps like Evia.

Cold Flashes

One lesser-known symptom is cold flashes, with or without hot flashes. These are sudden sensations of intense cold, often accompanied by shivering, chills, or goose bumps. They can happen on their own, or before or after a hot flash. Managing stress and limiting caffeine may be helpful in reducing their frequency and severity.

Symptoms: Weight Gain, Changes in Body Composition, Increased Belly Fat, Weight Fluctuations, Changes in Body Shape

The numbers on the scale are creeping up, and you're frustrated because you haven't changed how you eat or exercise. You're doing everything "right," but nothing's working, and you don't understand why. That was me too. When I was forty-six, I was twenty pounds heavier than my premenopausal self, and for the life of me, I couldn't figure out why.

Maybe you've gained weight, or your weight is fluctuating from one day to the next. Maybe it used to go to your butt, but now it's in your belly, and it's hard as a rock. Or you used to eat anything you wanted, but now, even though you're eating less, you're still gaining weight. Or maybe you're doing everything possible to eat and live a healthy lifestyle, including exercising, but you still can't lose a single pound.

There are at least seventeen different reasons we gain weight during perimenopause and menopause, including hormones, stress, muscle loss, lack of sleep, and gut health. I go into detail about each in Chapter 5.

Symptoms: Digestive Problems (Bloating, Gas, Constipation, Loose Stools, Indigestion, Cravings, Increased Hunger, Abdominal Pain, Heartburn, Fullness, Loss of Appetite, Etc.)

Nearly 50 percent of women in perimenopause and menopause experience digestive problems such as gas, bloating, loose stools, and constipation. Other digestive symptoms can include nausea, heart-burn, abdominal pain, feeling hungrier than before, craving certain foods, and feeling like food is sitting in your stomach for hours after you've eaten. On the other hand, you might be less hungry, feel full quickly, and eat less than you used to. I talk about digestion and gut health in the next chapter.

Symptom: Dryness (Vaginal, Skin, Eyes, Scalp, Ears, Mouth, Lips, and Nose)

As we enter perimenopause and menopause, dryness becomes a common issue affecting different parts of our bodies. The drop in estrogen impacts our body's ability to retain moisture, leading to dryness, including vaginal dryness, dry skin, a flaky scalp, a parched mouth, a dry nose, and dry, itchy ears.

Vaginal Dryness

Estrogen helps maintain the health, moisture, and pH of your vaginal tissues. As levels drop, along with lower levels of collagen and elastin, the vaginal lining and tissues become thinner, less elastic, and less lubricated, causing dryness and friction, which can lead to pain and discomfort on its own or during intercourse. Lower estrogen levels can also reduce blood flow to the vagina, which adds to the dryness and affects the health of the tissues. Some women experience atrophic vaginitis, or vaginal atrophy, where the vaginal wall tissues become dry, thin, inflamed, and irritated.

Our research shows that 40 percent of women in perimenopause and menopause experience vaginal dryness, and 50 percent of menopausal women have it, which is consistent with other research.

According to Dr. Anna Cabeca, DO, OBGYN, FACOG, The Girlfriend Doctor, and best-selling author of *The Hormone Fix*, *Keto-Green 16*, and *MenuPause*, vaginal dryness is one of the most common and distressing symptoms she sees in her clinical practice. "It's important for women to know they don't have to suffer in silence. Declining estrogen levels play a significant role, but we also need to consider the benefits of DHEA, which is a precursor to both estrogen and testosterone. Topical DHEA has been a game-changer for many of my patients, helping to restore vaginal tissue integrity, improve lubrication, and even enhance sexual satisfaction. Combining this with lifestyle changes, like a nutrient-rich diet and stress management, can make a profound difference." Dr. Cabeca has a topical DHEA cream called Julva that I use regularly and love. I talk more about my experience with Julva at www.nourishingmeno pausebook.com, under the Resources section.

Vaginal dryness and related changes are part of genitourinary syndrome of menopause (GSM), which I discuss in more detail later in this chapter.

Dry Skin and Other Skin-Related Symptoms

A recent study in *Nature Aging* found that biological aging speeds up dramatically at two pivotal points in our life: at about ages forty-four and sixty. At forty-four, the body goes through changes in how it processes fats, alcohol, and energy, which can affect metabolism and heart health. In our sixties, changes are more about managing blood sugar, fighting off infections, and kidney health. These changes also affect how much collagen we make, which is why many women notice changes in their skin, joints, and tissues during these years.

About fifteen years ago, I was in Venice Beach waiting at the cash register to pay for a pair of jeans when a woman standing in line complimented my skin. She told me that she used to have beautiful skin, but about five years into menopause, it completely changed. I asked her to explain what she meant, and she said her skin was now saggy, the texture was rough and dry, the color was dull and pale, and she had a lot of deep wrinkles.

What I didn't know at the time was that when estrogen drops, your skin feels it big time. Collagen is the most abundant protein in your body, and it keeps skin firm, plump, and flexible. Think of it as the scaffolding for your skin, bones, muscles, ligaments, and cartilage. But with age, you produce less of it, which can mean thinner, saggier, drier skin that is more prone to developing fine lines and wrinkles. We're born with a lot of collagen. That's why babies have beautiful, plump, firm, wrinkle-free skin. As we get older, collagen production slows, and we lose about 1 percent a year starting in our mid-twenties. By the time we reach our forties, we will have lost a significant amount, and once we reach menopause, we lose an extra 30 percent within the first five years. After that, the loss slows down but doesn't stop, and we continue to lose about 2 percent of our collagen a year.

As a result of collagen loss, your skin can start to feel delicate, so healing from cuts or scrapes may take longer than it used to. And this isn't just limited to your face. Your arms, legs, hands, and the rest of your body feel it too.

Elastin fibers, which give skin its ability to stretch and snap back, also lessen, leading to sagging skin, especially around the neck and jawline, giving rise to what some call "jowls" or "turkey neck." Whenever I hear the word *jowls*, I think of my teen years and my dad. I used to love pinching his jowls because I thought they made him look more endearing, but now that I have them, too, *endearing* isn't the exact word I'd use to describe them anymore.

Menopause can also make your skin more sensitive, and some women may notice breakouts (acne), often linked to changing hormones. Strong soaps or cleansers with fragrances or alcohol, cold weather, or sun exposure can worsen dryness and irritation or cause itching, redness, or rashes.

Dry Scalp

A decrease in estrogen levels can lead to less oil production, making your scalp feel dry and itchy. You might also notice increased flakiness, irritation, or thinning as the scalp becomes drier. A dry scalp can also make your hair look greasy or oily. This is because when the scalp is dry, it may produce more oil to make up for the lack of moisture.

Dry (Itchy) Ears, Nose, Eyes, and Mouth

Lower estrogen can mean less hydration in your skin and the mucous membranes in your ears, eyes, and nose. As a result, these areas can become drier and more prone to irritation, which may cause discomfort, itching, or flaking.

Ears

Are your ears itchy on the inside? Are you scratching them non-stop? In my opinion, this is one of the most annoying symptoms! In addition to being itchy, your ears may also feel a bit wet or damp. When the skin in the ear canal dries out and makes less natural oil, wax can build up more easily, and, in some cases, make hearing feel a bit muffled. Believe it or not, the inner ear is sensitive to estrogen, so changing estrogen levels may affect how well we can hear.

Nose

Dryness can make it harder to breathe through your nose, especially at night, and you might feel stuffed up because the inside of your nose is inflamed or swollen. Some women get nosebleeds because the nasal lining can become so dry that it cracks. Sinus problems may become more common, especially in the winter. And you may notice pain, discomfort, sinus headaches, or even infections.

Eyes (Dry and/or Watery)

Hormonal changes during perimenopause and menopause can cause dry, watery, burning, irritated, blurry, or red eyes. They can also make you more sensitive to light. Lower levels of androgens such as testosterone and shifts in estrogen affect eye tissue health and tear production. If you're told you have something called meibomian gland dysfunction, or MGD (like I was), it basically means the glands in your eyelids aren't making enough oil, so your tears dry up quickly. This can make your eyes feel dry, irritated, or watery.

Mouth

Dryness and soreness in your mouth, throat, tongue, or lips can make it harder to talk, taste, or chew your food. Your tongue or lips may hurt, or you might have a burning sensation in your mouth or tongue (commonly referred to as burning mouth syndrome) or notice a metallic taste. This could be due to dryness or digestive issues like bile or acid reflux.

You may also have less saliva production, and since saliva keeps the bacteria in your mouth in check, having less can lead to tooth decay, cavities, bad breath, infections, and receding gums.

In addition to a drop in estrogen, other potential causes for a dry mouth are an underactive thyroid (hypothyroidism), nutritional deficiencies, medications, allergies, nerve sensitivity, and infections in the mouth or mouth area.

One of the most effective remedies I've personally found for dryness-related symptoms are omega-3s. I talk more about them in Chapter 8.

Symptom: A Sensation of Bugs Crawling on Skin

Another skin-related symptom is feeling like there are bugs or insects crawling on or under your skin. Its official name is *formication* or tactile hallucination, a type of paresthesia (a nerve-related feeling of tingling or crawling). Women in our Morphus online and social media communities have said it can also feel like tiny bites all over your body or a strand of hair or piece of thread on your skin. It can happen when your brain thinks it's feeling something that isn't really there. This makes the crawling feeling seem real and may cause you to scratch or pick at your skin. It can happen for different reasons, but during perimenopause and menopause, these sensations are often linked to hormone changes, especially as estrogen levels fall. While the exact cause isn't clear, it may involve shifts in how nerves send signals or changes in blood flow. These crawling feelings can be accompanied by dry, itchy, or burning skin because lower estrogen can make the skin less hydrated and more sensitive.

Symptom: Period and Cycle Changes

Cycle and period changes are a telltale sign of perimenopause and are often one of the first noticeable ones. Your periods may be heavier or lighter, and your cycles may be shorter or longer than usual; some women miss periods altogether (like me), and some don't miss any at all and stay completely regular.

According to Dr. Fay Weisberg, MD, a gynecology and reproductive medicine specialist and the clinic director of First Steps Fertility and FemRenew, a clinic that specializes in women's vaginal health, "The main symptom I see repeatedly with perimenopause is irregularity of periods, both in timing and amount of flow. The predictability of regular cycles is gone, and there may be delays or more frequent cycles. This is related to the decrease in the quality of eggs that sometimes cannot complete a menstrual cycle."

Irregular periods are often linked to changes in the hormones estrogen and progesterone, which control the menstrual cycle. When ovulation doesn't happen, meaning the ovaries don't release an egg (called anovulation), the body doesn't make progesterone the way it normally would. Estrogen ends up acting alone, which can cause the uterine lining to build up and shed at unpredictable times. That's why bleeding can be lighter, heavier, or more irregular than usual.

According to Danielle Meitiv, a board-certified health coach and functional medicine practitioner who focuses on thyroid health, imbalanced thyroid hormones can also cause irregular periods and even fertility issues. Thyroid hormones regulate a protein called sex hormone-binding globulin (SHBG), which controls how much estrogen and progesterone is available in your blood. If you're in perimenopause and trying to conceive, it's important to monitor and manage your thyroid function carefully.

You can still be in perimenopause even if your periods are regular. This is important because many women have told me that their doctors dismiss them because their cycles are consistent from month to month.

Symptom: Low or Decreased Libido

As you saw from our research in Chapter 2, libido is the sixth-most-common symptom, and it affects nearly 60 percent of women in perimenopause and menopause, with more women in menopause experiencing it than those in perimenopause. Vaginal dryness can make sex uncomfortable or painful. (Refer to the section on genitourinary symptoms on page 62 for more information.) Painful intercourse can be a major mood killer, making those of us who suffer from it want to avoid sex and intimacy altogether. The frustration, embarrassment, or anxiety associated with vaginal dryness can cause problems within a relationship.

Dr. James Simon, MD, medical director and founder of Intim-Medicine Specialists' and past president of both the International Society for the Study of Women's Sexual Health (ISSWSH) and The Menopause Society, explains that "hormone fluctuations in perimenopause can either increase or decrease sexual desire, but once hormone levels drop in menopause, interest often lags." He adds that "sleep disturbance, heavy bleeding, premenstrual pelvic pain, breast tenderness, or moodiness can further lower libido, while relationship dynamics and certain medications can also play a major role."

In addition, testosterone, which sparks sexual desire, can drop to 15 percent of premenopause levels once you're in menopause. "Testosterone is the hormone of desire in both men and women," says Dr. Simon. "It's well documented to improve libido following menopause, and in my view, most women benefit from testosterone therapy when it's carefully monitored."

Dr. Ashley Alexis, ND, a licensed naturopathic medical doctor specializing in menopause care and founder of Golden Leaf Health Center, agrees. She believes testosterone often works best in combination with other hormones. "Testosterone can be very helpful for libido," she says, "but sex drive is also supported by estradiol and oxytocin. A combination can be especially effective for increasing desire while also boosting energy and stamina."

But libido is rarely about hormones alone. Dr. Weisberg notes that libido is "multifactorial, related to self-esteem, health, family dynamics, cultural factors, and even a partner's health and/or lack of erection. Many women think it's hormonal when in fact it can be relationship- or lifestyle-driven." She emphasizes the importance of addressing vaginal dryness, vestibular pain (burning, stinging, or irritation around the vaginal opening), pelvic pain, bladder concerns, medication side effects, or partner issues, as they all play a role. Treatments like vaginal estrogen, PRP (the O-shot), or behavioral adjustments can often help.

So, while hormones are one of the main players in this shift, a mix of physical and emotional factors, like stress, sleep, night sweats, mood, weight gain, body image, and relationship connection, can also contribute to your sex drive being on airplane mode. Low libido is complex, but understanding the underlying cause and working with the right practitioner can help improve it.

I spoke with Dr. Simon and Dr. Weisberg about sexual health and libido on my podcast, *Menopause Reimagined*. Listen to episodes #86, #87, #126, and #179 to hear more.

Symptom: Body Odor

It's not your imagination; you do smell worse than you used to. An increase in body odor is common during this time of life, even if the smell is only noticeable to you.

We tend to sweat more now because of hormonal fluctuations and vasomotor symptoms like hot flashes and night sweats. Many women have shared with me that they're sweating in places they never did before! Hormonal shifts (including estrogen and testosterone) can change how your sweat interacts with the bacteria on your skin, causing a funkier smell. We're also more prone to stress and anxiety in perimenopause and menopause, and when we're anxious or stressed, our sweat glands go into overdrive and release more sweat. And sweat from anxiety or emotional stress has a stronger, more pungent smell. For some of us, our sense of smell becomes more sensitive, making us think we smell bad even when we don't.

In some cases, menopause-related body odor has an acidic smell from urinary changes, dehydration, or UTIs that are also common during this time. If you notice a fruity smell, speak with your healthcare provider ASAP, especially if you also feel nauseous, fatigued, or extremely thirsty, as this can signal something beyond a typical infection.

I've found that layering two different types of deodorants during this time is very helpful for managing this symptom.

Symptom: Phantom Smells

Lower estrogen affects our sense of smell, causing us to smell things that aren't really there. This is also known as phantosmia and olfactory hallucinations. Women are more prone to phantom smells than men, and you may smell them in one or both nostrils. They tend to come and go, and for the most part, they disappear on their own.

Starting in my mid-thirties, I'd smell smoke, gasoline, and burnt toast out of nowhere. When I'd ask others around me if they smelled them too, the answer was always no. I spoke to my doctor about it and was referred to an ear, nose, and throat specialist (ENT), who said he couldn't find anything wrong. I had several tests, including an MRI, and the results always came back clear. Nobody could figure out what was causing them. My phantom smells disappeared once I was in menopause, and looking back, I realize they were one of my very first symptoms, but I had no idea they were related to perimenopause.

Our phantom smells survey, which has nearly 1,300 responses at the time of writing this book, shows that the most common phantom smells in perimenopause and menopause are smoke, fire, heat, and things burning. This includes cigarette or cigar smoke, bonfires, matches, electricity or overheated electronics, burnt wires, burnt plastic, burning rubber, hot pans, and burnt toast or coffee. Other phantom smells include mildew, body odor (BO), sewage, weed or cannabis, cat pee, poop (cat, dog, and human), garbage, sulfur, chemicals, sewage, bleach, rotten eggs, food or meat, cheap plastic (like flip-flops), skunk, metal, oily hair, cheap perfume, gasoline, and car exhaust. Some women smell pleasant things like baking (chocolate chip cookies, blueberry muffins, and freshly baked bread), chicken soup, and floral scents.

Other possible causes or triggers for phantom smells include sinus and nasal issues, a dry mouth, infections, migraines, stress, hypothyroidism (low thyroid hormone levels), medications, neurological conditions (like Parkinson's and head trauma), and vitamin deficiencies. In rare cases, they can be linked to seizures or stroke, which is why it's important to rule out other causes.

Note: If you smell something *before* someone else does, or you have a sensitive nose and the smell is actually there, then it isn't considered a phantom smell because it's a real scent.

Symptoms: Tinnitus, Dizziness, Vertigo

If you're experiencing ringing, humming, buzzing, throbbing, or even sounds like music or singing in your ears, all the time or once in a while, you may have tinnitus. Our research shows that 25 percent of women in perimenopause and menopause experience this symptom. Lower estrogen levels can affect the Eustachian tube and inner ear, which can lead to earaches, hot ears, itchy ears, blocked ears, hearing loss, and tinnitus. Hormonal changes during perimenopause and menopause can affect blood pressure and blood flow, which may play a role in conditions like tinnitus. Other possible contributing factors include loud noises, teeth grinding, low vitamin B12 levels, a buildup of earwax, side effects of medications, and old injuries to the head and neck. Tinnitus can also start or worsen during perimenopause, when estrogen levels fluctuate unpredictably.

Vertigo and Dizziness

Feeling lightheaded, off-balance, or like you might fall or faint? It can happen from changes in your hormones, like a drop in estrogen, which messes with your nervous system and blood flow.

If it feels like the room is spinning or tilting, this type of dizziness is known as vertigo. A common cause is something called benign paroxysmal positional vertigo, or BPPV, where tiny crystals in your inner ear move out of place. Estrogen plays a role in this condition, too, which is why vertigo tends to show up as a symptom for many women in perimenopause and menopause. Low levels of vitamin D are linked to more frequent recurrences of BPPV, so making sure your vitamin D levels are optimal can lower the risk of it coming back. I share what the recommended optimal vitamin D levels are in Chapter 10.

Other possible triggers for both tinnitus and vertigo include stress, anxiety, panic attacks, lack of sleep, migraines, ear infections, dehydration, and head- and neck-related movements like bending down, stretching your neck, or changing positions too quickly. Unstable blood sugar and long periods of sitting don't directly cause vertigo, but they can make you more sensitive to dizziness and balance problems in midlife.

Our Morphus research shows that 35 percent of women in perimenopause and menopause experience dizziness, and another 22 percent have vertigo. I had vertigo in my early forties, and it lasted about six weeks. My doctor at the time told me I had a virus called labyrinthitis, and looking back, I wonder if I was more susceptible because I was in perimenopause. It's something to ask your doctor about if you're experiencing any of these symptoms as well.

Symptom: Electric Shocks

This is a freaky symptom because it feels like your whole body lights up. When it happens to me, it usually feels like a jolt of electricity passes through my neck. I've also heard women refer to this symptom as "brain zaps."

As your hormones fluctuate and eventually drop during perimenopause and menopause, they can affect your nervous system and change the way your nerves send and process signals. That's why some women experience strange feelings like electric shocks, jolts, tremors, or zaps. Other possible sensations include pins and needles, numbness, pain, and tingling in extremities like hands and feet.

They can also happen because our connective tissues become less flexible as we age, and weight changes put extra pressure on nerves, leading to tingling, pins and needles, or even electric shock–like sensations. Hot flashes and night sweats can be accompanied by tingling sensations as blood flow and nerve sensitivity fluctuate. And heightened stress and anxiety can make you hyperaware of sensations in your body.

Other reasons for electric shocks can be low vitamin B12 levels and medical conditions such as fibromyalgia or multiple sclerosis, which may become more noticeable while your hormones are changing.

Symptoms: Burning Mouth, Scalp, Tongue, Feet

Does it feel like your mouth, tongue, lips, gums, or inner cheeks are burning? This symptom is known as burning mouth syndrome (BMS). Hormonal changes can affect the nerves inside your mouth, contributing to dry mouth (known as xerostomia), which can make the burning feeling even more intense. Foods or beverages may taste different to you now too. Lowered levels of estrogen can affect your taste buds, so your favorite bottle of red wine might suddenly taste off, even though it hasn't gone bad.

Some perimenopausal and menopausal women also feel burning or tingling sensations on their scalp and feet. Your feet may feel like they're on fire, often at night, but the only physical sign (if any) is some redness. In addition to hormonal changes due to a drop in estrogen, these burning sensations can be linked to nerve damage, nutritional deficiencies (like zinc, iron, and certain B vitamins like B1, B2, B6, folate, and B12), an underactive thyroid, diabetes, or local causes like allergies or infections.

Symptom: Bruises

Estrogen helps to keep our skin moist and plump. As our estrogen levels go down, our collagen levels go down too, making our skin thinner. Also, as we age, our blood vessels become more fragile, both of which make us more prone to bruising. Other possible causes of easy bruising include low platelets, certain nutrient deficiencies (like vitamin C or K), and underlying health issues such as diabetes or genetics.

Symptom: Restless Legs

This is one symptom I haven't experienced, but my friend described how it feels for her. She said it usually starts in the evening or once she gets into bed. Her legs start to buzz, tingle, or twitch, and she feels the need to move, stretch, or shake them. It interferes with her sleep and prevents her from getting a good night's rest.

Restless Legs Syndrome (RLS) is more common in women than

men and has been associated with hormonal fluctuations, especially lower estrogen during perimenopause and menopause, metabolic changes, and nutrient deficiencies such as magnesium, iron, potassium, and vitamin D. Also, women in perimenopause and menopause who have vasomotor symptoms, like night sweats, are more likely to have it.

Symptoms: Headaches and Migraine Attacks

During perimenopause, as hormones shift and fluctuate, headaches and migraines can increase in both frequency and intensity, even if they were well-managed before. Estrogen swings can influence neurotransmitters and other hormones, raising brain sensitivity and lowering the threshold for an attack.

After menopause, many women who experience migraine attacks notice fewer or milder episodes, and some say they stop altogether, although hormones often take a few years to stabilize. Women with chronic migraine (fifteen or more headache days a month for at least three months) may notice an improvement, while others may continue to have ongoing symptoms.

Common triggers reported by women in our community include stress; sleep changes; low blood sugar; alcohol; caffeine; dehydration; toxic relationships; changes in weather; sensory overload; skipping meals; food sensitivities; inflammation; processed meats (due to high sodium levels and/or nitrates); food additives (like artificial sweeteners, MSG, and artificial flavors); fermented foods like kombucha, kimchi, and tempeh; chocolate; gluten; oxalates found in spinach, beets, nuts and seeds, and nut butters; lectins found in beans, legumes, tomatoes, soybeans, and potatoes; and histamine-rich foods such as aged cheeses and leftovers.

Symptom: Hair Loss

When our hair starts thinning or falling out, as it does for many of us now, it affects more than just our appearance. It also affects our confidence and self-esteem.

Hair loss in women is called female pattern hair loss (FPHL) or androgenetic alopecia/female pattern alopecia, and it generally increases with age, especially after age forty, when many of us go into perimenopause. Women tend to find their hair thins or falls out at the top and the crown of the scalp (the top of your head toward the back), rather than receding at the hairline.

As estrogen and progesterone levels drop, the quantity and thickness of hair can drop, too, leading to slower growth and thinner strands. You also might notice changes in the texture of your hair (maybe it's curlier or frizzier now, or maybe the texture changes from one day to the next). At the same time, the relative increase in androgens (male hormones, particularly testosterone) can shrink hair follicles, resulting in hair loss on the scalp, but ironically, androgens can stimulate "peach fuzz" or coarse hairs in areas where we don't typically have hair, like the chin, upper lip, and nipples. Another possible reason for unwanted hair growth is insulin resistance (see Chapter 5).

Stress plays a huge role when it comes to hair loss, and research shows that chronic stress can prevent hair growth. Genetics (a family history of hair loss), inflammation of the scalp, illness, certain medications, nutritional deficiencies (such as low iron, protein, zinc, and more rarely biotin), environmental exposures to toxicants, pesticides, heavy metals, and thyroid problems can also lead to hair loss. One clue that your thyroid might be involved is if you notice that the outer third of your eyebrows is thinning.

Genitourinary Symptoms: Recurrent Urinary Tract Infections (UTIs), Vaginal Dryness, Vaginal or Urethral Burning, Burning with Urination, Pain During Sex, Urinary Urgency or Frequency, Leaking Urine, Vaginal Itching, Discharge or Odor, Loss of Elasticity, Difficulty Emptying the Bladder, Pelvic Pressure, and Mild Pelvic Organ Prolapse

I recently watched a viral social media post saying that our clitoris shrinks in menopause. This shook me and the thousands of other women who saw the video (hence the virality!).

What we all wanted to know was, is this true?

Unfortunately, it is. And this symptom falls under a broader term called genitourinary syndrome of menopause. GSM encompasses genital, sexual, and urinary symptoms. It used to be called "vaginal atrophy," but it was updated because, as Kim Vopni, a certified menopause support practitioner and vagina coach explains, the older term didn't include all the signs and symptoms that fall under the umbrella of GSM. GSM is mostly linked to the loss of estrogen.

According to Kim, genital symptoms could refer to physical changes to our external genitalia, or vulva, like thinning and drying of the tissues. For example, the labia can start to thin; the labia minora can shrink, flatten, or in some cases fully disappear; and the clitoral hood can become smaller or adhered (fused) over the clitoris. We lose that fullness and suppleness that the tissues typically have before estrogen levels fall. There may also be some itching, dryness, burning, and possibly bleeding with any sort of friction.

Then we have urinary symptoms, which could include urgency, frequency, burning, stress urinary incontinence, UTIs, and pelvic organ prolapse. There are also sexual symptoms, which could include decreased lubrication and painful sex. The pain could come from dry tissues or organs that have shifted out of place, or tight muscles. This isn't a full list, but these are the most common symptoms. I interviewed Kim on my podcast, *Menopause Reimagined*, on episode #139.

Urinary Tract Infections

UTIs are so common that approximately 50–60 percent of women will experience at least one in their lifetime. And as we age and go into menopause, that risk increases due to lower estrogen levels, which lead to shifts in vaginal bacteria, especially a decrease in protective lactobacilli and an increase in pH levels. Dr. James Simon and I had an in-depth conversation about UTIs (episode #101 on my podcast) and how the vagina has its own defense system against bacteria, fungi, and some viruses when it's kept healthy. But when the pH shifts from acidic to more alkaline, it makes it easier for pathogens to grow and move up into the urinary tract, increasing the risk of UTIs, bacterial vaginosis, and yeast infections.

Symptoms of UTIs include a strong urge to pee (and often with only small amounts of urine), pain or burning when you pee, cloudy urine or foul-smelling urine, lower-back pain, pressure in the pelvic area or the middle or side of your stomach, feeling unwell or fatigued, and blood in the urine.

I'd had a few UTIs as an adult, so I knew what they felt like. But as I've gotten older (which coincided with when I went into menopause), I find that my symptoms show up differently now. Instead of the usual signs, many of which I mentioned above, I can often tell I have a UTI because my memory is affected. I'd heard this could happen, so I dug into the research. I discovered that in older adults, UTIs can still come with the typical symptoms, but they can also show up as memory loss, confusion, fatigue, sudden changes in behavior, agitation, delusions, hallucinations, or paranoia. If symptoms like these appear unexpectedly, it's important to consider the possibility of a UTI.

I use at-home UTI test strips at least once a month, or more often if I suspect I have one. While they aren't a firm diagnostic tool, they can give you an indication of whether you should speak to your doctor about getting a proper urine test. And even if the test doesn't show anything, it's still worth speaking to your doctor if something feels off.

Here's an interesting and empowering perspective that my friend Jana Danielson, founder of Bloom Better and creator of the Cooch Ball, told me when it comes to pelvic health: Research from urogynecologist Dr. Bruce Crawford shows that 90 percent of pelvic floor dysfunction (PFD) is a fitness issue, not a medical one. He says that PFD often comes from poor breathing, poor posture, and less blood flow to the pelvic area. Adjusting these three key areas can help us pee, poop, move better, and have more comfortable sex because the pelvic floor supports all of those functions. Jana and I talked more about this on my podcast, *Menopause Reimagined*, episode #181.

Here's an important takeaway: When speaking to your healthcare provider about any symptoms you may be experiencing, mention that you're going through perimenopause or menopause (if you know you are) or suspect you might be so they can take this into account. You are your own best advocate.

4

Nourishing Your Gut: Menopause and Digestive Health

Any nutritionist, including myself, loves to talk about gut health because it's one of the foundations of our education, if not *the* foundation.

My own gut health issues inspired me to go back to school in my late twenties to study nutrition. I was experiencing gas and bloating every time I ate, and eventually I got tired of running around in circles trying to figure out why.

Digestion is a key part of understanding perimenopause and menopause because it plays a role in how your body regulates hormones, absorbs nutrients, and functions day to day. About half of us are experiencing digestive issues now, including gas, bloating, indigestion, loose stools (diarrhea), constipation, pain, and reflux after eating.

Does this sound like something you've been saying to yourself lately:

I don't understand . . . I was always able to eat or drink XYZ, but now I can't, and it causes me to [finish the sentence with your own symptom(s)].

This is why I say: What happens *before* perimenopause and menopause can (and probably will) change *after* you go into perimenopause and menopause, especially when it comes to digestion and gut health.

But *why* are things different now? Why do some of your favorite foods suddenly become a challenge to eat? Or why do you suddenly find yourself dealing with digestive issues that you never had before?

The answer includes a combination of several related factors, including changing hormones during this life stage; changes in digestion, which can make it less efficient; and the role gut health plays in absorbing nutrients, processing hormones, and keeping your immune system strong and healthy.

I know this isn't a simple topic, and I don't expect you to become an expert on gut health just by reading this chapter. However, understanding *how* your digestive system works can help explain *why* the way your body processes food changes as you go into peri-menopause and menopause. Once you know why, you can make adjustments to better support your digestive health.

Here are some things to keep in mind as you read through this chapter and the rest of the book:

1. You *can* make changes to your lifestyle that will improve your digestion, gut health, symptoms, and quality of life. In some cases, it may take a while to see the results, but rest assured, every change is a positive step forward.

2. Go at your own pace. Whether you decide to go slow, or do everything all at once, both ways are the right way.

3. If you're not already doing so, learn how to listen to your body; it's always communicating with you.

4. You're the boss. You know your body best, so listen to yourself when it comes to what foods are best for you. Others (no matter what their influence or credentials are) can offer ideas and suggestions, but you're the one who gets to decide what's right for you.

Digestion 101

The digestive system is made up of many parts that work together to break down food, absorb nutrients, and eliminate whatever it no longer needs. To understand what happens where, I'll take you on a journey through your digestive system.

But first, try this: Think about your favorite food. How does it look, taste, and smell? Is your mouth watering yet? Most likely, it is, because digestion starts even *before* you take the first bite. Just thinking about food triggers saliva production, which contains enzymes like amylase to start breaking down starches into sugars (ever notice how food tastes sweeter the longer you chew?). Chewing breaks food into smaller pieces, making it easier for your digestive system to do its job.

Once swallowed, food travels through the esophagus to the stomach, pushed along by muscle contractions called *peristalsis* (or gut motility). Think of it as a wave, or a conveyor belt, in your gut that moves food through your digestive tract. This motion helps your body take in nutrients and clear out waste.

In your stomach, food mixes with stomach acid, called hydrochloric acid, or HCl, and enzymes to break proteins into smaller pieces called peptides.

From here, other organs step in to help, and digestion becomes a team effort:

- The pancreas releases enzymes into the small intestine to digest proteins, fats, and carbs. It also produces insulin to regulate blood sugar (more on that in Chapter 5).

- The liver makes bile to help break down fats, and the gallbladder stores it and then releases it as needed. If you don't have a gallbladder, your liver continuously releases bile into your intestines to help your body digest food.

- The small intestine is the powerhouse of digestion and nutrient absorption. At about 20 feet long, it uses bile and enzymes from the pancreas to break down food into nutrients your body can absorb.

- At around 5 feet long, the colon, also known as the large intestine, absorbs water and electrolytes and prepares waste for removal by forming stool (aka poop).

- Together, the small and large intestines are known as *the gut*.

- Stool that's ready to go is stored in the rectum. The anus, with its sensors and muscles, ensures it's released at the right time.

The Gut Microbiome

Over the last fifteen years, gut health has received a lot of attention, and for good reason. Research shows that the types of microbiota living in your gut microbiome (bacteria, viruses, archaea, and fungi, both "friendly" and unfavorable) play a large part in supporting digestive, brain, mental, hormone, and immune health. When the microbiome is in balance, meaning all the microbiota are living in harmony, digestion works well, supporting your overall wellness.

However, when the microbiome becomes imbalanced, a state called dysbiosis, it can lead to health problems. This imbalance can be triggered by factors such as poor diet, ongoing stress, infections, alcohol, smoking, overuse of antibiotics, exposure to environmental pollutants, and hormonal changes during perimenopause and menopause.

The microbes living in your gut microbiome help you digest food and do much more than that. Chronic inflammation, which is linked to conditions like arthritis, cardiovascular disease, and others, has a strong relationship with gut health. Research also shows that the gut plays a role in other health issues like obesity, mental health, type 2 diabetes, brain health, liver disease, hormone imbalances, and more.

So protecting and nourishing your gut microbiome is essential for keeping your whole body healthy and your hormones in check.

The Gut-Brain Connection

The gut and the brain are constantly talking to each other, and they're connected through a two-way superhighway called the vagus nerve. This is the largest cranial nerve (a major nerve that carries signals between the brain and body). It runs from the brain stem (the base of the neck) down to the top of the large intestine. The gut and brain send important messages back and forth, and it's why the gut is also called "the second brain." When one is happy, the other is happy too, and when one is upset, the other is upset too.

Scientists refer to this communication system as the *gut-brain axis*. It's also called the *gut-brain connection*, and that's the term I'll use throughout this book.

While the vagus nerve is best known for its role in the nervous system and how we respond to stress, it also helps to regulate digestion by telling the stomach to release acid and trigger digestive enzymes that break down food. It also helps control appetite by sending signals from the stomach and intestines to the brain. Have you heard the phrase "rest and digest"? It refers to when the vagus nerve stimulates the parasympathetic part of your nervous system, which helps you to relax so you can properly digest your food. I talk about the vagus nerve in Chapter 6, where I go into detail about the sympathetic and parasympathetic nervous systems and the gut-brain connection.

Perimenopause, Menopause, and Stress

Now that you know the basics, let's look at the top digestive complaints for women in perimenopause and menopause and what you can do about them. At the top of the list are gas, bloating, loose stools, and constipation.

One of the main reasons these issues are popping up now is because your hormones are changing, and as estrogen levels fluctuate, how you respond to stress and how you digest food are affected. When we're stressed, cortisol (a key stress hormone) is released. When it comes to digestive health specifically, chronic stress and consistently high cortisol levels can negatively impact digestion by lowering the production of digestive enzymes as well as stomach acid, both of which are necessary for breaking down what we eat and drink. Stress can also slow peristalsis, which means food takes longer to move through your digestive tract. When this happens, food can sit there longer than it should, and start to ferment, which can lead to gas, bloating, cramping, or changes in bowel movements. It can also increase the likelihood of gut permeability (leaky gut).

When daily stressors such as bills, work, aging parents, and kids take their toll, they can create the perfect storm for digestive issues. Poor digestion can lead to nutrients not being absorbed properly. When this happens, undigested food moves into the large intestine, where it throws off the gut bacteria there, leading to bloating, diarrhea, and discomfort in the intestinal lining. Over time, this kind of stress on the digestive system can lead to inflammation. Higher cortisol levels during menopause can also contribute to this inflammation, potentially causing symptoms like loose stools, constipation, gas, bloating, nausea, heartburn, fatigue, abdominal pain or discomfort, gut permeability, and so on.

Also, for many women, food sensitivities, and sometimes existing allergies, can show up or get worse around this time. Again, this is primarily due to your changing hormones, which can impact the immune and digestive systems (more on this later in the chapter).

The Estrobolome

The gut microbiome plays an important role when it comes to regulating estrogen levels. Within the microbiome is a collection of gut bacteria with special genes called the estrobolome. These bacteria help to break down and metabolize estrogen so your body can process and clear it. Having a good amount of different types of beneficial bacteria is important for the overall health of the estrobolome. Research shows that menopause can lead to changes in the balance of bacteria in the gut microbiome and the estrobolome, which in turn can affect how we break down and clear estrogen from the body. In fact, some research also shows that the gut microbiomes of women in menopause start to look similar to those of men. Hopefully, more research will be done to confirm this pattern and learn what it means for long-term health.

If your estrobolome is out of balance and your gut is in a state of dysbiosis, it can disrupt how estrogen is broken down and cleared, causing levels to be either too high or too low. One potential side effect of an imbalanced estrobolome is an increase in the production of an enzyme called beta-glucuronidase. When high, this enzyme can reactivate the estrogen your body was trying to get rid of, putting it back into circulation in an active form, which can lead to potentially elevated levels of estrogen. Higher levels of estrogen, relative to progesterone, can increase the risk of blood clots and estrogen-dominant cancers such as breast and ovarian. Symptoms of a higher estrogen to progesterone ratio, often called estrogen dominance, include heavy bleeding, irregular periods, moodiness, acne, uterine fibroids, cysts, and breast tenderness. On the other hand, when beta-glucuronidase is too low, more estrogen is excreted than reabsorbed. This can lower estrogen levels and affect your mood, skin, hair, brain function, bone loss, and cardiovascular health.

As you can see, an imbalance of bacteria in your gut can affect your hormones, and changing hormone levels can affect your gut bacteria, creating a cycle where both problems feed into each other and can trigger or worsen perimenopause and menopause symptoms. A healthy gut microbiome, including a balanced estrobolome, helps support beneficial bacteria and the right amount of enzymes like beta-glucuronidase, which help regulate estrogen, and, in turn, can help alleviate symptoms.

So how can we support our estrobolome?

Research shows that eating more fiber is associated with larger stools and easier bowel movements, and potentially less reabsorption of the estrogen your body has already broken down (estrogen metabolites).

Eating a whole foods diet that includes fermented probiotic-rich foods (if tolerated*), soluble fiber, regular exercise, good-quality sleep, and stress management practices can all support gut health. In turn, this supports the estrobolome and hormone function and may help ease symptoms during perimenopause and menopause.

You can check your beta-glucuronidase levels with a gut test like Vitract (www.vitract.com).

---

* Those with histamine intolerance, dysbiosis, or yeast overgrowth, such as candida; a sensitivity to tyramine (a natural compound found in aged cheese, cured meats, and soy sauce); or FODMAP sensitivities may not be able to tolerate fermented foods. FODMAP is an acronym for certain types of carbs that some people have a hard time digesting. It stands for: fermentable oligosaccharides, disaccharides, monosaccharides, and polyols.

Common Digestive Complaints in Perimenopause and Menopause

Here's a more detailed list of the most common digestive complaints women in perimenopause and menopause experience and *why* they happen. In the next section, I'll provide some top-line tips for relieving them. I say "top-line" because, in some cases, digestive issues can be relatively simple to solve. However, they can also be complicated, so consult with your doctor or a gut health specialist to dig deeper into your personal experiences.

Bloating

As we get older, peristalsis can slow down, and food and waste move more slowly through the intestines. When food sits in the gut longer, bacteria have more time to ferment it, producing gas that often leads to bloating. Bloating can also happen when the stomach doesn't produce enough acid to properly break down food or when gut bacteria are out of balance. These changes can lead to a buildup of gas in your colon, making the belly feel swollen or hard. Bloating can be uncomfortable, sometimes painful, and it can happen once in a while or on a regular basis.

Gas (belching, burping, and flatulence)

We're gas-producing machines! Your digestive system releases gas from the stomach through the mouth (belching and burping) and through your intestines via the rectum (flatulence). We may not like to talk about it openly, but it's totally normal to pass gas anywhere from twelve to twenty-five times a day, but if you're passing gas too often, it can be annoying, embarrassing, and in some cases worrisome. We pass gas for different reasons: swallowing air when we eat, drink, or talk; bacteria in the gut breaking down leftover food and making gas; eating high-fiber or gas-producing foods like beans and cruciferous vegetables; digestive issues such as lactose intolerance or an irritable bowel (IBS); side effects from certain medications; and even stress.

Constipation

Chronic constipation can be frustrating, uncomfortable, and stressful. Keeping track of when you go and what your bowel movements look like can provide some insight into your bowel habits. Changing hormones can dry out stool, making it harder to pass, but there are many other reasons you get constipated, including a low-fiber diet or not drinking enough water, changes in your activity, quitting smoking, an underactive thyroid, certain medications, stress, or a weak pelvic floor.

Loose Stools or Diarrhea

Diarrhea is defined as having more than three loose, watery bowel movements a day. There are many reasons for having loose or watery stools at this stage of life, including intolerances to certain foods, additives, or supplement ingredients; too much fiber; greasy or fatty food; alcohol; caffeine; certain sweeteners (for example, high amounts of sugar alcohols like xylitol); or lower hydrochloric acid (HCl) levels. Other reasons include side effects of certain medications, infections, digestive disorders (like celiac, colitis, IBS, or inflammatory bowel disease), an overactive thyroid (hyperthyroidism), stress, and more.

Heartburn, Acid Reflux/Gastroesophageal Reflux Disease (GERD)

Heartburn, a burning sensation in your chest, is a common symptom of acid reflux or GERD. Other symptoms include food backing up into your throat, a bitter or sour taste at the back of your mouth, trouble swallowing, burping, bloating, and chest pain when you lie down or bend over.

Women are more prone to heartburn in perimenopause and menopause because lower estrogen and progesterone levels can weaken the muscle that prevents stomach acid from flowing back into the esophagus, called the lower esophageal sphincter (LES). Age; stress and increased cortisol levels; weight gain; certain medications, including nonsteroidal anti-inflammatory drugs (NSAIDs), like ibuprofen; lifestyle choices (such as eating too close to bed or smoking); and certain foods (like citrus, caffeine, onions, tomatoes/tomato products, alcohol, and greasy and spicy foods) can also trigger it. In fact, women in menopause are 3.5 times more likely to have GERD than women who are premenopausal.

A common misconception about heartburn is that it's caused by too much acid. While stomach acid is at the source of the issue, many experts believe it's triggered by having too little stomach acid. Stomach acid lowers with age, and low stomach acid (called hypochlorhydria) becomes more common after age sixty due to chronic stress, poor diet, nutrient deficiencies, and long-term antacid use.

Indigestion

Indigestion (aka dyspepsia) simply means you're experiencing some sort of digestive discomfort like stomach pain, a feeling of fullness, gas, nausea, or stomach gurgling after eating. Hormones and stress play a role. A drop in estrogen can slow down digestion, leading to these symptoms, and stress can worsen symptoms of indigestion.

Indigestion can range from mild to severe. Many symptoms can overlap with other digestive issues like heartburn or IBS, so watch for patterns or possible triggers that could be causing it.

Irritable Bowel Syndrome (IBS)

IBS affects about 10 percent of the world's population and is more common among women. Symptoms include diarrhea, constipation, or both (alternating), and often abdominal pain, cramping, gas, bloating, and mucus in the stool. Changing hormones and increased stress in perimenopause and menopause are contributing factors that can trigger or intensify IBS symptoms. Many women report that their IBS symptoms become more intense or severe once they're in menopause.

Small Intestinal Bacterial Overgrowth (SIBO)

Normally, the small intestine has only a small amount of gut bacteria, as the majority live in the large intestine. The small intestine's main roles are to digest food and absorb nutrients, so its bacterial population must be minimal and controlled.

During perimenopause and menopause, changes in hormones, especially lower levels of progesterone and estrogen, can slow digestion and interfere with a built-in mechanism that prevents bacteria from creeping into the small intestine. As a result, too many or the wrong kinds of bacteria can build up and overgrow in the small intestine, causing a condition called small intestinal bacterial overgrowth, or SIBO.

Many people have both SIBO and IBS. SIBO can also develop if there are structural issues in the digestive tract, past surgeries, or you're taking certain medications like proton pump inhibitors (PPIs). Current testing for SIBO isn't entirely reliable, but it's improving, and the condition can be managed with diet, antibiotics, probiotics, and herbal remedies. If you're experiencing ongoing digestive symptoms such as gas, bloating, diarrhea, nausea, cramping, fatigue, intense cravings for sugar or carbs, unintentional weight loss, stomach pain, or even constipation, ask your doctor to test you for it.

Increased Intestinal Permeability, or Leaky Gut

Increased intestinal permeability, more commonly known as leaky gut syndrome, is when the lining of the small intestine becomes more porous than it should be. A healthy gut lining, which is only one cell thick, is very intentional about letting nutrients through while keeping harmful substances out. When the lining becomes "leaky," small gaps can open, allowing tiny particles of undigested food, toxins, and bacteria to pass through and into the bloodstream. When this happens, it can trigger inflammation, fatigue, brain fog, memory loss, skin problems, and potentially many other symptoms. It's also been linked to medical conditions like type 2 diabetes and dementia.

Women in perimenopause and menopause are more likely to have a weaker gut lining because estrogen and progesterone normally help keep that lining strong. At the same time, we're more prone to higher cortisol levels, which can weaken the lining even further. And changes in gut bacteria can throw off the balance of beneficial and harmful microbes, weakening the gut's natural defense.

Infections

Lower levels of estrogen and progesterone can weaken the gut's built-in defense systems, making you more vulnerable to infections like *H. pylori* and candida. Infections in the digestive system can throw the gut microbiome out of balance and cause digestive problems. Medically, *H. pylori* is usually treated with antibiotics and sometimes probiotics to restore balance. If you suspect you have candida, a yeast overgrowth that can disrupt the balance of the gut and other areas of the body, the best approach is to work with a doctor or healthcare provider who can create a personalized treatment plan that may include antifungals, dietary changes, probiotics, or supplements.

Tips for Optimal Digestion and Gut Health

You've probably heard the expression "You are what you eat." While that's true, a more accurate saying is "You are what you eat, digest, and absorb." You can eat the most nutritious food in the world, but if you can't properly digest or absorb its nutrients, it doesn't really benefit you.

Here are some suggestions to help manage and improve digestion:

Adopt a whole foods diet. Eat foods that are minimally processed and as close to their natural state as possible. Limit ultra-processed foods, which contain empty calories; refined sugars and carbs; additives; unhealthy fats; and other ingredients that can disrupt your gut microbiome and, in turn, your hormones. Refer to Chapter 11 for a sustainable, long-term eating plan.

Take enzymes. When it comes to digestion, your body makes special proteins called enzymes. Enzymes help your body break down food and nutrients into smaller, more digestible pieces (or, more accurately, molecules) so your body can absorb them and use them for energy, to build muscle, and to repair itself. As you age, your body's ability to produce certain digestive enzymes may decrease, and this tends to become even more common in midlife, which may affect how well you break down and absorb some foods. Raw fruits and vegetables, raw honey, and fermented foods like kimchi, sauerkraut, and tempeh contain naturally occurring enzymes. There are different types of enzymes, each designed to break down specific foods. The more common ones include protease, amylase, lipase, and lactase, which help to break down protein, carbohydrates, fats, and lactose, respectively. Raw foods contain more enzymes than cooked foods, as cooking above 117 degrees Fahrenheit (47 degrees Celcius) destroys them.

If you need extra support, you can buy digestive enzymes in supplement form, and you can get them for specific conditions. For example, if you don't have a gallbladder, you can take a digestive enzyme that has lipase and ox bile (or bile salts) to help break down fats, as well as amylase and protease for overall digestive support. If you're lactose intolerant, taking lactase pills can help prevent gas and discomfort when eating dairy. If you're looking for overall digestive support, you can take a full-spectrum digestive enzyme right before a meal, especially a larger meal. Choose a brand that includes a variety of enzymes specific to your digestive needs. If you shop at a health food or natural product store, ask a staff member to help guide you as to which digestive enzyme supplement may be right for you. You can also speak to a health professional who specializes in digestion, like a nutritionist, and always consult with your doctor or healthcare provider before taking anything new.

Get bitter. Bitter plants (like arugula, bitter melon, Brussels sprouts, and dandelion) stimulate bitter taste receptors on your tongue, telling your brain to release digestive enzymes in the gut (the gut-brain connection at work!). Digestive bitters (not to be confused with cocktail bitters, which evolved to flavor drinks) have been used for centuries in herbal traditions around the world, including traditional Chinese medicine. They stimulate your taste buds to produce more saliva, helping to kickstart the production of digestive juices in your stomach. Bitters can be purchased in liquid form. Take them ten to fifteen minutes before you eat a meal. In order for bitters to work their magic, you have to *taste* them, so don't just swallow them quickly! Be sure to savor their bitter taste.

Boost your acid. If you don't have digestive enzymes with hydrochloric acid, or HCl, handy, use a small amount of fresh-squeezed lemon juice or apple cider vinegar to help stimulate digestion. Add one to two teaspoons of lemon juice or apple cider vinegar to one-quarter cup of room-temperature water and drink it about ten minutes before a meal or when you start eating. The acidic nature of the lemon or apple cider vinegar may help support digestion, especially protein digestion, in the stomach. While this idea is widely accepted in the natural health world, keep in mind that it's based on theory and anecdotal evidence rather than solid scientific research.

Drink wisely with meals. Drinking large amounts of liquid while you're eating a meal is a habit that many of us learned as kids or as part of a weight management approach. If you have digestive issues, try sipping small amounts of liquid instead, or drink between meals, and stop drinking a minimum of thirty minutes *before* you eat to give the liquids time to clear your system before you eat any food.

Slow down. Eating slowly, putting your cutlery down between mouthfuls, and taking smaller bites give your mind and body an opportunity to communicate. The body sends its satiety signals to the brain about twenty minutes after you start eating, which is why it's so easy to overeat. By eating more slowly, you give your body a chance to catch up to your brain so it can recognize the signals that you've had enough.

Chew, chew, chew. Chewing is the first step in the digestive process, and it's the *only* part of digestion that you have full control over. When you chew, larger food particles are broken down into smaller ones, making it easier for nutrients to be absorbed. Saliva contains digestive enzymes, and chewing cues your stomach to make more HCl. When you don't chew properly, swallowing large pieces of food makes it harder for your body to digest, which can lead to gas, bloating, constipation, and other digestive discomforts. Also, chewing thoroughly allows you to savor the flavor, texture, and aroma of each bite.

Note: If you're like 27 percent of women in perimenopause and menopause who have a dry mouth or tongue, you might notice you don't have as much saliva as you used to. Less saliva means fewer enzymes for breaking down your food, so pay extra attention to chewing your food thoroughly and drinking enough water during the day to help move your food through your digestive tract. If you have trouble chewing, stick to a soft-food diet consisting of foods that are easy to chew and swallow. Greek yogurt, cottage cheese, mashed fruits and vegetables, pureed soups and stews, scrambled eggs, soups, smooth nut butters, smoothies, and protein shakes are all good, nourishing options. You can also blend your food before eating it.

Eat enough fiber. Both the U.S. Department of Agriculture and Health Canada recommend getting 21–25 grams of fiber a day, yet most of us fall short of this goal. As a nutritionist, I like to see that number somewhere between 25 and 30 grams. Fiber, a nondigestible carbohydrate found in plant foods, comes in two forms: soluble (dissolves in water) and insoluble (doesn't dissolve in water).

Fiber helps support a healthy gut microbiome. It helps to keep you regular, improves peristalsis, and adds bulk to stool, helping it to move more easily through your intestines, reducing the risk of digestive disorders like hemorrhoids, diverticulosis, and constipation.

Eat the right carbs. All carbohydrates are not created equal, nor are they the enemy. Choose your carbohydrates wisely. Quality carbs such as vegetables, low-glycemic fruits, and whole grains are necessary for physical and mental performance, energy, moods, and mental health. They're also important for thyroid health, sleep, and helping to make hormones. If you severely restrict or eliminate carbohydrates altogether, you'll miss out on important nutrients and fiber. I talk a lot more about carbohydrates in Chapters 8 and 10.

Eliminate distractions. Try eating without distractions. When you put away your phone and remove yourself from screens at mealtimes, you can pay closer attention to your food and its taste, smell, and texture. This helps your body start the digestion process, prevents overeating, and stimulates your parasympathetic nervous system ("rest and digest" mode) so you're primed for digestion.

Eat smaller meals, and more often. If you have acid reflux or your digestion is slow, try eating smaller meals more often. This way of eating can help take some of the stress off your digestive system, especially the lower esophageal sphincter, which allows acid to flow back into your esophagus when it's weakened.

However, it's important to note that eating too often, especially when your meals and snacks are high in ultra-processed and refined carbohydrates and sugars, can lead to consistently high glucose and insulin levels. And over time this may lead to insulin resistance, weight gain, and a sluggish metabolism. I dive deeper into this topic in Chapter 5.

Do what feels right for you and your body.

Sleep smart. If you have acid reflux or heartburn, especially at night before bed, try lying on your left side with your head slightly lifted. Research shows that this position can lower your exposure to acid by up to 71 percent. Avoid sleeping on your right side, because it can increase your chances of having reflux by allowing stomach acid to enter the esophagus. This doesn't work for everyone, but give it a try and see how your body responds. You can also try sleeping with your head and chest higher than your stomach (raise the head of your bed about six inches higher than the rest of your body using risers, an extra pillow, or sturdy objects). If you don't get heartburn at night, sleeping on your right side is best (more on sleep positions in Chapter 7).

Manage your weight. Increased fat around the midsection can have a negative impact on digestion by putting extra pressure on the organs around your belly. It can also promote inflammation and interfere with gut function by slowing peristalsis and changing the balance of the microbes that live there. In Chapter 11, I discuss principles that support a healthy metabolism, which can help with weight loss and weight maintenance.

Consider prebiotics, probiotics, and postbiotics. *Probiotics* are live microorganisms found in certain foods and supplements that can support your microbiome. The most common types of probiotics are bacteria or yeast, for example, *Lactobacillus acidophilus* and *Bifido-bacterium bifidum* (bacteria) and *Saccharomyces boulardii* (yeast). Research shows that certain probiotics can have a positive effect on your mental health, digestion, and immune system. Some probiotics have anti-inflammatory properties, which can help support vaginal health, weight control, and a reduction in systemic inflammation, all of which can be affected when you're in perimenopause and menopause. You can find probiotics in fermented foods like yogurt with live and active cultures, kimchi, sauerkraut, kefir, miso, pickles (raw lacto-fermented), and tempeh. You can also take them as a supplement. If you choose to take probiotics as a supplement, choose brands that offer specific bacterial strains targeted for your individual health needs.

Tip: Don't take probiotics with a piping-hot beverage, as the heat can kill the beneficial bacteria (wait thirty minutes before and after drinking something hot to take them). Follow the directions on the bottle for best results.

Prebiotics have become so popular that food companies are adding them to foods and beverages like sodas, gum, smoothies, and bars. Prebiotics are types of plant fiber that travel to the lower digestive tract, where they feed the good bacteria (probiotics) in your gut. Think of them as food for the probiotics, helping them grow so they can keep your microbiome and body healthy. Like probiotics, prebiotics have many health benefits. They support digestion and mental health as well as bone health and immune function by enhancing the absorption of minerals like calcium and magnesium. Some of the best food sources of prebiotic fiber include garlic, onions, jicamas, Jerusalem artichokes, leeks, apples, asparagus, dandelion greens, konjac, burdock root, carrots with the skin on, and yacón (you can find this as a sweetener as well. I love using it in recipes that call for liquid sugar). Prebiotic fiber is also available as a supplement.

Postbiotics are made when the good bacteria in your gut break down fiber. Think of them as the waste products of probiotics, essentially "probiotic poop." Postbiotics may help ease menopausal symptoms by supporting gut and hormone health, and calming inflammation. They're also being studied for their potential to improve postmenopausal osteoporosis (PMOP) by promoting bone growth and reducing bone loss, strengthening the immune system, supporting healthy blood sugar balance, and helping to curb hunger. Postbiotics include short-chain fatty acids like acetate, butyrate, and propionate, as well as enzymes, amino acids, and more.

You can naturally increase postbiotics by eating foods rich in probiotics and prebiotics, as well as plant-based foods like vegetables, low-glycemic fruits, whole grains, fermented foods, and legumes. Lifestyle plays a role too. Reducing stress (Chapter 6) and improving the quality of your sleep (Chapter 7) helps keep your gut healthy, which supports the production of postbiotics. They're also available as supplements.

- *Probiotics*: Live beneficial microorganisms, including beneficial bacteria and some yeasts, that support gut health.

- *Prebiotics*: Food (fibers) for probiotics that helps them grow.

- *Postbiotics*: The beneficial compounds that probiotics produce.

A balanced gut microbiome relies on all three working together to create a healthy environment for digestion, strong immunity, and overall optimal health.

Movement: Exercise has a ton of incredible health benefits, including digestion! It improves the diversity of gut bacteria and helps move things along the digestive tract to keep you regular. Walking, swimming, low-impact aerobics, pickleball, and tennis are all excellent options.

Medications: If you're taking medication, check whether its side effects include any digestive issues like constipation, loose stools, heartburn, or indigestion.

Food Allergies, Intolerances, and Sensitivities

Do you find that certain foods affect you differently now? For example, you used to eat dairy all the time, but now even the thought of a grilled cheese sandwich or pizza makes you feel bloated, gassy, or nauseous. Or your signature BBQ beef or tofu dish that you survived on in your thirties now gives you a stomachache and headache every time you eat it. This is frustrating, uncomfortable, and sometimes painful. New sensitivities can show up seemingly out of nowhere, and reactions that were once mild can suddenly feel more intense.

Why are food intolerances, sensitivities, and allergies an issue specifically now? For many of the reasons I already mentioned: Changing hormone levels can cause your digestive system to slow down, which means food stays in your system longer, giving it more opportunity to cause irritation. Lower estrogen may contribute to reduced stomach acid (HCl) and a lower number of digestive enzymes being produced, which can lead to gas, bloating, indigestion, or other unpleasant symptoms. Stress, along with a drop in estrogen, can affect your immune system, making you more susceptible to food sensitivities. And your liver may not work as efficiently as it once did because of hormonal changes, stress, and age, which can influence digestion and detox pathways. It's a perfect storm.

Reactions to food can include some of the more common digestive symptoms, like gas, bloating, loose stools, and constipation. However, they may also trigger other responses, like headaches; migraine attacks; fatigue; tingling fingers and toes; flushing; heart palpitations; brain fog; itchy throat; bad breath; body odor, or B.O.; skin eruptions like acne, rashes, and hives; anxiety; moodiness; irritability; aches and pains; sleep issues; and more.

The most common foods that trigger reactions include gluten, wheat, sugar, dairy, soy, eggs, fish, seafood, sesame, shellfish, sulfites, peanuts, and tree nuts, as well as food additives found in ultra-processed foods, such as preservatives like nitrates, sulfites, and benzoates. You can also react to seemingly "healthy" foods like kale or broccoli.

The terms *food allergies*, *intolerances*, and *sensitivities* are sometimes used interchangeably, but they're very different and are their own distinct conditions.

Food Allergy

A true *food allergy* happens when your body's immune system overreacts to certain proteins in foods and mistakenly thinks they're harmful. When you ingest something you're allergic to, it triggers an immediate, or near-immediate, immune response usually minutes to a few hours after eating, drinking, or even being exposed to certain foods or beverages.

The first time, or first few times, you eat something you're allergic to, your body might mistake it for a threat, so it makes antibodies called IgE. These antibodies attach to specific cells in your immune system to prepare them to react the next time you're exposed to that food. Then, when you eat that food again, those antibodies recognize it and tell your immune cells to release chemicals, including histamine and cytokines to "fight" the offending food. It's your body's way of trying to protect you, even though the food itself isn't actually dangerous. Your body just sees it that way.

Allergic reactions can show up in different ways and can affect multiple systems in the body, including digestion, skin, breathing, mouth and throat, or even your heart and circulation. Possible reactions include vomiting, stomach cramps, hives, itching, eczema, swelling, shortness of breath, wheezing, trouble swallowing, swelling of the tongue, a weak pulse, pale skin, dizziness, and, in severe cases, anaphylaxis. Anaphylaxis can be life-threatening and always needs immediate emergency medical care.

Food Intolerance

A food intolerance, on the other hand, does not involve the immune system. It usually affects the digestive system, and it's very common. Symptoms can appear right after eating or drinking or be delayed for up to forty-eight hours.

Common food intolerance symptoms include stomach pain, bloating, gas, diarrhea, headaches, migraines, runny nose, and fatigue. They can also affect the skin and can show up as eczema, flushing, hives, and acne.

Unlike food allergies, where even a tiny amount of the allergen can trigger a reaction, food intolerance symptoms usually depend on how much of the triggering food you eat. In other words, for many people, the more you consume of that food, the more intense your symptoms might be.

Certain intolerances are related to a lack of the specific enzyme(s) needed to digest certain nutrients. Some of the most common intolerances are lactose intolerance, fructose intolerance, and gluten intolerance.

Lactose intolerance affects 25 percent of North Americans and 65 percent of people worldwide. When you experience gas or loose stools after eating dairy, it often means you produce less lactase, the enzyme needed to digest lactose, the sugar in dairy. You may also be genetically predisposed to it, like I am. Research shows that probiotics (refer to the foods I mentioned earlier) can help with lactose digestion. One example, kefir (a type of fermented milk drink that you can find in most grocery stores) contains a variety of beneficial microbes that can help break down lactose. These microbes can help support and rebuild the population of beneficial bacteria in your gut involved in digesting dairy, depending on the underlying cause of your symptoms.

A *histamine intolerance* happens when histamine builds up in the body because your body can't break it down quickly enough. Histamine is a natural chemical made by your body that plays an important role when it comes to your brain, appetite, digestion, and immune system. It's also found in certain foods, including aged cheeses, fermented foods, cured meats, red wine, beer, and leftovers.

When histamine builds up, it can trigger symptoms that often affect the digestive system, like gas, bloating, loose stools, or constipation, but it can also cause issues like dizziness, anxiety, heart palpitations, headaches, runny nose, congestion, sneezing, sinus issues, an itchy or inflamed nose, and flushing.

Estrogen and histamine are closely related: Higher estrogen can stimulate the release of histamine, histamine can influence estrogen levels, and too much estrogen may weaken the effectiveness of the enzyme (diamine oxidase or DAO) that breaks histamine down, leading to symptoms that feel a lot like perimenopause or menopause.

I interviewed Dr. Tania Dempsey about histamine intolerance in perimenopause and menopause on episode #66 of my podcast, *Menopause Reimagined.*

A *chemical sensitivity* is when you react to naturally occurring or added chemicals in foods. Some examples include monosodium glutamate (MSG), caffeine, sulfites (found in dried fruits, condiments, and red wine), artificial colors, and so on.

Food sensitivities or *hypersensitivities* are catch-all terms often used to describe reactions to foods, which can include allergies, intolerances, and autoimmune diseases like celiac. Sensitivities can happen for many reasons, including genetics, environmental factors like pollution, a weakened immune system, challenges with our gut microbiome such as leaky gut, or changes in the bacteria living in your gut.

The Importance of Rotating Your Food

Something to keep in mind is that we can unintentionally make our symptoms worse by eating the same foods every day (I ate eggs every morning for years until my throat became itchy, and I had to stop). This is why I recommend rotating the foods you eat and not eating the same things several days in a row. Changing up what you eat on a regular basis helps to feed your gut with different kinds of beneficial bacteria, supporting a more diverse microbiome. According to Linta Mustafa, cofounder and CEO of Vitract, "The more diverse your gut microbiome is by eating different types of foods, the better you're setting your terrain up to promote health." Linta describes the gut microbiome as a jungle of different bugs that all live together in perfect harmony. When that harmony is thrown off, it can have detrimental effects on your health. She goes on to say, "Gut microbiome science is very complex, but it can be boiled down to understanding that different bugs in your gut prefer different food sources. This means that when we consume certain foods, we are directly dictating which bugs will colonize in the gut." The good news is that Linta believes that harmony can be restored by eating a wide variety of colorful veggies and fruits (which contain prebiotic fibers), spices, herbs, legumes, complex carbohydrates, and fermented foods like kimchi, sauerkraut, sour pickles, miso, tempeh, and kefir, and by following many of the other tips discussed in this chapter and book.

Managing Food Sensitivities

Here are some tips for managing food sensitivities. If you have a severe allergy or anaphylaxis, please follow your doctor's advice.

Keep a food and symptoms journal. Track what you eat and drink and write down any symptoms you experience or foods you suspect may be an issue. Share this information with your doctor or health-care provider so they can help you identify potential trigger foods or ingredients. They can also create a plan to manage, minimize, or eliminate them. My team and I created a Food and Hydration Journal to help. You'll find it under the Resources section at www .nourishingmenopausebook.com. *Note:* If you suspect you have a food allergy, I recommend seeing an allergist as soon as possible.

Go pro. Eat a variety of probiotic- and prebiotic-rich foods, as they feed the entire ecosystem in your gut, also known as your micro-biota, which includes bacteria, fungi, viruses, archaea, and other microbes.

Love your liver. The liver is one of your body's major detoxification organs. Supporting its efforts to eliminate metabolized estrogen, medication(s), alcohol, and other substances that can potentially trigger food sensitivities is key. Eating a whole foods diet with a focus on cruciferous vegetables and bitter foods and staying well-hydrated is important. I talk more about the liver and its role in digestion later in the chapter.

Manage stress. Stress can worsen food sensitivities by throwing off the balance of gut bacteria (increasing the risk of dysbiosis), lowering stomach acid and the production of digestive enzymes, weakening the immune system, thinning the gut lining (making it more "leaky"), and increasing inflammation.

Try an elimination diet. This type of diet involves avoiding a specific food, or foods, for a limited time to see if you're still experiencing symptoms.

An elimination diet can be helpful for identifying foods that may be triggering your digestive issues. The underlying cause could be a food allergy, intolerance, digestive disorder, genetic abnormality, or a combination of these factors. For the best results, work with a qualified healthcare provider to ensure an elimination diet is right for you, and try it for four to six weeks.

Registered holistic nutritionist (R.H.N.) Julie Daniluk specializes in this process. In her book *Meals That Heal Inflammation*, she explains, "An effective elimination plan is a clear, short-term experiment. During that time, simplify meals to nourishing basics that calm the gut and steady blood sugar, focusing on quality protein, cooked colorful vegetables, and healthy fats, while removing the most common irritants such as gluten, dairy, refined sugar, alcohol, and seed oils (e.g., canola, corn, cottonseed, grapeseed, safflower, sunflower, and soybean). Keep a daily log of foods, symptoms, sleep, and stress to help patterns stand out. When you feel consistently better for at least two weeks, reintroduce one food you don't believe you're currently reacting to by consuming two servings in one day, then wait forty-eight to seventy-two hours to watch for changes in digestion, skin, pain, energy, or mood. If a food flares your symptoms, set it aside, rebuild with food that loves you back, and make practical swaps, like using ground flaxseed instead of wheat flour in crackers or using wraps made from egg whites instead of cornmeal."

The Art of Pooping in Perimenopause and Menopause

How often do you poop? Whatever that number is, consider it your baseline. According to a Healthline survey of over two thousand responses, 50 percent of the respondents reported that they go at least once a day, 28 percent go twice a day, and 5.6 percent said they go once or twice a week.

When you poop is governed by your circadian rhythm, so people tend to *go* around the same time of day. A bowel movement can also be stimulated by your eating habits, for example, *when* and *what* you eat. Sixty-one percent of the survey respondents said they go in the morning, 22 percent go in the afternoon, and 2.6 percent reported that they go late at night.

How often should you be pooping? According to Bonnie Wisener, registered holistic nutritionist (R.H.N.) and founder of the Shift Your Gut Therapy Method™, "Daily bowel movements are ideal for optimal digestion and gut health. However, what's considered normal can vary, with three times a week to three times a day generally falling within the healthy range. The key is consistency and how you feel." Bonnie explains that "it's not just about how often you poop, but how well you're evacuating. Healthy stool should be soft, well-formed, and easy to pass. Straining or incomplete evacuation are signs that something might be off, even if you're having regular bowel movements."

Once we go into perimenopause and menopause, it's important to have regular bowel movements, because it helps your body clear estrogen as well as other hormones. Estrogen is processed by the liver and then removed from the body through our bowels. If our digestion is sluggish and we go to the bathroom less often, our gut bacteria can reactivate some of that estrogen, and it could be reabsorbed back into the bloodstream, potentially worsening certain symptoms like bloating, mood swings, and breast tenderness.

Pooping is a natural part of life. We all do it. It's important to go to the bathroom when you feel the urge. Holding it in every once in a while isn't an issue, but making a habit of it can lead to constipation because as you use your anal and rectal muscles to push the stool back into your large intestine, water from the stool is absorbed, making your poop dry and hard. Also, you may feel nauseous or unwell, or you may not have the urge to go again until the next day. More serious consequences of holding in your poop are impaction (stool becomes stuck in the colon), hemorrhoids, and anal fissures or tears.

Have you heard of the term *poop-phoria*? The term was coined by Josh Richman and Anish Sheth, MD, authors of *What's Your Poo Telling You?*, and they explain, in a very entertaining way, that pooping makes us happy because it stimulates the vagus nerve and relaxes muscles, both of which may promote the release of endorphins and feelings of euphoria. During perimenopause and menopause, hormonal changes can disrupt both digestion and moods, making that "poop-phoria" feeling harder to come by. Given the connection between the gut and brain, supporting gut health is important not only for digestion, but also for our mental health.

Other than feeling a euphoric boost and helping to steady your mood, why else do I want you to poop at least once a day?

- Helps to remove waste from the body;

- Improves gut health, as it helps to balance the bacteria in your colon;

- Helps to alleviate discomfort from gas and bloating;

- Minimizes irritation of the gut lining;

- Reduces the potential for inflammation and sensitivities; and

- Helps to reduce stress and anxiety (the stress of not pooping is very real!).

Mastering the Art of Pooping

If you're having trouble going to the bathroom at least once a day consistently, even after trying everything I've recommended so far, try these suggestions:

- Take a magnesium supplement. Try magnesium citrate, oxide, or glycinate. Citrate draws water into the intestines, softening stool and stimulating peristalsis. Oxide works more slowly than citrate, and it also draws water into the intestines. Bisglycinate, or glycinate, is also great because it relaxes the muscles of your intestines, calms the nervous system, and gently softens stool with less risk of urgency or diarrhea. It's also gentle on the stomach.

- If you're severely constipated, try eating some prunes. Prunes provide fiber and sorbitol, a sugar alcohol that has a laxative effect. While prunes are rich in nutrients, they are also concentrated in natural sugars, so if that's a concern for you, be mindful of portions.

- Move to move your bowels. A study published in April 2024 in *The Lancet* found that an inactive lifestyle was linked to an increased risk of different gastrointestinal conditions, including reflux, irritable bowel syndrome (IBS), ulcers, Crohn's disease, and fatty liver, while those who were moderately active or very active had a decreased risk of these conditions. Try walking, hiking, yoga, swimming, pickleball, strength training, or anything else that helps to increase your physical activity.

- Do daily digestion stretches (upon waking and before bed). Try Knees to Chest (Apanasana) and Cat-Cow (Marjaryasana-Bitilasana).

- While sitting on the toilet, intentionally relax your abdominal and rectal muscles to help release stool from the colon. I learned this technique from my pelvic floor therapist: Close your eyes and breathe in and out slowly. Picture a flower opening while relaxing your pelvic floor muscles at the same time. I know it sounds funny, but it works!

- In an ideal pooping situation, you should feel like you completely emptied your colon. You should also be able to pass the stool easily, without straining or pushing and without discomfort or pain. Straining or sitting on the toilet for too long can lead to hemorrhoids and contribute to more serious issues like a prolapsed rectum, something we're more prone to now that we're in perimenopause and menopause. Hormonal changes can weaken pelvic floor muscles, slow digestion, and reduce the elasticity of tissue in the rectal area. If you don't have success the first time around, get off the toilet and try again later.

- Massage your belly clockwise starting at the lower right corner, next to your hip bone. Gently work your way up toward your rib cage and across your upper abdomen just below the ribs, then down your left side toward your hip bone. I did this massage for my kids whenever they'd have problems going to the bathroom. Apply a heating pad and some oil to help it work even better. Try this on yourself, or work with a massage therapist or pelvic floor specialist who can show you how to do it or do it for you.

- Sip on warm water with lemon or herbal teas like dandelion, fennel, ginger, or chamomile in between meals. Staying hydrated helps digestion, and many of these herbs have been used for centuries to calm the gut and help reduce bloating.

- Set yourself up for pooping success by making sure you're positioned properly on the toilet. Use a toilet stool (like the Squatty Potty®) or books to raise your feet, mimicking a squatting position. This posture helps to straighten your colon, making it easier to empty.

What Should Your Poop Look Like?

Now that you've mastered the art of pooping, what should it look like? Ideally, it should be medium to dark brown and formed like a snake or sausage.

Not all stools look the same, but there's a general guideline that divides them into seven categories according to shape and consistency. The Bristol Stool Chart is commonly used to identify digestive issues like constipation, IBS, and diarrhea. My team at Morphus created a Bristol Stool Chart you can download. Visit www.nourishing menopausebook.com and click on the Resources tab.

What About Smell?

Stools generally don't have a pleasant smell, but a major change in odor could be caused by a medication you're taking or something you ate. Certain foods like eggs, garlic, onions, red meat, cruciferous veggies, dairy, ultra-processed foods, alcohol, greasy meals, and coffee can make stools smell more pungent. Strong-smelling stool can also be a sign of lactose intolerance, IBS, inflammatory bowel disease (IBD), an infection, a sluggish bowel (meaning food sits in the colon for a longer-than-normal period before it's eliminated), or too few beneficial microbes in the gut.

If it only happens once in a while, it usually isn't anything to worry about. But if the smell is always awful, and you also have diarrhea, pain, blood, or unexplained weight loss, please mention it to your doctor.

Gut Bacteria and Hormones

Researchers at Arizona State University have discovered that the bacteria and hormones in our gut talk to each other, exchanging messages about our metabolism (yup, they play a role in weight), how our brain functions (our capacity to learn and remember), and our immune system.

The study found that when women go into menopause, that communication is interrupted and gut bacteria change, which may lead to a number of health issues, including changes in cognition and your health as a whole.

According to one of the authors of the study, Professor Rosa Krajmalnik-Brown, "What happens in the gut doesn't stay in the gut." What she means by this is that our gut bacteria affect other parts of our body too, which is exciting because it opens up the opportunity for more research to look for treatment options that address both mental and physical health in perimenopause and menopause.

Liver Health and Menopause

Your liver is located in the upper-right part of your abdomen, just below your ribs and diaphragm. It's an incredible multitasker as it deals with everything you eat, drink, inhale, and put on your skin once it enters your bloodstream. It deserves a ton of respect, as it works tirelessly to perform hundreds of functions. It truly is a hero organ.

When it comes to digestion, the liver does a lot, including breaking down and storing nutrients like glucose, vitamins, and minerals; converting fats, carbs, and proteins into energy or storing them for later use; and making bile to help with the digestion of fatty foods in the small intestine. It also helps in maintaining a proper balance of fluid in the tissues throughout the body and filters out harmful waste that could potentially interfere with digestion.

Remarkably, it can regenerate itself if parts are damaged or removed.

One of the liver's many important jobs is clearing out excess estrogen and cell-damaging substances. This task is important throughout life and continues to be important in perimenopause and menopause because of its impact on symptoms, hormones, and your health in general.

Estrogen helps to keep your liver healthy, so when levels drop, it can become more prone to stress and damage.

The size of your liver and its blood flow typically peak around the age of forty-four, right around perimenopause, then decrease after fifty, with more significant changes after seventy-five. Research shows that aging can contribute to the liver shrinking by up to 40 percent, and this loss of volume becomes more pronounced as women get older. As we age, the liver goes through changes because of different stressors, which can increase the risk of inflammation and fatty liver.

Metabolic Dysfunction-Associated Steatotic Liver Disease (MASLD)

As we go into menopause, we're more prone to developing fatty liver. Fatty liver used to be called non-alcoholic fatty liver disease, or NAFLD, but it's been renamed to metabolic dysfunction-associated steatotic liver disease, or MASLD. The reason is that in the past, liver damage and disease were often associated with heavy alcohol consumption. However, we now know that most cases of fatty liver are driven by metabolic changes (hence its new name) rather than alcohol. In fact, MALSD is now one of the most common liver diseases and it often shows up in people who drink very little or no alcohol at all.

With MASLD, fat builds up in the liver, which can lead to scarring, known as cirrhosis. Too much fat prevents the liver from doing its job properly.

MASLD tends to affect people with obesity, high belly fat, type 2 diabetes, high blood pressure, high cholesterol, and insulin resistance, all of which are common features of metabolic syndrome, a set of health issues that includes high blood pressure, high blood sugar, extra fat around the waist, and abnormal cholesterol and triglyceride levels. When you have insulin resistance, your cells can't use glucose (sugar) properly. As a result, the extra sugar in the bloodstream gets converted into fat, which can build up in the liver over time and lead to inflammation and scarring.

MASLD is more common in women who are in menopause, and the risk is even higher for women who go into menopause before the age of forty-five. One major reason is that lower estrogen affects metabolism, leading to more belly fat, higher insulin resistance, cholesterol changes, and less muscle mass, all of which increase the risk of MASLD. However, women who have healthy cholesterol, triglycerides, glucose, and insulin levels, even in menopause, have a lower risk for developing it.

Other important risk factors for women, especially for those between thirty-five and sixty-five, include high liver enzymes (alanine aminotransferase [ALT] and aspartate aminotransferase

[AST]), high uric acid levels, and a high ratio of triglycerides to HDL (TG/HDL). And 2024 research in perimenopausal and menopausal women found that those with moderate to severe hot flashes and night sweats were three times more likely to have MASLD than those who had only mild symptoms.

There's also an association between thyroid health and MASLD. Studies show that hypothyroidism (a low or sluggish thyroid) is more common in people with MASLD than in those without it, and women with MASLD are more likely to have an underactive thyroid.

Many people with MASLD have no symptoms, especially in the early stages. When symptoms do appear, they can include fatigue; nausea; loss of appetite; and vague pain or discomfort in the upper-right abdomen, sometimes with an enlarged liver. Ask your doctor about annual tests and imaging to be proactive, and review the advice under "Love Your Liver" earlier in this chapter. MASLD is often reversible with diet, exercise, and lifestyle changes.

Understanding how your digestive system affects your health during your perimenopausal and menopausal years helps you take the necessary steps to improve and manage many of your symptoms.

When your gut microbiome is in balance and well-nourished, you might notice you have better energy, your mood feels more steady, and your anxiety is more under control. Digestion also affects another area that many women find frustrating at this stage: weight. How your body breaks down food, keeps blood sugar stable, and manages hunger signals all play a role in how we gain, lose, or maintain weight. In the next chapter, I'll share the different reasons we experience weight changes, and in Chapter 11, I share what can be done to address them.

5

Why We Gain Weight in Perimenopause and Menopause

When I was going through perimenopause, my weight fluctuated up and down for years, and I was hungry all the time. My cravings were out of control, and I gained twenty pounds. My boobs grew two bra sizes, most of my clothes didn't fit me anymore, and I couldn't even button up my pants or get some of my favorite tank tops over my chest. My belly was as hard as a rock, and I felt like I gained weight just by looking at food.

I had no idea what was happening to my body, or why, because I hadn't changed anything that I was doing (I was eating and exercising the way I always did!). I struggled to accept how I felt and looked. My weight often dictated my mood, and my mood caused me to eat more. It was a vicious cycle and an old habit I carried with me from when I was young.

Looking back, I wish I had known or understood that it wasn't about willpower but rather biology, because my body was entering a new phase and responding in ways I didn't recognize.

Now I do understand. And I want to share what I've learned so you can understand the changes your body is going through as well.

To be clear, this chapter isn't about how to get your "old body" back. Instead, it's about empowering you with information so you can love and feel confident in the body you have now.

Does my story sound a lot like yours? The cravings. The weight gain, especially around your belly. The clothes that no longer fit. It's real. And it's not your fault.

According to our Morphus research, more than half (53%) of women in perimenopause and menopause reported changes in their metabolism, and 50 percent said their body had changed shape. Although women in both phases said they were experiencing weight-related symptoms, these two in particular were more common among the women in menopause. A third issue, weight fluctuations, impacted both groups equally, with 38 percent of women experiencing it.

But here's what we're not told: The weight changes aren't just about calories in and calories out. They're about hormonal shifts, metabolic changes, and body composition. They're about stress levels, lack of sleep, and gut health. They're about many different factors, some within your control, but many that aren't. The important thing to know is that you're not powerless. Once you understand why these changes in your body are happening, you can adapt your lifestyle, your food and supplement choices, and how you manage stress to support your body so you can feel better.

I put a lot of thought into writing this chapter. As real and frustrating as weight gain is during this time, many of us still carry decades of diet culture baggage. If you grew up in the 1980s and 1990s, like I did, you know what I mean. We were taught that our worth was tied to our weight. That thinness was a goal, a virtue, a requirement.

I fell for it too. One of my earliest memories of wanting to be thin was working out to Jane Fonda's Workout VHS tape. I was twelve, and I believed being skinny would make me happier. And that belief didn't disappear when I got older; it followed me into adulthood.

Fortunately, today's younger generation of women has access to more diverse and healthy role models than many of us Gen Xers or baby boomers had when it comes to body shape. Let's take a page out of their book and unlearn and reframe what we've been taught about weight and our worth. I know, it's not an easy process, and it can take time. Heck, I'm still working on it! But here's one powerful truth I've learned:

Living in the past, trying to fit into the jeans we wore at twenty-five, no longer serves our body or mind. It keeps us stuck. And it takes energy away from the version of who we are today and who we're becoming. Being in perimenopause and menopause is no longer about chasing skinny. It's about being strong in all areas of our life. We're at a pivotal point because what we do now will impact our future mental, physical, and emotional health. We're laying the foundation for the next thirty, forty, fifty, or more years, and it's now time to nourish ourselves. To mother ourselves. To nurture ourselves.

As my friend Marci Warhaft, a body image expert, creator of Fit vs Fiction, and author of *The Good Stripper: A Soccer Mom's Memoir of Lies, Loss and Lap Dances*, puts it: "As we get older, our bodies change; of course they do; it would be weird if they didn't. With every experience, we change emotionally and psychologically, so how could we not change physically as well? The problem isn't our ever-changing bodies; it's our fear around the changes that leads to unhealthy diets that can negatively impact our overall health. We've spent so many years working against our bodies instead of working with them. We can't achieve the bodies we want if we're constantly critiquing them. Hating our bodies won't make them skinny, but loving ourselves and understanding that we deserve to be healthy and happy WILL inspire us to make positive choices when it comes to food."

So buy the size that fits you now. Because putting on an old pair of jeans that no longer fits is a daily reminder of how your body has changed, and it can stir up negative self-talk. Choosing the right size for your body can help you shift your perspective. Plus, they're a lot more comfortable!

I was speaking with Caren Lettiere, the founder and president of Democracy Clothing, and she said something that really stuck with me. She said that as women, "we need to find our comfort zone, not just from a size perspective, but also from a place of self-acceptance. How we present our bodies in the clothes we're wearing determines the energy we project to the world and how we're reciprocally received."

To help with this process, ask yourself, *What's one kind, nourishing thing I can do for my body this week, not to change it but to honor it?*

Note: If body image issues are causing you stress or mental health problems, please see Chapter 12 for a discussion of tools you can use to help create a healthy self-image.

The Facts

Many women in perimenopause often start to see changes in how their bodies burn energy and store fat. We store less fat in areas like the thighs, butt, and hips, and more around the belly. In menopause, these shifts continue, and many women see an increase in total body fat, especially visceral (abdominal) fat. As a result, our waist gets thicker and the amount, type, and distribution of fat changes.

There's a lot of discussion about what really causes weight gain and an increase in body fat as we get older. Is it age, menopausal status, genetics, hormones, lifestyle choices, environmental factors, or all the above? Most research shows that women tend to gain weight for all these reasons as they age, regardless of whether they're going through "the change" or not. Menopause itself plays a bigger role in *where* the body stores fat rather than *how much* weight is gained. While our metabolism doesn't suddenly slow down when we go into menopause, these contributing factors can make it feel that way.

Subcutaneous Fat Versus Visceral Fat

Subcutaneous fat is located just under your skin, and you can pinch it on your arms, stomach, hips, and legs. It plays a role in regulating body temperature, acts as a shock absorber (e.g., if you fall, it helps to protect your internal organs from damage), and it is involved in the production of leptin, a hormone that regulates appetite and how much energy your body uses or stores. Having subcutaneous fat is normal and necessary, and it's generally not harmful unless there are excessive amounts, especially around the belly, which can eventually lead to health risks.

Visceral fat, on the other hand, is more concerning for us. But *what* is it, and *why* does it matter?

Estrogen influences where fat is stored in the body. Before menopause, many women tend to store more fat on their hips and thighs, leading to a "pear-shaped" figure. As we go into perimenopause and then menopause, when estrogen levels fluctuate and fall, fat starts to redistribute to the stomach area, which is often referred to as a "meno belly," or "menopause belly." This type of abdominal fat is different because it includes visceral fat, and unlike the softer, squishy subcutaneous fat that lies just under the skin, visceral fat accumulates deeper, beneath the muscle layer, and feels harder to the touch. Visceral fat wraps around your abdominal organs, including the liver, pancreas, stomach, and intestines, and it's referred to as "active fat" or an "endocrine organ" because it releases hormones and inflammatory substances that influence key body functions, including insulin sensitivity, inflammation, and cholesterol levels. Visceral fat can increase your chances of developing insulin resistance (I explain it in detail later in this chapter) and other health problems, like type 2 diabetes and heart disease. Women with more belly fat often have high blood pressure and abnormal cholesterol levels, which can increase their chances for heart disease, stroke, and metabolic syndrome. Visceral fat is a key factor in metabolic syndrome.

Research published in July 2024 in the *International Journal of Women's Health* looked at the connection between how long women were in menopause and its impact on metabolic syndrome. The study compared women between the ages of forty-five and sixty who were in menopause for one to five years versus six to ten years. The results showed that women who were in menopause longer tended to carry more fat around their belly and had a more than six-fold higher risk of developing metabolic syndrome. The researchers concluded that our risk for developing metabolic issues increases over time, which is *why* I'm so passionate about sharing what I've learned about nutrition, lifestyle, and supplements.

As you can see, visceral fat has a significant effect on our health. To put things into perspective, before we're in menopause, this type of fat makes up about 5–8 percent of a woman's total body fat. After menopause, that percentage rises to 15–20 percent.

Why We Gain Weight in Perimenopause and Menopause

There are at least seventeen major reasons why we gain weight in this stage of life:

- Hormones
- Fatigue
- Sleep
- Stress
- Inflammation
- Nutrition
- Nutritional deficiencies
- Not eating enough
- Muscle loss
- Physical activity
- Gut health
- Vasomotor symptoms
- Genetics
- Dehydration
- Mental health
- Environmental pollutants and toxicants
- Blood sugar issues / insulin resistance

Let's go through these one by one.

1. Hormones

Since hormones influence so many body changes during perimenopause and menopause, it makes sense to start here.

Estrogen

When estrogen levels fall, you may find that you're hungrier than usual, and the way your body stores fat is shifting from your hips and thighs to your belly. A drop in estrogen can also make your cells less sensitive to insulin (the hormone responsible for regulating blood sugar), so you might have more cravings, or gain weight more easily.

During perimenopause, while estrogen is fluctuating, progesterone is usually the first hormone to decline, leading to a greater discrepancy between the two. Once estrogen starts to fall as well, it can lead to an accumulation of belly fat, even if you're eating and exercising the same way you always have. Add in genetics, lower muscle mass, and aging, and it becomes clear why you're more likely to store fat.

Surgical Menopause

If you've had your ovaries surgically removed (oophorectomy), research suggests you may have a 78 percent higher risk of becoming obese, a threefold increased risk of severe obesity, and an increased risk of metabolic syndrome compared to those who go through menopause naturally. In addition, the sudden loss of estrogen from surgical menopause can lead to intense symptoms, like hot flashes, sleep issues, mood changes, and fatigue, which can make physical activity more challenging and it can shift how fat is distributed in the body, as I've previously mentioned.

Androgens

During perimenopause, androgen hormones, like testosterone, DHEA, and DHEA-S, don't drop as quickly as estrogen and progesterone. This shift in hormone balance can lead to weight gain and/or more visceral belly fat.

This is particularly true if you have a condition like polycystic ovary syndrome (PCOS), which already involves hormonal imbalances, such as high androgens, low or irregular progesterone, imbalanced estrogen, and insulin resistance. Research has found a strong relationship between PCOS, metabolic syndrome, and type 2 diabetes before and after menopause, all of which are linked with weight gain.

Cortisol

Increased cortisol levels, from biological stress or other stressors in your life, can contribute to weight gain, especially around the belly. Chronically higher cortisol levels can make you hungrier, interfere with your sleep, and affect your mood, gut health, and metabolism, adding to weight management challenges.

Research shows that women have higher cortisol levels in the later stages of perimenopause and the early stages of menopause.

Leptin and Ghrelin

Leptin and ghrelin, two hormones that help to regulate hunger and fullness (satiety), can shift once you go into perimenopause and menopause.

Leptin regulates how much you eat (appetite control) and how full you feel (satiety). It also influences metabolism and how your body uses and stores energy. In nonobese women, leptin levels tend to rise from premenopause to (post)menopause, although it's different for everyone. When leptin is out of balance, or when the brain doesn't respond to it properly (leptin resistance), it can lead to obesity, increased hunger, food cravings, and other metabolic problems.

Ghrelin has almost the opposite effect on appetite as leptin. It's nicknamed the "hunger hormone" because it makes you feel hungry. Ghrelin naturally rises before you eat and falls afterward, which is why it plays a key role in triggering eating. A small study of women in different menopausal stages found ghrelin levels were higher in perimenopause, which may explain why some women feel hungrier than usual during this phase. Interestingly, a 2020 study found that (post)menopausal women with high levels of ghrelin were more likely to have hot flashes than those with lower levels.

The way I remember the difference between the two hormones is that ghrelin makes your stomach "gr-owl."

Thyroid

As we age, thyroid disorders, especially an underactive thyroid (hypothyroidism), become more common. Since estrogen plays a role in how your body uses thyroid hormones, lower estrogen levels can throw off the balance. Women are more likely than men to develop an underactive thyroid.

Many symptoms of thyroid problems can overlap with those of perimenopause and menopause. Some of the more common ones include fatigue, brain fog, sleep issues, mood swings, low libido, heart palpitations, sensitivity to temperature, hair changes (thinning, loss), irregular cycles, depression, and weight gain.

So how does the thyroid affect weight gain? One of its main jobs is to regulate metabolism, so an underactive thyroid can slow it down, making it harder to burn calories.

Another way a sluggish thyroid can affect your weight is by interfering with how your body uses insulin.

According to Danielle Meitiv, MS, a board-certified health coach and functional medicine practitioner who focuses on thyroid health, "Hypothyroidism can significantly impact blood sugar balance by disrupting how the body uses insulin and glucose. Thyroid hormones are essential for cells to respond properly to insulin. When thyroid levels are low, as in hypothyroidism, metabolism slows down and cells become less responsive to insulin. Over time, this can lead to insulin resistance, where the body needs more insulin to keep blood sugar in check."

The thyroid plays an important role in overall metabolic health, from regulating body temperature to influencing how your body uses the calories you eat, how well you metabolize carbs and fats, and how your body builds and maintains muscles and other protein-based tissues like hair, skin, and nails.

To learn more about thyroid health in perimenopause and menopause, listen to my podcast interviews with Danielle (episode #85) and Dr. Amie Hornaman (episode #102).

As you can see, our changing hormones can make managing weight during perimenopause and menopause more challenging because they affect how our bodies produce and respond to hormones that help regulate appetite and fat storage. It's no wonder weight management can feel like an uphill battle for so many of us during this time!

2. Fatigue

There are many reasons you might be feeling exhausted now. Some come from what's happening in your body, and others from what's going on around you.

Let's start with sleep. The insomnia and disrupted sleep that often start in perimenopause have a huge impact on your energy levels and metabolism. I'll discuss this more in the next section (#3).

Then there are physiological changes that may be happening inside your body, which can take a toll on your energy levels. For example, you may have an underactive thyroid or low iron levels, both of which can leave you feeling drained, and lower levels of certain essential nutrients like B vitamins (especially vitamin B12), magnesium, and vitamin D can interfere with your body's energy-making processes.

Diet also has a huge impact on your energy levels. In a perfect world, most of your calories would come from whole, nutrient-dense foods that supply the enzymes, nutrients, electrolytes, antioxidants, and hydration your body needs to fuel your cells, keep your energy steady throughout the day, and keep your weight, blood sugar, and body fat where you want them to be. But because you live in the real world, this isn't always possible when time and energy are limited. Or perhaps you don't live in a neighborhood with easily accessible high-quality, unprocessed foods. Add in the exhaustion-plus-hormonal combo, and you may be eating empty calories with ingredients that can trigger inflammation and digestive issues, making it harder for your body to absorb nutrients.

As you saw in Chapter 4, digestive health can change now due to shifts in hormones. A slower digestive system, gut inflammation, blood sugar swings, bloating, and in some cases a reduced ability to absorb important nutrients like vitamins, minerals, and amino acids can all drain your energy levels and make mental and physical fatigue feel more intense.

We hear so much about the consequences of stress, like headaches, muscle tension, or digestive issues, but stress can really take a toll on your energy levels as well, both physically and mentally. Stress depletes nutrients such as B vitamins, vitamin C, magnesium, and zinc, leaving you feeling worn down and burned out. I go into more detail about stress in reason #4 and the depletion of nutrients in reason #7.

All the above, and more, can drain your energy and lead to weight gain.

3. Sleep

Think of your body as an orchestra, where sleep is the conductor. It keeps every part of your body in tune, from your immune system to your brain function to preventing chronic disease. But as many women reach perimenopause and menopause, sleep often becomes a struggle, throwing off that beautiful harmony.

A lack of sleep can mess with your metabolism, making it harder for your body to handle sugar and respond to insulin. When you haven't slept well or enough, you're less likely to make healthy eating choices, and more likely to crave junk food like cakes, cookies, and fast food, as they provide a quick boost of energy.

Poor sleep can throw off your appetite hormones, leptin and ghrelin. These hormones work with your circadian rhythm, so if you don't get enough sleep, you may feel hungrier and have an increased appetite.

When you don't sleep enough, you may feel more emotional and stressed. You're more likely to get sick, you may feel forgetful, and your body may start holding on to more fat, especially around your belly.

Why? A lack of consistent high-quality sleep stresses the body, can cause cortisol to rise and, in many cases, stay elevated. Chronically high cortisol can promote inflammation and interfere with how your body uses energy, making it harder to use and burn fat efficiently. As a result, you may have less energy and feel more tired. Higher cortisol can also make you feel hungrier, which can lead you to eat more, especially when you're feeling stressed. All of this and more can make weight gain more likely.

4. Stress

In addition to stress from a lack of sleep, other stressors in our lives can cause weight gain as well. When you're stressed, your body produces cortisol. While cortisol is important for how your body responds to stress, consistently high levels can make you hungrier and may increase cravings for comfort foods. High cortisol levels can promote fat storage, especially around the belly.

Stress can also lead to emotional eating as a coping mechanism, leaving you feeling tired, less motivated, and in turn less active.

During perimenopause and menopause, we're even more sensitive to the effects of stress, as you saw in Chapter 2. Because it's such an important topic, I dedicated all of Chapter 6 to it.

5. Inflammation

We tend to associate inflammation with pain, not with weight gain. Chronic low-grade inflammation can contribute to hormonal imbalances, increased fat storage, and metabolic changes that make losing weight harder.

Estrogen generally helps to keep inflammation in check. As levels fluctuate in perimenopause and then drop in menopause, you may experience an increase in, or worsening of, chronic low-grade inflammation.

But what does inflammation have to do with weight gain? Visceral fat releases inflammatory proteins called cytokines, like TNF-α and IL-6, and these can disrupt how your body uses insulin. This disruption can make it easier for your body to store fat, especially around the belly. Inflammation is also a big contributor to metabolic syndrome because it messes with how your body regulates blood sugar.

When inflammation goes up and you gain weight, your brain can become less responsive to leptin, the hormone that signals fullness. After a while, you can develop or worsen something called leptin resistance, where you still feel hungry after you've finished eating, making it harder to manage your weight.

Unfortunately, your body ends up in an ongoing loop of cause and effect: Weight gain, especially visceral fat, leads to inflammation, and that inflammation makes it easier to gain more weight.

So what can you do?

There's a lot of good evidence supporting an anti-inflammatory diet, especially the Mediterranean diet, to reduce inflammation in the body. These diets focus on fatty fish, fruits, vegetables, whole grains, legumes, nuts, and olive oil, and they're rich in good-quality fats, like omega-3 fatty acids, fiber, vitamins, minerals, and antioxidants. There's also evidence that plant-based, especially vegan, diets are associated with lower inflammation. You can check your levels of inflammation by asking your doctor for a high-sensitivity C-reactive protein (hs-CRP) blood test, which is often used as a marker for low-grade systemic inflammation. Some doctors may also want to order an erythrocyte sedimentation rate (ESR) test, which can be an indication of general inflammation.

6. Nutrition

How and what you eat in perimenopause and menopause is important, not just when it comes to weight but also for energy, mood, and overall health. The body and mind thrive when they're nourished.

Your cells, hormones, and brain depend on the nutrients you ingest to function well. What you eat or drink can work either for you or against you with respect to how you feel and move.

Not getting enough of the essential nutrients your body needs on a daily basis, especially protein, fiber, and quality fats like omega-3s from fish, nuts, and seeds, can leave you feeling unsatisfied, which in turn can lead to cravings. Cravings can lead to increased snacking, overeating, or reaching for convenient but less nourishing options, which, over time, can result in weight gain and low energy.

This is the time to focus on nutrients rather than calories.

Making nutrient-dense foods a priority ensures your body receives the nourishment it needs. When planning meals, prioritize protein, fiber, nonstarchy vegetables, healthy fats, and complex carbohydrates. Protein helps balance blood sugar, and fiber supports healthy digestion. Both can reduce hunger and help you feel full. Healthy fats, like omega-3s, reduce inflammation. Limiting ultra-processed foods, refined grains, added sugars (including sugar-sweetened beverages), and alcohol can help reduce the risk of weight gain and support hormone health. While you can't control everything that affects weight gain now, you *can* choose how you fuel your body.

7. Nutritional Deficiencies

As you get older, your need for certain nutrients, including vitamins and minerals, stays the same or increases once you go into perimenopause and menopause.

Deficiencies and insufficiencies in micronutrients such as vitamin D, magnesium, vitamins B6 and B12, folate, and iron are common in women in perimenopause and beyond. These imbalances are associated with an increased risk of health problems such as heart and metabolic diseases (e.g., metabolic syndrome), osteoporosis, anemia, mood and memory issues, and potentially more serious conditions.

As far as weight is concerned, research shows that vitamin D may support metabolism and body composition. Meaning, those with higher levels have more success with weight management than those with lower levels. Also, low levels of vitamin D are linked to how your body uses insulin, which may influence blood sugar regulation and fat storage, particularly around the belly.

Another aspect of vitamin D that's important to consider is its influence on mood, energy levels, and mental health. Low levels of vitamin D are is associated with low energy levels, depression, and mood disorders, all of which can affect your motivation for being active. Women in menopause are at an increased risk for vitamin D deficiency, partly because biology and lifestyle habits tend to shift with age, so making sure you're getting enough of this nutrient is a priority.

Iron is another important nutrient. It's essential for carrying oxygen, making DNA, and producing energy. While having low iron levels doesn't directly cause weight gain, it can lead to symp-

> **Did you know?** Iron and vitamin D are interconnected. Healthy vitamin D levels may lower the risk of iron-deficient anemia.

toms that may indirectly contribute to weight changes, because iron helps your body produce energy. Low ferritin levels (a measure of your iron stores) can cause fatigue, and when you layer on other symptoms like headaches and joint pain, your energy and motivation for physical activity can take a back seat.

Low ferritin can, in some cases, affect your thyroid, especially when ferritin is really low, which can then affect your metabolism. Low iron levels are also common in people with Hashimoto's thyroiditis. Hashimoto's is an autoimmune condition that can lead to an underactive thyroid (hypothyroidism). In perimenopause and menopause, dropping estrogen and progesterone levels, poor sleep, stress, and low nutrients can throw your immune system off-balance, triggering flare-ups of autoimmune issues like Hashimoto's in women who are already predisposed, even if they were dormant until now.

Vitamin B12 helps make red blood cells and supports the way your body turns food into energy. Low vitamin B12 can cause fatigue and weakness, which makes it harder to stay active. B12 plays a role in mood and brain function, and low levels can result in depression or brain fog.

B12 is primarily found in animal products like eggs, salmon, and dairy. Vegetarians or vegans should look for fortified foods or supplements. Before supplementing, ask your doctor to check your levels with a blood test. In some cases, additional markers like methylmalonic acid (MMA) or homocysteine may give you a clearer picture of your B12 levels.

Note: Certain medications, like some birth control pills, can deplete important nutrients like B vitamins and magnesium, so be extra mindful about replenishing them if you're on the pill.

I expand on minerals and vitamins in Chapters 9 and 10.

8. Not Eating Enough

Something I hear over and over again from the women in our community and my friends is that they don't understand *why* they're not losing weight because they're eating *much less* than they used to and exercising the same, if not more. I asked myself the same question for years.

While logically it makes sense that eating less would lead to weight loss, this line of thinking can actually backfire on us now.

Here's why: Consistently not eating *enough* shifts your body into "energy conservation mode," slowing down your metabolism to preserve energy. It's your body's protective mechanism so you don't burn through too many calories. Over time, this way of eating makes it harder for your body to burn calories efficiently, even if you're not eating or doing very much.

And as you just saw in reason #7, cutting back on calories without paying attention to the quality of the foods you're eating can lead to nutrient deficiencies or insufficiencies that can slow your metabolism, disrupt hormones, and make it harder to maintain a healthy weight in the long run.

Undereating also increases cortisol, which over time can cause your body to store more fat, especially around the belly. In addition, not eating enough might cause you to feel tired, moody, and hungrier later on, which could lead to poor nutrition choices.

The real goal is to have a nourished, healthy body, whatever that looks like for *you*, so focusing on foods that fuel you should be front and center. I talk more about how to figure out if you're eating enough in Chapter 11.

9. Muscle Loss

Having more muscle mass and strength impacts weight management because it helps to keep your metabolism active so you burn more calories, even when you're not physically active. But once you go into perimenopause and menopause, hormonal changes, including lower estrogen, can affect how quickly you lose muscle and strength. This gradual loss of muscle mass and function is referred to as age-related muscle loss, or sarcopenia.

How do you know if you're losing muscle? You might notice changes in your strength, recover more slowly, or it might feel more challenging to do movements that used to feel easy.

Bottom line: The more muscle you have, the better your overall metabolic health.

I dive deeper into exercise and building muscle mass and strength in Chapter 13.

10. Physical Activity

When the number on the scale starts to creep up and your waistline starts to expand, the natural first instinct is to exercise more and move your body. But when you're exhausted and your energy levels are low, finding the motivation to exercise or stay active isn't exactly at the top of your priority list; rather, just making it through the day is! So around and around we go: Low energy leads to a lack of movement, and lack of movement contributes to low energy, both of which can lead to weight gain.

While physical activity is critical at any stage in life, once we go into perimenopause and menopause, symptoms such as fatigue, lack of motivation, joint pain, and a lack of sleep, as well as injuries, can prevent us from being consistent.

A sedentary lifestyle can mess with cortisol levels, make your body less sensitive to insulin, and slow your metabolism. It weakens bones and muscles, affects mental and emotional health (which can show up as depression or mood swings), and leads to stiffness, less flexibility, and poorer balance, all of which can make weight gain more likely.

My good friend Lisa Tsakos, weight-loss coach and my coauthor of *Unjunk Your Junk Food*, shared that many of her female clients who struggle to lose the weight they gained in perimenopause and menopause are overly focused on burning calories through high-intensity cardio rather than lifting weights. Once they start incorporating resistance training into their routines, they notice positive changes in their strength, shape, and weight.

11. Gut Health

The conversation about weight often centers on energy balance (cal-ories in vs. calories out), exercise, and hormones, but the digestive system plays a surprisingly large role in weight and metabolic health.

Research shows that obesity is linked not only to *what* or *how much* you eat but also to the mix of bacteria living in your gut. Gut bacteria play a key role in *how* your body uses and makes energy to help it function. They help break down what you eat, absorb nutri-ents, and influence how much energy you get from food. A study in the *International Journal of Obesity* found that women who had more of a mix of different types of bacteria in their gut and ate a high-fiber diet tended to gain less weight over time than women with less gut diversity and lower fiber intake.

The diversity of your gut microbiome tends to increase through early to mid-adulthood, and then level off. From mid-dle age onward, the composition of your gut microbiota becomes more and more unique to you. Interestingly, people who live exceptionally long lives, like those in their nineties and beyond, often have diverse, distinct gut microbiomes compared to younger adults. I talked about how to increase your gut diversity in the previous chapter.

12. Vasomotor Symptoms

Research suggests that women who have more body fat or gain weight in midlife may have a higher chance of experiencing vasomo-tor symptoms (VMS), like hot flashes and night sweats, than those who don't. As fat moves from the hips and thighs (subcutaneous fat) to the belly (visceral fat) during perimenopause and menopause, some studies have linked changes in how the body stores fat and reg-ulates blood sugar with more frequent or more intense symptoms.

Vasomotor symptoms like night sweats often lead to poor sleep quality and insomnia, which can disrupt appetite-regulating hor-mones and make it easier to gain weight over time. As I've already explained, poor sleep can increase levels of the hunger hormone ghrelin and decrease levels of the satiety hormone leptin, leading to increased appetite and potential weight gain. And speaking from personal experience, hot flashes and night sweats can be debilitating, making it harder to sleep, exercise, work, or go about your daily routines. They can lower your motivation to move or do much at all, making it easier to gain weight.

13. Genetics

Genetics play a role in the levels of hormones you produce, such as leptin, the satiety hormone, and adiponectin, a hormone produced and released by fat tissue. Your genes also impact how your body responds to these hormones. This means that some bodies may be predisposed to feeling less full after eating and to hanging on to fat more easily.

14. Dehydration

When you're dehydrated, you may feel tired because your body, both physically and mentally, needs water to keep your energy levels up.

We sometimes confuse thirst with hunger because both sensations are regulated in the hypothalamus. When you're not well-hydrated, you may feel like you want to eat when what you really need is water, so drinking a glass of water first can help you tell the difference.

In menopause, changes in estrogen and progesterone levels can affect the balance of fluids in your body, possibly leading to dehydration or water retention, but for different reasons. Estrogen helps to regulate fluid balance, so when it decreases, it can make it harder for your body to manage fluids properly. This can lead to dehydration and imbalances in electrolytes. Electrolyte imbalances can cause muscle cramps, weakness, fatigue, and nervous system symptoms like headaches, confusion, and dizziness. Lower progesterone can affect how your body holds on to fluids, so you may feel bloated or puffy.

As we get older, our sense of thirst isn't what it used to be, and we may not feel the need to hydrate, even after we've lost fluids through exercise, hot flashes, night sweats, hormonal changes, heavy periods, sweating, or as a response to stress. This could mean we aren't drinking as often as we should be, making us more likely to become dehydrated.

Two very important things to consider when it comes to hydration are stress and sleep.

When we're stressed, our adrenals release cortisol, and if we're not well-hydrated, our body may release more cortisol than they normally would. And when we're dehydrated, we're more likely to feel the effects of stress, so not drinking enough and feeling stressed can feed into each other. Even mild dehydration can raise cortisol levels.

When you sleep, your body naturally loses fluids, especially if you have night sweats. A lack of hydration can affect sleep in different ways. It can result in a dry mouth, which may increase the chances of snoring and worsen sleep apnea symptoms. Interestingly, getting less sleep, specifically less than six hours, is linked to a higher risk of dehydration. Also, proper hydration helps to regulate body temperature and reduce the likelihood of waking up thirsty. One tip is to keep a glass of water on your nightstand to drink as soon as you wake up.

How can you tell if you're dehydrated? In addition to what's been mentioned, look for signs that include feeling very thirsty; brain fog; headaches; mood changes; morning sinus congestion; constipation; dark, strong-smelling urine; dizziness; dry skin; muscle cramps; and feeling tired.

Drinking enough water throughout the day can minimize many of the issues related to dehydration. Aim to drink half your body weight in ounces every single day. For example, if you weigh 140 pounds, that's roughly 70 ounces, or about 8¾ cups. Drinking hydrating fluids like water or herbal teas (decaffeinated without added sugar), replenishing with electrolytes after exercise or major sweat loss, and eating high-water-content vegetables (cucumbers, zucchini, lettuce, radishes, cauliflower, spinach, celery, etc.), low-glycemic fruits like berries and green apples, and soups can all help.

I carry around a big mug everywhere I go. I bought one that holds 4 cups of liquid, keeps them hot or cold for hours, and fits into the cupholder in my car.

15. Mental Health

Mental health can play a big part in weight changes during peri-menopause and menopause. As hormone levels shift, they can affect your mood, mindset, and emotional balance, which can change how and what you eat, how much you crave certain foods, and whether you reach for comfort foods when you're feeling down or stressed. Your mental health can also affect motivation and how your body handles stress. Stress can make you crave comfort foods that are often high in refined sugars and trans fats, and it can change how your body controls hunger and fullness. It also raises cortisol levels, which can increase appetite and encourage fat storage, especially around the belly. Reaching out to a trusted friend or therapist can help support your mental and emotional health during this time. I go into more detail about mental health in Chapter 12.

16. Environmental Pollutants and Toxicants

I'm very familiar with this topic because it was a big part of my work at Naturally Savvy (www.naturallysavvy.com). Over the years, I met some incredible experts who've dedicated their careers to educating us about toxicants. Toxicants show up in many forms: pesticides and herbicides in agriculture, heavy metals in water and food, industrial chemicals like per- and polyfluoroalkyl substances (PFAS) and bisphenol S (BPS), plasticizers such as bisphenol A (BPA) and phthalates, and mold toxins and contaminants formed during food processing. Many also hide in personal care and household products, from parabens and synthetic fragrances to flame retardants and antibacterial agents like triclosan.

I interviewed Amy Ziff, the founder of MADE SAFE (www.madesafe.org), for my podcast (episode #94), and we talked about some of the more common toxicants found in our environment. She shared how these chemicals have serious consequences for our health. They can accumulate in our body, mess with our hormones, affect nerves, interfere with how our immune system works, and raise the risk of chronic disease.

Industrial chemicals, such as BPA, phthalates, and PFAS, also known as forever chemicals (with more than thirteen thousand identified types!), are particularly insidious because, in addition to disrupting hormones, they may also affect our metabolism and promote fat storage. These harmful substances are known as obesogens.

Obesogens are chemicals that can mess with our hormones in ways that make us more likely to store fat and gain weight. They can affect how the body manages weight by creating more fat cells, causing existing fat cells to hold on to even more fat, influencing gut bacteria, interfering with appetite hormones like leptin and ghrelin, and affecting our metabolism, all of which can make weight harder to manage.

Unfortunately, you don't even have to eat these chemicals to be exposed to them. Many are absorbed through the skin or inhaled, and obesogens can be found in everyday items like personal care products. Phthalates, parabens, triclosan, and other hormone-disrupting chemicals are used in makeup, moisturizers, shampoos, conditioners, styling products, perfumes, scented body sprays, antiperspirants, and deodorants. Certain sunscreens may contain oxybenzone and other chemical filters that can act as obesogens. Nail polishes and removers can contain obesogens like dibutyl phthalate (DBP), along with other potentially harmful substances such as acetone, toluene, and formaldehyde.

Obesogens are also found in aluminum cans, clothing, furniture, computers, pesticides, and food packaging (e.g., plastic bottles, takeout containers, etc.). Even cash receipts are a common source of BPA and BPS, both obesogens.

To minimize exposure to these types of chemicals, check ingredients and look for products labeled phthalate-free, paraben-free, acetone-free, and so on. Companies that make toxicant-free products will proudly mention it on their labels or websites. The best way to avoid touching cash receipts is to ask for a digital copy, or manually fold them inward to avoid touching the coated side.

This topic can feel overwhelming, and you don't live in a bubble. Given we're exposed to a plethora of toxicants on a daily basis, it comes down to doing what you can to lower your exposure as much as possible. A good place to start is to switch to personal care products that don't contain parabens or phthalates. If you're still menstruating, choose organic tampons and pads whenever possible or a reusable menstrual cup, bring your own products to nail and hair salons, and once you finish a cleaning product, buy a new one that's safer for you and the environment.

Look for businesses and brands that offer organic or better-for-you ingredients, and check out madesafe.org for its list of certified products. You can also use apps like Think Dirty, Yuka, INCI Beauty, CosmEthics, and the Environmental Working Group's Skin Deep database to give you an idea of the safety of the ingredients in personal care products.

17. Blood Sugar Issues / Insulin Resistance

I've mentioned the term *insulin resistance* a few times already, but *what* does it mean, and *why* does it affect us, particularly now? And *how* does it relate to weight gain in perimenopause and menopause?

First, let me explain *how* insulin helps to regulate your blood sugar.

How Insulin and Blood Sugar Work

Insulin and blood sugar work together to keep each other in balance. Here's a quick explanation:

- When you eat carbs, your body breaks them down into glucose. For example, when you eat a piece of bread or pasta, the complex carbs, or starches and sugars, are broken down into glucose (sugar) during digestion.

- That glucose goes into the bloodstream, raising blood sugar levels. As blood sugar levels go up, the pancreas releases the hormone insulin.

- Insulin helps the glucose in your bloodstream get into your cells so it can be used for energy.

- Once the glucose in your bloodstream moves into the cells, blood sugar drops, and your pancreas slows down the production of insulin.

- If there's more glucose in your blood than your body can use immediately for energy, insulin tells the liver and muscles to store it as glycogen to use at another time.

- When your blood sugar levels drop (like between meals or when you're fasting), your pancreas releases glucagon. That signals your liver to release some of the stored glycogen into the bloodstream to help keep your energy levels steady.

What Happens When You're Insulin Resistant

However, when there's consistently too much glucose in the bloodstream and your blood sugar levels are always high, the entire system I just described starts to struggle to do its job.

- The pancreas produces more and more insulin to move the excess glucose into the muscle, liver, and fat cells.

- Over time, these cells stop responding to this big push of insulin, and they become "insulin resistant." Meaning, it takes even more insulin to do the *same* job.

- The pancreas works overtime to produce more insulin to try and force glucose into the resistant cells to keep your blood sugar balanced.

- Eventually, the pancreas can't keep up with making so much insulin, and your blood sugar levels increase.

Chronic insulin resistance, which can happen in both smaller and larger bodies, usually leads to chronically high insulin levels as your body tries to maintain normal blood sugar levels. This is called *hyperinsulinemia.* Hyperinsulinemia, or too much insulin in the blood, is often an early sign of insulin resistance. A fasting insulin blood test can provide you with some useful insight into the risk of insulin resistance, especially when it's interpreted together with other markers like fasting glucose, HbA1c, liver enzymes (ALT, AST, GGT), HOMA-IR (a formula combining fasting insulin and fasting glucose), and sometimes other tests, like an oral glucose tolerance test (OGTT) or lipoprotein insulin resistance index (LP-IR), rather than being used as a stand-alone test.

To be clear, when you have insulin resistance, your cells are *less sensitive* to insulin (known as insulin insensitivity), so your blood sugar stays high. There are different degrees of it, as some of us are more or less sensitive than others. When you don't have insulin resistance, your cells are *more sensitive* to insulin (known as insulin sensitivity).

Insulin resistance is the first step in a long process that, if left untreated or unmanaged, can lead to prediabetes and then ultimately type 2 diabetes. It often starts decades before the high blood sugar levels characteristic of diabetes show up. Over time, the pancreas can't keep up with the increased demand for insulin, and blood sugar levels stay high, eventually leading to type 2 diabetes.

Perimenopause, Menopause, and Insulin Resistance

Okay, ladies, here's the reason this topic is so important. Women in perimenopause and menopause can be more prone to developing insulin resistance due to:

- Hormonal shifts (as estrogen drops, your body's cells become *less* sensitive to insulin),

- Higher cortisol levels,

- Thyroid imbalances (generally, hypothyroid),

- A diet high in refined and ultra-processed carbs and sugars,

- Poor sleep,

- Higher stress levels,

- Increased (visceral) belly fat,

- Less physical activity, and

- Loss of muscle mass (sarcopenia).

And if you have polycystic ovary syndrome (PCOS), chances are you already had some degree of insulin resistance by the time you got to perimenopause.

Remember how I talked about visceral fat being inflammatory? Well, chronic inflammation caused by visceral fat can contribute to insulin resistance, and insulin resistance can further promote inflammation, creating a harmful cycle.

Then there's the stress factor. We know that chronic stress is a major issue now. Cortisol sends messages to the liver that your body needs quick fuel to handle a stressful situation. In response, the liver releases glycogen, which is then converted to glucose to give you energy. As a result, your blood sugar rises, even if you haven't eaten anything, and insulin rises too. If you're living in a constant state of stress, your body is continuously producing cortisol, which eventually can lead to insulin resistance, weight gain, and fatigue, and interfere with your ability to lose weight. Stress also affects sleep, and poor sleep raises cortisol and blood sugar levels, making us *less sensitive* to insulin.

A sedentary lifestyle is another contributing factor because it lowers how much glucose your muscles use throughout the day. At any age, when you eat carbs (like pasta, cereals, rice, oatmeal, fruit, baked goods, juices, sodas, etc.), your body breaks them down into glucose to give you energy. Insulin helps to move glucose into your muscles, liver, and fat cells so it can be used right away or stored as glycogen to use at a later time. When you're physically active, your muscles are constantly using stored glycogen, helping to keep blood sugar and insulin levels in a healthy range. But if you spend most of the day sitting and your glycogen stores are already full, extra glucose is more likely to be sent to the liver, where it can be converted into fat (triglycerides) and stored in fat tissue.

This can lead to two things:

- Weight gain. Eating more sugar than your body can use leads to it being stored in fat cells, increasing body fat.

- Type 2 diabetes. Eventually even the fat cells become resistant to insulin, leading to consistently high blood sugar and insulin levels.

As I mentioned earlier, during perimenopause and menopause, cells can become less responsive or less sensitive to insulin, so insulin production increases to keep blood sugar levels stable. As a result, this makes managing blood sugar even harder than it was before your hormones started shifting. High insulin levels encourage your body to store more fat, create more fat, and slow down fat burning, which ultimately leads to weight gain. At the same time, lower estrogen and aging increase visceral fat, further raising the risk of insulin resistance and type 2 diabetes. See the cycle?

Insulin resistance is associated with many serious health concerns that affect women in perimenopause and menopause, like weight gain, heart disease, high cholesterol, fatty liver or metabolic dysfunction-associated steatotic liver disease (MASLD), type 2 diabetes, and more. It's also associated with memory problems. In fact, researchers use the term type 3 diabetes to describe insulin resistance in the brain, and it's been linked to cognitive issues and Alzheimer's.

Multiple studies have found that women who go into menopause early have a higher risk of developing type 2 diabetes. According to one study, women with premature menopause (before age forty) are at high risk of developing diabetes or prediabetes, and women entering menopause between the ages of forty and forty-four have a higher risk of developing diabetes.

In general, perimenopausal and menopausal women are at a higher risk for developing insulin resistance because lower estrogen makes us *less insulin sensitive*.

Now that you understand this better, there's a lot you can do to help manage insulin more effectively. Research shows that diet and lifestyle adjustments, as well as regular movement, improve insulin sensitivity.

In addition, a 2024 meta-analysis showed that menopause hormone therapy (MHT) "significantly reduced insulin resistance in healthy (post)menopausal women without metabolic diseases, including diabetes, hypertension, and cardiovascular diseases."

To reduce your risk of developing health problems associated with insulin resistance, Ben Bikman, PhD, author of *Why We Get*

Sick, recommends living a "low insulin lifestyle." This approach focuses on managing blood sugar through diet, exercise, sleep, and stress management.

Signs and Symptoms of Insulin Resistance

Aside from testing, how would you know you have insulin resistance? You may not always experience symptoms, especially in the early stages, but here are some to be aware of (as you'll see, many of them overlap with perimenopause and menopause symptoms):

- Increased thirst and urination
- Fatigue or feeling sleepy, especially after meals
- Belly fat (visceral)
- Hard time losing weight regardless of a healthy diet and exercise
- Skin tags (acrochordons), usually found behind the neck or armpits, upper chest, or groin. A higher number of skin tags is often associated with higher fasting insulin levels.
- Dark, velvety patches of skin called acanthosis nigricans
- Fatty liver (MASLD)
- Polycystic ovary syndrome (PCOS)

If you have a family history of heart disease or a family member who has it or who has type 2 diabetes, please speak to your doctor and make sure you're on top of your blood work.

If you've tried everything in your power to lose weight or lower your blood sugar and insulin levels, even if you're at a healthy weight, and nothing will budge, consider speaking to your doctor about other options, such as medications like metformin and GLP-1 agonists.

GLP-1 is a hormone made in your gut that helps keep blood sugar and appetite in check. Medications like Ozempic and Wegovy (semaglutide), along with newer options like Mounjaro, are used to manage blood sugar, treat type 2 diabetes, and in some cases support weight loss by acting on these same pathways in the body. Mounjaro (tirzepatide) also works on an additional hormone called GIP, which adds another layer of support for blood sugar control and how the body handles fat.

Speak to your doctor about whether these medications are right for you, as they're meant to be used under medical supervision.

I reached out to Nathalie, host of the *Longevity with Nathalie Niddam* podcast, to share her perspective on this topic on my podcast (episode #83, *Menopause Reimagined*).

The Big Takeaway

As you can see, weight gain during perimenopause and menopause isn't about willpower. The pounds aren't random. It's your body's natural way of adjusting to hormonal shifts and finding a new balance that supports your health through these changes. Gaining weight during this time isn't something to feel ashamed about. It's not a sign of failure, even though it might feel like it when you're doing everything you can to change it. Instead, it's a symptom of many different factors at play. This chapter covered several of the root causes, and in the next chapter, I'll talk about one of the main drivers, stress.

6

Stress and the Menopausal Nervous System

Anxiety has a way of stealing your peace. It sneaks into your thoughts without your permission, takes away your happiness, and fills your days with worry and fear. It prevents you from living in the moment because you're constantly thinking about the past and/or future. It makes you less productive and prevents you from doing things you love. And it doesn't just affect you; it impacts your relationships too. If you suffer from it, then you know exactly what I'm talking about, and there's a good chance your anxiety is worse now than it was before. If anxiety is new for you and you're experiencing it for the first time now that you're in perimenopause or menopause, I know it can feel scary. I understand how you're feeling, and I'm going to share practical ways to manage it.

I've already touched on stress quite a bit, but I wanted to go deeper and pull it all together in one chapter so you can revisit it anytime you need to.

My Anxiety Story

I'm no stranger to anxiety. I suffered with it for much of my teenage and adult life. Until now, I haven't really talked openly about it, but over the years, and throughout different points in my life, I suffered from many different forms, including panic attacks, obsessive-compulsive disorder (OCD), and post-traumatic stress disorder (PTSD). It was a daily struggle, and I tried hard not to let it take over my life. But when it did, it was awful. I would shut down, stop eating, stop socializing, and ruminate.

I've been dealing with anxiety on and off for the past forty years, and it surfaced again more recently. This time it also came with major depression. I had severe heart palpitations, my voice got hoarse, and I lost twenty pounds in two months. I could hardly function and struggled to get out of bed. On top of the mental and physical symptoms, I felt guilty about how it was affecting my kids and husband. The underlying issue turned out to be Hashimoto's thyroiditis, an autoimmune condition that affects women more than men and most often develops between the ages of thirty and fifty, although it can happen at any age. I've had hypothyroidism since my twenties, but I can't remember if my antibodies were ever tested, so I didn't realize at the time that it was autoimmune. Thankfully, my doctor figured it out and adjusted my medication. Once my levels stabilized, my symptoms started to improve fairly quickly. That's why I'm so passionate about staying up-to-date on blood work and getting annual (or biannual) tests (refer to the Resources section at www.nourishingmenopausebook.com for a list of the tests I recommend speaking to your doctor about). Listen to your body, because you know it best. If you feel something is off, please speak to your doctor or healthcare practitioner.

Gender Differences and Stress Coping Mechanisms

As we learned from our Morphus Signs and Symptoms research survey, mental/cognitive health symptoms can represent up to 50–90 percent of the top ten most common perimenopause and menopause symptoms, with anxiety coming in at number five. And our Stress and Anxiety survey showed that 66 percent of us are more stressed now than before (Chapter 2).

Unfortunately, for many of us, high stress levels and less ability to cope don't make for a great combination.

Beyond hormonal shifts, we have a lot on our plates! Many of us are managing family responsibilities, taking care of aging parents, dealing with health challenges (our own or a family member's), or any of the 103+ symptoms. Around the same time, we may start reflecting on or evaluating our lives, relationships, financial matters, and career changes.

Add the physical changes on top of the psychological, and it's no wonder women experience anxiety, depression, and other mental health challenges at this time.

It can feel like a lot.

Women often feel more stress on a daily basis than men. One reason is because we manage multiple roles and responsibilities at the same time. Men and women go through similar life events, but women tend to feel the effects of those events more strongly. Research also shows that women are more likely to be caregivers, and while caregiving is important and meaningful, it adds another layer of responsibility that can increase mental stress and take a toll on our physical health.

Here are a few other interesting facts about women and stress:

- Women are more prone to depression. Women tend to dwell on negative thoughts more than men, and rumination can be a precursor to depression.

- Women are more prone to PTSD.

- Women often talk about their thoughts and feelings more, which may lead some women to dwell on things longer.

- Women going through perimenopause and menopause may feel alone and/or lack resources or effective ways to cope with the changes they're facing, which can increase their stress levels and affect their coping mechanisms.

All this stress puts a strain on the nervous system and the brain.

Both women and men are affected by stress, but research shows that it can impact women differently. Hormones are a big reason for this: The female brain is strongly influenced by estrogen and progesterone, while the male brain is influenced more heavily by testosterone and other androgens, although all three of these hormones are present in both sexes. Estrogen helps the brain use glucose properly, which supports focus, memory, and mental energy. Progesterone has a calming effect and supports emotional balance, stable moods, and deeper sleep. During menopause, when both estrogen and progesterone are lower, many of us become less resilient to stress, so we feel it more, and it can take longer to recover than before.

According to Dr. Lisa Mosconi, PhD, estrogen, "estradiol in particular, is the master regulator of women's brains. It pushes the neurons in the brain to make more energy." A decline in estrogen results in reduced brain energy and activity, "putting women more at risk for suffering more from the effects of stress." Sleep problems, depression, mood swings, brain fog, mental fatigue, hot flashes, anxiety, lower self-esteem and confidence, and forgetfulness are all possible symptoms of this hormonal decline. Some research suggests that menopause-related brain changes may also be linked to a long-term risk of dementia, including Alzheimer's disease.

Dr. James LaValle, founder of LaValle Metabolic Code Enterprises and chief science officer at Life Time, says that few people realize that women have a "more exaggerated response" to stress than men do. This may help explain why women are more prone to issues like anxiety, panic attacks, mood issues, and irritable bowel syndrome, which are all linked to the nervous system.

Other research shows that, on average, women remember emotional situations more deeply and vividly than men, and according to some studies, remember them more quickly. They also feel them more intensely. Together, these factors can translate into higher stress levels.

Internist and gender-medicine specialist Dr. Marianne Legato, MD, founder and director of the Partnership for Gender-Specific Medicine at Columbia University, is a pioneer in this area and has conducted in-depth research on how women's and men's brains work and how they respond differently to stress. You can check out her website at gendermed.org.

Your Nervous System

To explain what's happening in your body when you feel stressed, let's start by understanding how the nervous system works.

Almost everything your body does is connected in some way to your nervous system. It's your body's main command center. It's made up of your brain, spinal cord, and nerves, and it works by sending messages between your brain and the rest of your body.

The nervous system is divided into two main parts:

- The *central nervous system* (CNS), made up of the brain and spinal cord.

- The *peripheral nervous system* (PNS), made up of all the nerves that branch out from the brain and spinal cord to the rest of your body. The PNS has two parts:

  » The *somatic nervous system*, which manages your voluntary movements (exercising, chewing, speaking); and

  » The *autonomic nervous system*, which deals with involuntary functions (heartbeat, breathing, blinking, digestion). The autonomic nervous system has two main branches: the *sympathetic* and the *parasympathetic*. These two systems are the key players in *how* your body responds to stress. The sympathetic nervous system manages the "fight-or-flight" response (aka the acute stress response), and the parasympathetic is responsible for the "rest and digest" state.

    Imagine you're late for an important event or appointment and you can't find your keys. How would you react? Does your heart start racing? Do you move faster? Are you fully alert? Are you freaking out? If you answered yes, this is what it feels like to be in a sympathetic state.

    Now think about how good it feels to get into bed or a warm bathtub after a long day, finish a delicious meal at your favorite restaurant, or go for a long walk in nature. Do you feel safe and calm? Does your breathing slow down? Do you feel your muscles and body relaxing? The parasympathetic state is responsible for those peaceful feelings.

    Both states are important, and your body is constantly balancing between the two.

Another system that also gets in on the action is the enteric nervous system (ENS), nicknamed "the second brain" because it controls the gastrointestinal system. The ENS is a huge network of neurons in the walls of the gastrointestinal (GI) tract that run from the esophagus all the way down to the rectum. The ENS contains more neurons than the spinal cord, so when you feel stress, your ENS feels it too, and it can mess with how your body digests food when things get tense. This is the gut-brain connection in action!

Sympathetic Nervous System: "Fight, Flight, Freeze, Fawn," or "SAFE" Response

When you're stressed, scared, or feel threatened, your body springs into action. Your nervous system can react in four different ways: defend yourself (fight), run away to safety (flight), become still (freeze), or appease and accommodate others to feel safe (fawn).

I call it the "SAFE" response, because each reaction is rooted in survival instincts designed to keep you safe:

S: Survival through action (Fight). Fighting back to defend yourself.

A: Avoidance (Flight). Escaping to safety.

F: Fawn. Seeking protection by engaging or appeasing.

E: Escape within (Freeze). Your body shuts down and conserves energy.

This survival response is triggered by a surge of hormones that starts in the brain and prepares your body to react.

There are three main stages to these responses:

The alarm stage: When your senses perceive stress or danger, they send signals to the brain's hypothalamus, which activates the sympathetic nervous system. Within seconds, your sympathetic nervous system signals your adrenal glands to release the hormones adrenaline (epinephrine) and noradrenaline (norepinephrine), and your heart rate, breathing, and blood pressure increase. Your focus becomes sharp so you can quickly respond to the threat, and you may also experience sweats or chills.

The hypothalamic-pituitary-adrenal (HPA) axis is part of your stress response. Think of it as your body's stress switch. Your brain tells your adrenal glands to release cortisol, flipping your body into survival mode, so you're ready to face the danger, whether it's real or perceived. The entire process is meant to be short-lived and can last anywhere from a few minutes to several hours. When the stress is over, your body relaxes and goes back to its normal state (where it was before the response was triggered).

During the SAFE response, cortisol and other stress hormones increase the amount of sugar (glucose) in your bloodstream to make sure your muscles and brain have enough glucose to deal with the situation at hand. Digestion and all other nonurgent functions slow down. The amygdala, the part of your brain responsible for fear, emotional processing, and behavior, also activates this response. When the SAFE stress response is triggered, our rational thinking can temporarily be overridden by irrational thinking. This is known as the "amygdala hijack." Have you ever been in a heated argument and tried to reason with the person in the moment? Or have you ever received an email that really upset you? Were you able to immediately defuse the situation in a rational way? Probably not. That's because emotions take over; we may overreact, and our ability to think and act reasonably goes out the window. When that happens, it's a good idea to let some time pass (implement the "24-hour rule") before discussing the argument or replying to that email. Taking time to process what happened gives your body time to calm down, collect your thoughts, and let the stress response pass. This processing time allows your pragmatic thinking to come back, preventing you from saying things you may regret later.

The resistance stage: In this phase, your body starts to recover from the alarm stage and tries to restore balance, but it's still on high alert. Adrenaline goes back to normal levels, but cortisol can stick around in case the stress continues.

How do you know if you're in this stage? First, you'll feel tired.

Unlike stage one, where you were wired and jumped out of bed every morning, now you're more likely to struggle to wake up, and you may drag your feet all day.

Your muscles may feel tense, and you might notice changes in your appetite, either completely losing it or wanting to eat all the time. Then there are the cognitive challenges, like brain fog and forgetfulness, where you can't think straight enough to make a good decision. And the emotional ones: feeling on edge, feeling like you're about to fall apart, and experiencing fits of rage.

But in a frustrating twist, when it's finally time for bed, instead of falling into deep sleep, you lie there wide awake for hours, or you fall asleep quickly only to wake up in the middle of the night with your mind racing.

In this stage, because you're tired all the time, you may turn to caffeine and sugar for energy, or alcohol to help you relax. And because you're feeling overwhelmed, instead of taking time for self-care, you might end up overworking or hyper-focused on completing tasks as a form of stress management, which may end up being counterproductive.

In today's world, stressors like unexpected bills, constant meetings, never-ending emails, taking care of kids, family fights, money issues, relationship problems, job or health concerns, traffic, and so on are repeatedly triggering the stress response. However, our bodies can't cope with high levels of stress hormones (like cortisol) long-term. If the resistance stage continues for a long time without a break, the stress response stops working the way it should, and gradually becomes dysregulated. Over time, the stress can become chronic.

The exhaustion stage: This is the point in time when you've been dealing with stress for so long that your body can't handle it anymore, and it begins to break down. In this stage, cortisol levels are out of balance, your energy tanks, and you feel physically, mentally, and emotionally drained. You may struggle to find your spark, and very little brings you joy. Your cognition is affected too. You find it hard to concentrate, remember anything, or make decisions. This is what many people describe as "burnout," and it's real.

The SAFE response is a good thing. It helps us during times of danger. This response helped our ancestors survive threats like wild animals and other predators. (When you're confronted with a saber-toothed tiger, you either freeze, run for your life, or stay and fight).

However, when stressors don't let up and your response system stays activated for extended periods, the stress becomes chronic. Over time, chronic stress can wear your body down. While you may not be running from wild animals, your brain still responds in similar ways. Chronic stress keeps stress hormones like cortisol high, putting you in a constant state of high alert.

We've heard how chronic stress isn't good for us, but why? How exactly does it affect us?

Stress can cause your muscles to tense up, so you may feel tightness or pain around the shoulders and upper back, which can lead to headaches, migraines, a sore jaw, and pain or tightness in other parts of your body. It can also cause heart palpitations, and breathing issues like shortness of breath, heavy breathing, or hyperventilation, and can make existing conditions like asthma or chronic obstructive pulmonary disease (COPD) symptoms worse. What's even scarier is that stress increases inflammation in your arteries, raises heart rate and blood pressure, and increases the risk of heart attack or stroke. Continuous stress can lead to chronic fatigue, depression, trouble sleeping, immune system problems, and metabolic changes (like blood sugar imbalances and weight gain). Digestive issues such as acid reflux, heartburn, loss of appetite, loose stools or constipation, pain, and bloating are common. And moods and cognition can also be affected. In women, stress can contribute to irregular menstrual cycles, lower sex drive, fertility and pregnancy issues, and more severe menopausal symptoms.

Parasympathetic Nervous System: "Rest and Digest"

While the sympathetic nervous system controls the SAFE response, the parasympathetic nervous system helps us to relax and calm down after experiencing stress.

It controls many of the body's slower "rest and digest" functions, with the vagus nerve playing a key role.

As I explained in Chapter 4, the vagus nerve is the body's information superhighway. It starts in the brain and travels down through the neck, chest, and abdomen, all the way to the colon. *Vagus* means "wandering" in Latin, and it connects the brain to nearly every major organ, including the heart, lungs, and digestive tract. The vagus nerve is also the main pathway of the parasympathetic nervous system. It helps slow down your heart rate, calm your breathing, stimulate digestion, and regulate blood pressure and blood sugar, and it keeps inflammation in check, giving your body the chance to relax and recover from stress.

Most of what the vagus nerve does is pass messages (or signals) from your organs to your brain (75–80 percent). The rest involves sending messages from your brain down to your organs and muscles.

Gut-Brain Connection

The enteric nervous system, which I mentioned earlier, is closely linked to the vagus nerve. As such, the vagus nerve plays an important role when it comes to gut health. This two-way highway connects your brain and gut, allowing them to constantly communicate with each other. To appreciate this connection, think of a time when you fell in love. Do you remember feeling butterflies in your stomach whenever you saw, spoke to, or even thought about the person you were in love with? Or how about when you feel nervous or anxious? Do you get the runs, have stomach pains, or feel nauseous? I do!

These reactions happen because the gut and brain are always talking to each other through nerves, gut bacteria, and chemicals in the bloodstream (for example, neurotransmitters like serotonin).

Vagal Tone and HRV

Vagal tone refers to how well your vagus nerve is working and how it affects different functions in your body. A common way to estimate vagal tone is by looking at heart rate variability (HRV), which you might have heard of from popular wearables that track different body functions, like certain smartwatches, fitness trackers, smart rings, and medical-grade devices. HRV is measured in milliseconds, and it shows how well your body can adapt to and recover from stress by measuring the variation in timing from one heartbeat to the next.

Poor vagal tone has been associated with many symptoms that are common in perimenopause and menopause, including depression, anxiety, moodiness, hot flashes, and sleep issues. Newer research also shows possible links to changes in blood pressure, inflammation, and pain. And emerging research suggests it may also influence how the body manages hormones and metabolism, including thyroid health, liver health, bone health, and blood sugar, although more research is needed.

It's important not to worry about a single HRV number, as stress itself can lower it. Instead, *focus on tracking your personal trends over time.* If you notice it's lower than usual, it's something to pay attention to. Maybe you're experiencing more stress than usual, not sleeping well, coming down with a cold, or dealing with other health issues. A higher HRV typically means you're adapting and recovering well to stress, while a lower HRV can suggest the opposite. *What matters most is how your HRV changes over time for you, not how it compares to someone else's.* For this reason, and the fact that HRV values vary depending on the tool or device you use to measure them, I didn't include any specific data ranges. Again, I want to emphasize that HRV is very personal and specific to your body. According to Navaz Habib, a chiropractor and functional medicine practitioner, and author of *Upgrade Your Vagus Nerve,* "A good HRV score is relative to your personal baseline. What's considered optimal for one woman may be suboptimal for another. Factors such as age, fitness level, stress, sleep quality, and overall health all play a role in determining your unique HRV profile." I've personally noticed that when I'm feeling under the weather, my average HRV plummets. And once I start feeling better, it starts to climb back and eventually returns to baseline.

HRV values can also be influenced by hormones (lower estrogen and progesterone levels during perimenopause and menopause can lower scores); genetics (some people naturally have a lower HRV); chronic diseases (which put physiological stress on the body); air quality; altitude; room temperature; lifestyle choices such as eating late, drinking alcohol, and strenuous exercise; dietary habits like too much caffeine; dehydration; certain medications; and high stress levels.

I share tips on how to support your vagus nerve and overall stress management at the end of this chapter.

I recommend listening to episodes #63 and #105 of my podcast, *Menopause Reimagined*, where Navaz and I discuss stress, anxiety, HRV, and the vagus nerve.

Cortisol and Menopause

Once you're fully menopausal and your ovaries stop producing large amounts of estrogen, your adrenal glands (and to a lesser extent, your ovaries) act as a backup by producing small amounts of hormones, like DHEA (dehydroepiandrosterone) and other androgens, which can be converted into estrogen and testosterone in other parts of your body, such as your fat cells, liver, brain, and skin. However, it's important to note that your ovaries don't stop producing hormones overnight (unless they've been removed surgically). It's a gradual decrease, and they can still produce small amounts of estrogen and androgens, but they're no longer the main source.

The adrenal glands also make cortisol. Cortisol affects almost every cell in your body, and when levels are in a healthy range, it helps manage inflammation, gives the brain more energy by increasing blood sugar, keeps blood pressure stable, and helps the body deal with stress better. It also helps your body use proteins, fats, and carbohydrates; supports your immune system to fight bacteria and viruses; and helps you get a good night's sleep.

This is how cortisol levels are supposed to flow throughout the day:

For most people, cortisol is naturally highest in the morning and reaches its peak around thirty to sixty minutes after you wake up. This is known as the "morning peak," or cortisol awakening response

(CAR). It's what helps you feel awake, focused, and ready to face the day. Higher levels of cortisol in the morning help support energy, metabolism, and stable blood sugar levels.

As the day goes on, cortisol levels gradually fall until they reach their lowest point, usually around bedtime. At the same time, melatonin rises to help you sleep. This daily cycle is called the cortisol curve, and it impacts our energy levels and how we respond to and cope with stress.

However, chronic stress, poor sleep, imbalanced blood sugar levels, and certain health conditions can all disrupt your daily cortisol levels.

For example:

- If cortisol is low in the morning you might find it hard to get out of bed and feel mentally sluggish.

- If it's high at night, you might have trouble falling asleep or going back to sleep.

- If it's low overall but spikes during the day, this can lead to short bursts of energy followed by longer stretches of fatigue and brain fog.

The cortisol curve can be affected by lifestyle choices such as drinking too much caffeine, late-night snacking, exercising too close to bed, or not getting enough physical activity, and (you guessed it!) perimenopause and menopause.

Progesterone is a calming hormone, and it helps to relax the nervous system by interacting with gamma-aminobutyric acid (GABA) receptors in the brain, buffering your body from stress. It's also part of a pathway that your body uses to make cortisol, so when your stress levels are constantly high, progesterone levels may fall, leaving you more susceptible to the negative effects of stress. And as progesterone naturally decreases during perimenopause and stays low in menopause, your body becomes more sensitive to stress, making it harder to manage and maintain a sense of calm.

Remember the HPA axis we talked about earlier and how it

kickstarts your SAFE response? An easy way to think of it is as the master switch that tells your adrenals when to make cortisol, and how much. But when stress is chronically high and the HPA axis is working on overdrive, the signals between your brain and adrenal glands can get mixed up, causing cortisol to be released at the wrong times or in the wrong amounts. In the wellness and functional medicine world, this is referred to as "adrenal dysregulation" or "adrenal fatigue," which is different from adrenal insufficiency, a diagnosed medical condition where the adrenal glands are damaged and can't make enough hormones, especially cortisol. Addison's disease is the best-known example of adrenal insufficiency. While adrenal dysregulation and insufficiency share some of the same symptoms, they're not the same thing.

As you go through perimenopause and menopause and depend more on your adrenal glands to produce small amounts of androgens, chronic stress can make it harder for your HPA axis and adrenals to keep up. Years of stress can throw off the signals between your brain and adrenals (the HPA axis), so the hormones your adrenals release can become more unpredictable, and as a result, your perimenopause and menopause symptoms can feel more intense.

Either way, when cortisol is too high for too long, it can impact almost every system in your body.

Common symptoms of chronic stress and imbalanced cortisol include blood sugar spikes and fluctuations, increased inflammation, weight gain (especially around your belly), cravings (typically for high-calorie sugary or salty foods, or carbohydrate-rich foods),

---

Do you feel burned out, or have you been told you have low cortisol levels? This can happen when your stress response is always working and doesn't turn on and off the way it's meant to (in other words, it never gets a break). When that happens, your stress response system (the HPA axis) can become dysregulated and may stop sending strong enough signals to make the cortisol your body needs.

insomnia and poor sleep (often waking up between 2 a.m. and 4 a.m.), fatigue, and mood swings. It can also make general and morning anxiety worse, disrupt your immune system, raise blood pressure, and mess with digestion.

Research shows that higher cortisol levels are linked to more severe hot flashes, along with thinning hair or loss, acne and other skin problems, period changes, frequent urination, and low libido. It can also influence other hormones, like androgens, which may lead to increased hair growth under your chin.

It's important to manage stress as best you can, not only because of the symptoms I just listed but also because chronic stress can take a toll on your body and raise the risk of heart disease, osteoporosis (due to increased bone loss), type 2 diabetes, and mental health issues such as depression.

Cortisol and the Menopause Brain

High cortisol levels from chronic stress can affect brain cells (neurons) and are linked to changes in the hippocampus, the part of the brain that helps with memory. They also impact the front part of your brain, called the prefrontal cortex, which helps with planning, focus, learning, and judgment. When the prefrontal cortex is under prolonged stress, it may not work as well as it should, making it harder to learn new information or think clearly.

Cortisol also affects the amygdala, the part of the brain that processes strong emotions like fear and anxiety, so over time you may feel stress more intensely, get upset over things that never bothered you before, or react more quickly and strongly than you used to.

Cortisol affects women's brains differently than men's. In women, high cortisol has been linked to changes in how certain parts of the brain use glucose (the brain's main source of energy). Researchers believe this may help explain why women have a higher risk of developing Alzheimer's, though research is still ongoing. This tells us that long-lasting stress can have a stronger effect on women's brains, so managing it in ways that benefit female bodies and hormones may help protect our brain health as we age.

As you read in Chapter 2, many women notice changes in how their brain works during perimenopause and menopause. This can show up as memory issues, forgetfulness, a lack of focus and concentration, trouble finding the right words or learning new ones, and feeling slower when thinking or speaking. While these issues are usually temporary, they can be stressful and add to feelings of uncertainty, stress, and anxiety.

If you suspect you have a cortisol imbalance, speak to your doctor or healthcare provider about testing your cortisol levels. You can also look into twenty-four-hour urine and saliva testing.

I interviewed Aron Gonshor, PhD, DDS, and CEO of FluidsIQ, about different testing options to consider. I also spoke with Emaline Brown, ND, who works with Vibrant Wellness. You can listen to both conversations in episodes #137 and #180 of my podcast, *Menopause Reimagined*.

Rethinking Stress in Perimenopause and Menopause

One secret to managing stress successfully is to embrace it rather than see it as the enemy or something to be afraid of, which only adds to your mental and emotional stress and discomfort.

I know it sounds funny, but hear me out.

There's a great TED Talk called "How to Make Stress Your Friend" by psychologist Kelly McGonigal, PhD. She discusses a Harvard study that followed thirty thousand adults for eight years and found that people who were experiencing a lot of stress and believed it was bad for their health had the highest risk of dying. On the other hand, those with high stress levels who didn't see it as harmful had no increased risk of dying. The study suggested that changing *how you think about stress may influence your body's response to it*. Dr. McGonigal suggests using the following mantra during stressful times to reframe your thoughts:

"This is my body helping me rise to this challenge."

Try it next time you're feeling overwhelmed. I printed it out and put it in my office. You can also keep it on your phone or in your bathroom to read out loud when you're getting ready for your day.

Another study looked at 179 (post)menopausal women (with an average age of about fifty-one) and found that the most common ways they coped with stress included expressing their emotions, taking direct action, and seeking social support. Stressful events included family issues, menopause symptoms, work problems, daily hassles, and other health concerns. The study found that what matters most is *how* women see and think about stress, not their age, menopause symptoms, or even how much stress they have. This means that their *perspective on a stressful event* can help determine *how they handle it* in menopause.

A situation is first perceived by our senses, including sight, hearing, smell, touch, and taste. But the ultimate decision-maker is the brain, and it decides whether the situation is stressful or not. Some events, like trauma or intense pain, cause instant and sometimes unavoidable stress. However, most of the time, it's not the situation itself that causes the stress but rather *how we see it* or *what we think it means*. And since we can change *how* we *see* things, research shows that reframing our thoughts can help change *how we react* or *respond* to them.

You and I both know that managing stress isn't as simple as taking a yoga class, getting an extra half hour of sleep, or me suggesting you do it. It involves supporting the systems and organs involved in the stress response, plus, as the research shows, having the right mindset. This is how you build resilience. Resilience is the process of adapting well and the ability to bounce back from adversity, trauma, tragedy, threats, or significant sources of stress. The more tools you have in your toolbox, the more resilient you are and the better prepared your body is to recover from and cope with whatever stress comes your way.

Actionable Tips for Managing Stress

Now that you understand how stress affects your body and brain during perimenopause and menopause, learning how to manage it is really important. Think of it as one of the most valuable gifts you can give yourself. By incorporating the following strategies into your daily routine, you'll nourish your nervous system and strengthen your overall mental and physical health. By focusing on daily habits that help you recognize, manage, and reduce stress, you may notice changes in your symptoms. They might become less severe, or some may even disappear altogether.

Let's start with nutrition because it sets the stage for a calmer nervous system and better resilience to stress.

Eat whole foods. Nourishing your body with nutritious foods can make a big difference in how you feel. What you eat and drink can either give you energy and help you handle stress or leave you feeling more stressed and tired.

Focus on whole foods and limit alcohol, excessive caffeine, and ultra-processed foods. Also, check out the Mediterranean diet, as research from May 2024 shows that people who follow it experience fewer symptoms of stress and anxiety.

And make sure you eat enough. Chronic stress can change the way your body uses calories and nutrients. When your adrenal glands are continuously responding to stress, your body burns through nutrients more quickly or uses them less efficiently, which can leave you feeling tired, drained, or cranky.

Consider nutrients. Think about a time in your life when you were under pressure, maybe during exams, a big work deadline, or while caring for family. Once it was over, did you get sick? That happens because by the time stress runs you down, your body may change how it uses or stores key nutrients, and together with other possible contributing factors (like less sleep), it can leave you and your immune system run-down.

Many nutrients support your nervous system and overall stress response (HPA axis) and help your body regulate cortisol levels, which can help you better cope with the effects of stress. These include:

- **Protein,** including both animal and plant-based options.

- **Vitamins and minerals** such as magnesium, vitamin C, selenium, iron, copper, B vitamins, and zinc. These nutrients can be found in leafy greens (spinach, Swiss chard, and kale), berries (strawberries, blueberries, and raspberries), meat (beef, pork, chicken, and lamb), and legumes (chickpeas, lentils, and beans).

- **Omega-3 fatty acids** support brain health and have been shown to help reduce the effects of stress in the body. These include fatty fish like salmon, sardines, and herring, as well as vegan sources like chia, hemp, and flaxseeds.

- **Potassium** helps with hydration (electrolyte balance) and over-all nerve and muscle function. Foods include sweet potatoes, lentils, Swiss chard, white beans, and avocados.

- **B vitamins** support adrenal health by helping the body build resilience and cope with stress. Certain Bs, like B5, B6, B12, and folate, are especially important for making stress hormones and helping the body handle stress. B vitamins also support mood and energy production, and each B vitamin helps your brain make the brain chemicals (neurotransmitters) that regulate stress, mood, and cognition.

  Food sources of B vitamins include dark leafy greens for folate (raw and cooked), animal-based foods like salmon, eggs, poultry, and meat, and whole grains and legumes. Include these foods often in your diet during low-stress periods. During high-stress periods, consider adding a B complex supplement. Take it earlier in the day with breakfast or lunch and start with a lower dose (around 25 to 50 mg of the key B vitamins such as B1, B2, B3, B6, and B12). For some people, higher doses can overstim-ulate the nervous system, making them feel jittery or on edge. Avoid taking B vitamins, especially B6 and B12, too close to bedtime, as they can be energizing, and may interfere with your sleep. Choose brands with methylated forms, like methylcobal-amin for B12, and methylfolate for folate.

  Note: A small percentage of people might feel wired, anx-ious, or irritable on higher doses of methylated B vitamins. In that case, try hydroxocobalamin (for B12) or folinic acid (for folate) and see how you feel. If needed, work with a qualified practitioner to help guide you.

- **Magnesium** is known as the "anti-stress mineral." It helps to keep your stress and anxiety levels in check by supporting your nervous system and helping you feel more relaxed.

  When you're stressed, your body tends to burn through magnesium faster, and when your levels drop, you become more stressed and less able to cope, creating a vicious cycle.

  You can get this mineral from leafy green vegetables like spinach, kale, collard, and mustard greens; nuts and seeds like almonds, cashews, pumpkin, and sunflower; legumes like lentils and chickpeas; whole grains; fatty fish like salmon; avocados; and dark chocolate.

  When taken as a supplement, all forms of magnesium can help to some degree during periods of stress, but magnesium bisglycinate (or glycinate) is my personal go-to, and it's an excellent choice for perimenopausal and menopausal women. It can be taken during the day to help manage stress and to calm your mind. It can also be taken thirty to forty minutes before bed to help you get a better night's sleep, as it's attached to the amino acid glycine, which helps your body and muscles relax. Magnesium bisglycinate is easily absorbed and gentle on the stomach.

- **Vitamin D** is important for stabilizing mood. A 2024 study found that higher levels of vitamin D were associated with lower levels of anxiety and sleep disorders in physically active adults.

- **Adaptogenic herbs, or adaptogens,** help your body handle stress better by supporting your overall stress response (HPA axis) and improving *how* you cope with different types of stressors (physical, mental, emotional, and environmental). There are many types of adaptogens; some have stimulating effects, while others are more calming. They've been used for centuries in Traditional Chinese Medicine and Ayurveda. Examples of adaptogens include holy basil (tulsi), ashwagandha, rhodiola rosea, Siberian ginseng (eleuthero), schisandra, and cordyceps.

  Note: If you're taking prescription medications, it's a good idea to double-check with your healthcare provider before starting any new herbs, as they can interact.

Test for nutritional deficiencies. Since stress can deplete important vitamins and minerals from your body, including B vitamins, magnesium, vitamins C and D, iron, potassium, iodine, selenium, zinc, amino acids, and omega-3 fatty acids, you may feel tired, inflamed, moody, dizzy, or experience other symptoms that are also common in perimenopause and menopause, making it hard to differentiate between the two. If you're feeling off, talk to your healthcare provider about identifying any nutritional deficiencies and then work together to replenish them.

Increase your antioxidants. Chronically high levels of stress increase the production of free radicals, which can damage cells and fuel inflammation, aging, and chronic diseases. And remember what cortisol does? It helps to reduce inflammation in the short term, but long-term stress makes the body less sensitive to cortisol, allowing inflammation to increase again. A good way to lower free radicals and inflammation in your body is to eat a diet filled with brightly colored, antioxidant-rich vegetables and low-glycemic fruits, like red peppers, artichokes, and berries; herbs and spices, like sumac (a Middle Eastern spice), oregano, rosemary, garlic, and ginger; dark chocolate; and nuts like almonds, pecans, and walnuts, which are all ranked high on the antioxidant scale.

Manage blood sugar. Stress affects your blood sugar levels, and the opposite is true as well: *Blood sugar levels have a profound impact on your stress hormones.*

When you're stressed, your body makes sure it has enough sugar or energy available to deal with the circumstances at hand, so blood sugar levels and stress hormones like cortisol and adrenaline go up. However, high cortisol levels over time make it harder for insulin to control blood sugar, making you less sensitive to insulin and more prone to insulin resistance.

Refer to Chapters 5 and 11 on effective ways to manage blood sugar levels.

Simplify digestion. When you're stressed, your body activates the sympathetic nervous system and increases cortisol levels, which makes digestion less important (it takes a back seat). Eating when you're stressed can cause stomach problems like heartburn, gas, bloating, and irritable bowel syndrome (IBS) flare-ups.

Natural nutrition coach and nutritionist Lisa Tsakos has worked with many clients experiencing adrenal dysregulation. She recommends the following tips when you're feeling anxious, overwhelmed, or have a lot on your plate:

Take at least three deep breaths before eating to stimulate the parasympathetic nervous system. Eat smaller meals and make sure a meal is digested before you eat again. Chew carefully and eat slowly, and take digestive enzymes or take a teaspoon of apple cider vinegar before meals to support digestion and blood sugar. Also, eating a soft-food diet (pureed, mashed, and blended foods) helps take the pressure off the digestive system.

Support your gut microbiome. Chronic stress can disrupt the balance of bacteria in your gut. Because the gut and brain constantly communicate, those changes can affect mood and mental health. Support your gut health with probiotic and prebiotic foods, as well as enough fiber.

Refer to Chapter 4 on how to support your gut microbiome.

Stick to a routine. The body operates on biological rhythms. It likes routine, and routine is key for recovery from stress. Try to eat and go to sleep around the same time every day. Start your day with a protein-rich breakfast, like eggs or a protein shake. Eating breakfast helps to keep blood sugar levels and energy more balanced, and helps you handle whatever stressful situations might come your way throughout the day.

Cut down on caffeine. Be mindful of how much caffeine or coffee you drink when you're stressed or when you expect to have a busy day. On very stressful days, eating a meal and having a lot of caffeine can raise cortisol levels even higher. You may want to think about reducing or eliminating caffeinated beverages and foods on those days, particularly when consuming them on an empty stomach.

If you can't go without caffeine, limit it to first thing in the morning and try half caff (half caffeinated and half decaf). This is a good time to try coffee substitutes or herbal teas.

Limit alcohol and smoking (cigarettes). Chronic drinking and smoking can increase cortisol levels in the body. Although both can help you relax, that feeling is temporary and can lead to higher anxiety over time.

Move. Physical activity has many health benefits, and one of them is improved HRV. Research shows that exercise improves HRV not only in people with heart problems, which become more common after menopause, but also in healthy (post)menopausal women. Simply put, exercise lowers stress and protects your heart. A 2024 study published in the *Journal of the American College of Cardiology* found that regular exercise lowers the risk of heart disease, mainly by helping the brain handle stress better. This effect was greatest in people who have depression. How the brain handles stress is connected to heart disease and mental health problems like anxiety and depression. Moderate-intensity exercise like walking, hiking, gardening, dancing, golf, pickleball, tennis, volleyball, leisure bike riding, and strength training help to lower stress, support heart health, and improve overall life expectancy. Doing yoga helps to activate the parasympathetic nervous system and supports healthy blood flow, digestion, and heart rate.

I'll be discussing exercise in Chapter 13, but for now, keep in mind that high-intensity interval training, sprinting, and spinning can temporarily spike cortisol. If your overall stress levels are already high, these forms of exercise may affect your recovery and leave you feeling wiped out or run-down, so allowing more time between workouts can be helpful.

Sleep. Getting enough sleep is critical when it comes to managing and recovering from stress, and research proves it. Many studies have found that lack of sleep significantly raises cortisol levels and can have a negative effect on blood sugar levels. I cover sleep in detail in the next chapter.

Connect. One theory about why friendships and close relationships are good for our health is that the support we get from social connections can shield us from the negative physical effects of stress, and extend our lifespan. These relationships don't have to be romantic in nature. Establishing closer connections with family, friends, religious groups, clubs, coworkers, partners, and others can be just as fulfilling (and even more so in some cases). If you've never read Anita Diamant's book *The Red Tent*, I highly recommend it. It shows what happens when women come together and support one another.

Get touchy. Physical touch releases the "love hormone" or "love drug," oxytocin. Oxytocin—similar to endorphins, serotonin, and dopamine—is a feel-good hormone. When you give someone a massage, cuddle, have sex, or hug someone, it increases oxytocin levels (theirs and yours), which leads to happier and more content feelings. And hugging is good for your heart! It makes you happier, reduces pain, enhances intimacy, and reduces stress. A 2021 study involving nearly 1,500 people found that lack of intimate touch from close family and partners was linked to higher levels of anxiety and loneliness. Regular, intimate touch can have lasting positive effects on mental health.

Listen to sounds of nature or other calming music. Sound can have a profound effect on our nervous system; it can either stimulate it or calm it. Sounds of nature, like birds singing, crickets chirping, or ocean waves crashing at the shore, can help shift your body into a parasympathetic state of relaxation. Research shows that a combination of calming sounds can help slow your heart rate, lower stress hormones like cortisol, and make you feel more relaxed.

Practice self-love. Practicing self-love and self-compassion is important for dealing with stress and difficult situations. A 2021 review found that people with more self-compassion used healthier ways to cope, while those with less self-compassion turned to harmful methods. The research showed that self-compassion is particularly important for helping people avoid unhealthy coping methods. Since self-love is such an important topic, I dedicated an entire chapter to it (Chapter 12).

Avoid multitasking. Leave yourself longer blocks of time to accomplish a task. Trying to get too much done in a short amount of time creates unnecessary stress.

Help others. Helping others boosts your sense of connection and gives you purpose. This can make you feel better emotionally, which helps lower your stress, reduces cortisol, and can even lower your blood pressure. Plus, doing good deeds can make you feel like you belong and aren't alone, which also helps reduce stress. So not only does helping others make a difference in their lives, but it also brings big benefits to your own mental and physical health.

Volunteer. People who volunteer often report better health and longer lifespans, and they experience lower rates of anxiety and depression. The Mayo Clinic notes that "volunteering reduces stress and increases positive, relaxed feelings by releasing dopamine."

Get help. Seeing a therapist or other mental health professional, trusted family member, or friend(s) can help you acknowledge your anxious feelings and process them.

Limit exposure to media and social media. Limit the time you spend watching the news, social media, or even scary, intense, or emotionally charged shows, especially before you go to bed.

If social media makes you feel anxious or overwhelmed, unfollow accounts that add to that stress.

Set boundaries. Setting boundaries helps you keep your stress levels in check. Identify situations, events, or people that cause you stress. Take a moment to ask yourself *how* and *why* they trigger feelings like anxiety, fear, and frustration, then decide what you can do to mitigate them by setting boundaries that feel right for you.

Fight fair. People with stressed partners tend to have higher cortisol levels throughout the day, especially after disagreements. And the impact is worse if the couple argues in a combative way. On the other hand, those with less stressed partners have healthier cortisol patterns. This shows how your partner's stress can affect your own stress levels and health, especially during fights or disagreements.

Meditate or unmeditate. A 2020 study found that mindfulness meditation can improve HRV. Another study found it can help to improve insomnia and sleep quality. And in yet another study, those who practiced loving-kindness meditation for six weeks showed an improvement in vagal tone. Even a short five-to-ten-minute meditation session can help reduce stress levels. Whenever possible, start and end your day by meditating in a comfortable, quiet space. If you have a hard time meditating, try "unmeditating," like my friend Lisa Borden, adviser and mentor for curious thinkers and purpose-driven entrepreneurs and founder of The Wellness Intelligence Collective (TWIC), suggests: "Instead of trying to force yourself into stillness, try moving, writing, humming, breathing, or simply being aware of what's happening around you in real-time . . . no pressure, no app, no timer. Just you, tuning in." Lisa teaches that "stress relief and meditation don't have to look like a monk on a mountaintop." It can be something as simple as closing your eyes for thirty seconds, doing a balancing yoga pose while the water boils, or noticing your breath while waiting in line.

Sing or hum. Using your voice, whether singing, humming, or chanting, activates the parasympathetic nervous system, slows breathing, and can increase HRV. As clinical psychologist Dr. Glenn Doyle explains, "The vagus nerve is deeply plugged into our heart, our guts, and our voice. . . . When we speak, shout, sing, the vagus nerve is lit up like a Christmas tree, which is one of the reasons why those activities can be so cathartic and emotional for so many of us."

Gargle. Gargling activates the muscles in your throat that are connected to the vagus nerve, which is why some health experts believe it may help lower stress and promote relaxation.

Try deep-breathing exercises. Research shows that practicing deep, slow breathing can improve vagal tone and reduce anxiety. It's one of the fastest ways to activate the parasympathetic nervous system, shifting your body into a calmer, more relaxed state. Try taking a few deep breaths and making the exhalation twice as long as the inhalation whenever you feel anxious, nervous, or overly excited, and also before you eat, as the digestive system works best in the parasympathetic state. Do whatever breathing method you enjoy most.

Relax. Calming activities can help improve vagal tone. Whether it's watching a good (low-stress) movie, socializing with friends, reading a good book, or spending time with people you love, relaxation supports your parasympathetic nervous system and helps your body reset.

Practice shinrin-yoku. This Japanese practice, also known as "forest bathing," involves spending time in nature, whether it's strolling in a park, taking a hike, walking on a trail, bird-watching, or just sitting next to a lake, ocean, creek, or stream. Many studies have shown that it can help reduce stress and cortisol, improve HRV, lower blood pressure, and support heart health and general well-being.

Spend time near the ocean. Whenever possible, walk, swim, or sit by, in, or near the ocean. If you're unable to be near water physically, listen to sounds of crashing waves, watch videos of the ocean, or visualize water to calm your brain and nervous system. Walking barefoot on the sand helps you feel more grounded, which has positive effects on stress. Meditating near or in (shallow) water helps to enhance that sense of calm.

Get a massage. Getting a massage or massaging yourself can help to activate your parasympathetic nervous system. Add a drop or two of your favorite essential oil(s) to your fingertips. Massage the oil in a circular motion behind your ears, up to your earlobes, around the front of your ears, on your shoulders, and behind your neck. Once you're done, inhale the oils, as they contain terpenes, plant chemicals that calm the nervous system and help you relax.

Journal. Writing down your thoughts, dreams, goals, and interpretations of life events can be healing. Studies prove that journaling is an effective outlet and tool for managing and reducing stress and improving well-being. Journaling before bed can help you process your emotions and resolve any tension and stress you may be feeling. Physically writing something down on paper reinforces and solidifies your emotions and ideas.

Laugh. A small pilot study found that a twenty-minute laughter yoga class (including breathing, chanting, and meditation) improved HRV and mood.

Smell something nice. Smell plays a big role in how we feel and handle stress. Scents from plants, vegetables, and fruits, as well as certain essential oils, may help influence brain chemicals like GABA and dopamine, which can support mood and relaxation and help reduce anxiety. If you like essential oils, try calming ones like lavender, clary sage, chamomile, rose, eucalyptus, lemon, lemongrass, rosemary, coriander, patchouli, jasmine, and frankincense. Add them to massage oils or a bath, inhale, or diffuse them.

Take a bath. Adding Epsom salt (magnesium sulfate), or magnesium chloride flakes, to your bath can help you absorb some of it through your skin. Since magnesium is crucial for helping to relieve stress, it's another way to get more magnesium into your body. A bath is also relaxing right before bed.

Cool yourself. Applying cold air or water to your face or neck for fifteen to thirty seconds can improve HRV in the short term. Doing this consistently once or twice a day may help you feel calmer and more relaxed, although more research is needed to understand its long-term benefits.

Practice gratitude. Research shows that practicing gratitude can improve mood, reduce stress and anxiety, lessen rumination, and improve mental health. Think of three things you're grateful for right now, big or small. Try this exercise every night before bed or when you wake up. I find it helps to put things into perspective. You can also keep a gratitude journal and write in it every morning and/or night.

Give yourself permission to rest. Chronic stress can lead to an imbalance of cortisol, inflammation, and body pain. Rest lowers stress and cortisol levels and gives your stress response system (the HPA axis) time to reset.

Do something you love. Life can be hectic, so carving out some time to do something you love is important. It will make you happy and help you relax, because it helps your brain release feel-good chemicals like endorphins, dopamine, and serotonin.

Say no. Do you find it hard to say no when someone asks you to do something you really don't have time for or don't want to do? Saying yes when you should say no can lead to a buildup of anxiety, resentment, and added stress. Remember, it's okay to say no. As I heard Jane Fonda say in an interview, "No is a full sentence."

Don't stress over "what ifs." We often add to our worry by thinking of many "what if" situations that may never happen. Worrying about *possible* outcomes raises cortisol levels and some of its negative effects. Shifting your focus to what you *can* control may help you manage the situation with less anxiety and stress. One of my husband's favorite mantras is "Don't stress over what you can't control."

Make a list. When I was in perimenopause, even simple responsibilities felt daunting and stressful. What helped me was making lists and then tackling one task at a time, rather than focusing on everything all at once. This "one by one" approach was helpful because I felt a sense of accomplishment every time I got through my list, and I wasn't locked in overwhelm or fear.

Be artistic. If you loved to color as a child or even enjoy it now as an adult, studies show that making art can boost dopamine and lower cortisol levels in just forty-five minutes. Try coloring, sketching, using a pottery wheel, painting, or whatever gets your creative juices flowing! You can also explore the option of taking art classes or working with a licensed art therapist. Engaging in creative projects is a fun way to feel better and lower stress.

Choose color. Building on my point above, whether you're coloring in a coloring book, painting your house, or getting dressed in the morning, certain colors may play a role in how stressed, or not, you feel. Blue, for example, has the most calming and soothing effect and has been shown to lower stress levels. Other calming colors include soft pink, soft yellow, white, beige, soft purple (violet), gray, and green. Bright and highly saturated colors, like red, yellow, and orange, may have the opposite effect. Listen to your body and experiment with different colors.

Download apps. Try stress-relieving meditations and games by downloading apps on your phone or iPad. Search for terms like "calm," "mindfulness," "stress relief," or "meditation" in the app store to find a variety of options.

Try tech. There are wearable devices that can help reduce stress. Some track signals in your body and give you instant feedback, so you can slow your breathing, calm your mind, or refocus. Others gently guide your body to relax with soft vibrations, changes in temperature, or built-in mindfulness exercises. One thing to pay attention to is whether tracking your stats stresses you out instead of easing stress. If you notice yourself getting too caught up in the data, it might be a good idea to take a break, use it less often, or use it only when you feel it will be helpful.

Take omega-3 fish oil. Research suggests that the omega-3 fatty acids found in fish oil may improve HRV. Omega-3s help reduce inflammation and improve the overall health of your heart and blood vessels. By supporting your heart and nervous system health, fish oil may help promote healthier vagal tone. When the vagus nerve is working better, your body can relax more easily, and you're better able to manage stress.

Consider hormone therapy. Speak to your doctor about the option of hormone therapy if you're open to it. Research shows that estrogen-based therapy can improve the health of blood vessels and help regulate blood pressure in postmenopausal women. Some studies show that it may also support vagal tone, but the results are mixed.

Perimenopause and menopause stress is real and can affect your mental and physical health, but it doesn't have to control your life. By using many of the strategies in this chapter, you can start managing stress in a way that feels doable, one step at a time. Since sleep is one of the most powerful tools for managing stress, let's dive into *how* to support it.

7

What's Happening to Our Sleep?

How much sleep did you get last night?

Would I be right if I guessed *not much*?

For many of us, sleep is elusive.

Changes in our sleep habits are among the first symptoms that show up in the early stages of perimenopause and continue well into menopause.

When I asked women in our community if their sleep has changed and what it's like for them now, I got these responses:

"Menopause sleep = no sleep at all."

"It's brutal. I maybe get four hours of sleep at a time."

"I wake up with sweaty legs and damp pants. I thought I had an accident."

"Every night for five and a half years I've had the worst sleep ever."

And the comments go on and on and on . . .

Sleep deprivation is so common in this phase of life that it ranks third on our list of 103+ symptoms. Other research has shown that deficient or disrupted sleep severely interferes with women's daily activities.

Women tend to have more sleep issues than men throughout their lives, and these sleep issues affect us in different ways. For example, you might find it hard to fall asleep or stay asleep. Or you may wake up more often during the night, can't fall back asleep, wake up too early, or maybe you're in and out of sleep all night because of night sweats.

Let's start with the basics: What does sleep look like, what are the different stages, and why does our sleep get so disrupted at this stage of life?

What Sleep Looks Like

When you're sleeping, your body cycles through four distinct stages, and they repeat several times a night depending on how many hours you sleep. Like all natural body rhythms, the way your body moves through these stages is influenced by signals from the environment, such as light, darkness, and sound.

What are the different stages of sleep?

Stage 1, Light Sleep: This is the lightest stage. Your brain and muscles begin to relax, and your heartbeat slows. You're still breathing normally, and you're just starting to nod off. This stage typically lasts only a few minutes. Overall, you spend about 2–5 percent of your sleep in this stage, and you can easily be woken up.

Stage 2, Light/Intermediate Sleep: During this stage, you're moving into a deeper sleep. Your body continues to relax, and your breathing slows. You spend about half of your total sleep in this stage.

Stage 3, Deep Sleep or Slow-Wave Sleep: Also known as restorative sleep, this is one of the most important stages because it's when your body does most of the healing and recovery from the wear and tear of your day. Your heart rate and breathing are at their lowest, and your muscles are deeply relaxed. This is also the stage where your glymphatic system kicks in (more on that shortly). You get more deep sleep in the first half of the night, and the more you get, the more energy you have the next day. On average, healthy adults spend about 15–20 percent of their total time asleep in this stage, and it decreases with age.

REM Sleep: REM sleep is often referred to as active sleep or dream sleep. REM stands for rapid eye movement, and although it's not the only time you dream, it's when your dreams are the most vivid and detailed. REM sleep is interesting because the brain is almost as active as when you're awake, and if you looked at it on an electro-encephalogram (EEG), the activity would look very similar. REM sleep is important because it helps your brain sort and store what you learned during the day, a process called memory consolidation. It also helps you think more creatively, solve problems, and remember things better.

REM sleep is the most well-known stage of sleep, mainly because of its link to dreaming. The other three stages are non-REM sleep.

REM sleep accounts for about 20–25 percent of your total sleep, and non-REM accounts for 75–80 percent. Each cycle typically takes anywhere from an hour and a half to two hours to complete. When you get a proper night's sleep, your body should go through four or five of these sleep cycles. This is typical for someone who sleeps seven to nine hours a night.

Sleep and Circadian Rhythm

You're probably familiar with the term *circadian rhythm*. It's your body's natural internal twenty-four-hour clock. There are many circadian rhythms in the body, and one of the most well-known is the sleep-wake cycle. Others help regulate hunger, digestion, metabolism, fertility, mood, body temperature, immunity, blood pressure, blood sugar regulation, and more. At the center of these systems is the hypothalamus, which helps synchronize these rhythms in response to environmental signals like light and darkness.

Light and darkness have the biggest impact on your circadian rhythm, but it's also affected by your sleep habits (including shift work), what and when you eat, when you exercise, travel (especially to a different time zone), stress levels, inside and outside temperatures, mental health, genetics, neurological diseases like Alzheimer's and Parkinson's, major illnesses or surgery, and certain medications.

When your circadian rhythm is in sync with your other natural rhythms, it helps you get deep and restorative sleep. But if it's out of sync, you might have trouble falling asleep, wake up more often during the night, or wake up too early in the morning.

During perimenopause and menopause, changing hormones can disrupt the circadian rhythm of your sleep-wake cycle. Declining estrogen and progesterone can interfere with the production of melatonin, while hot flashes and night sweats can throw off your body temperature, and cortisol can rise at the wrong time. These changes can mess with your sleep, making you wake up more often during the night, so your sleep feels choppier, and you wake up exhausted.

When your sleep-wake cycle is out of sync, it can lead to lower-quality sleep, less total sleep, and a higher risk of health problems.

How Much Sleep Are You Getting?

The amount of sleep you need changes throughout your lifetime, and so do your sleep patterns. For example, you need more sleep when you're younger and a little less as an adult. As far as patterns go, you'll have less deep and REM sleep as you age compared to when you were a child.

Both the National Sleep Foundation and the U.S. Centers for Disease Control and Prevention (CDC) recommend that most adults get seven to nine hours of sleep a night, and that adults sixty-five and older get between seven and eight hours a night.

If you're getting between seven and eight hours of sleep a night, and you feel refreshed and alert the next day, you're in a healthy zone.

On average, women tend to sleep a little bit longer than men, about ten to fifteen minutes more per night. But even though we get more sleep and prioritize sleep more, we tend to have poorer quality sleep and more sleep problems. We also wake up more during the night because of stress from work, family responsibilities, pregnancy, perimenopause and menopause, and partners who snore. In addition, we're more likely to have anxiety, insomnia, and restless legs syndrome, all factors that can mess with our sleep. For many of us, sleep quality tends to drop right before our periods because of PMS symptoms, and the chance of developing sleep apnea, which is when our breathing stops and starts when we're sleeping, goes up once we're in menopause, most likely because of changes in hormone levels.

Gen Xers grew up in a culture that valued hard work, independence, and a "do it all" mentality, often neglecting sleep. According to a 2019 YouGov survey reported by Statista, Gen Xers have the lowest average sleep of all generations, with an estimated nightly average of six and a half hours.

Why We Need Sleep in Menopause

Sleep is very important for keeping your body and mind healthy, especially now that you're in perimenopause and menopause.

Here's why:

Research from 2024 in *Frontiers in Endocrinology* showed that sleeping too little or too much makes us more prone to depression.

Not getting enough sleep can also weaken our immune system. Poor or short sleep is linked to chronic low-grade inflammation, a higher chance of catching colds, and an increased risk for developing inflammatory and autoimmune conditions.

Research shows that women are at an increased risk for cardiovascular disease (CVD) once we're in menopause, and poor sleep in this phase of life is a contributing factor. Even if we feel healthy now, a lack of sleep is tied to hidden early stages of heart disease that raise the risk of serious problems later in life.

For many menopausal women, even one poor night's sleep can increase anxiety, trigger stress hormones like cortisol, and mess with our mood and appetite. As we learned in the last chapter, cortisol levels should be highest in the morning, but when we're sleep-deprived, our body can cause cortisol to rise at the wrong time (usually between 2 a.m. and 4 a.m.), waking us up and making it hard to fall back to sleep or stay asleep.

A lack of sleep also puts us at risk for metabolic issues like obesity, insulin resistance, and type 2 diabetes. And as we saw in Chapter 5, not getting enough sleep can also lead to weight gain.

Brain Waste Management

Our body has its own trash-removal system, a way to clean waste products from the brain and central nervous system. This system is known as the glymphatic system. It works similarly to the lymphatic system (which removes waste and toxins from your tissues).

Animal studies show that while they sleep, the spaces between brain cells expand by about 60 percent, making it easier to clear metabolic waste that accumulates during the day. This built-in cleaning process is most active during stage 3 deep sleep and slows down by about 90 percent when the brain is awake. Newer studies suggest that humans use a similar cleaning system when we sleep too!

Researchers believe that because the glymphatic system clears away neurotoxic waste products, or "brain trash," including proteins like beta-amyloid that are associated with Alzheimer's disease, and tau, which is linked to cognitive decline and dementia, it plays an important role in long-term brain health. Scientists are still learning how this brain-cleaning system works and how it can possibly open the door for new treatments or ways to prevent brain diseases in the future. A 2013 human study showed that getting enough good-quality sleep might help prevent Alzheimer's, especially in people who have a certain genetic risk (the apolipoprotein E gene). The researchers said that helping older people get enough sleep could possibly help prevent this disease.

Since sleep is a major issue for many of us now that we're in perimenopause and menopause, getting consistent restorative deep sleep can be more challenging. Because the glymphatic system is most active during deep sleep, getting less of it may mean this brain-cleaning process doesn't work as efficiently as it once did. As a result, a buildup of "brain trash" may be linked to brain fog, memory issues, and mental fatigue, all common symptoms of perimenopause and menopause. Making sleep a priority is one of the most important things we can do to protect our brain in the long run.

How Your Brain Clears Itself

Removing waste from the brain is critical, but how can you support this natural cleansing process? The most effective way is to consistently lead a healthy lifestyle that includes the following habits, in addition to getting enough good-quality sleep:

- **Sleep on your side rather than on your back or stomach.** When scientists watched how the brain clears waste in sleeping rats, they noticed it worked better when they slept on their sides compared to their backs or stomachs. Human research is still limited, but it suggests that the position you sleep in may influence how well your brain's glymphatic system gets rid of harmful waste. Some experts think that sleeping on your right side may help the glymphatic system work more efficiently, since the right internal jugular vein is often larger and drains more blood from the brain than the left. Sleeping on your side (either one) may also be better for you if you have sleep apnea, as it can help reduce snoring.

- **Reach for anti-inflammatory foods.** Diets rich in polyphenols (plant chemicals), omega-3s, fiber, and antioxidants have been shown to lower brain and systemic inflammation. The Mediterranean and MIND diets, more specifically, have been shown to promote better brain health and lower levels of cognitive decline. A 2024 study titled "Enriching the Mediterranean Diet Could Nourish the Brain More Effectively" found that adding more brain-friendly foods to your diet may help support better brain health. Like my book title suggests, this is powerful proof that the foods you eat during perimenopause and menopause can truly nourish your body and mind.

    Focus on eating fresh low-glycemic fruits and veggies, whole grains, beans and legumes, healthy fats (olive and avocado oil, nuts, seeds, and salmon), spices and herbs, fermented foods, and bone broth. Avoid or significantly reduce foods with added sugar, ultra-processed and fast foods, alcohol, caffeine, and conventionally raised meat and dairy (if you can find grass-fed or organic meat from your local farmer, and it's in your budget, that's a great option).

- **Exercise.** Exercise may help your body clean out waste from your brain, and it also lowers stress, which can help you sleep better. *Note:* See page 186 for more on how exercising right before bed may impact sleep.

- **Try intermittent fasting.** Intermittent fasting (IF) is when you switch between scheduled periods of not eating (fasting) and eating (commonly referred to as an eating window). Intermittent fasting can be approached in different ways. The most common or popular plan is 16/8: sixteen hours of fasting and eight hours during which you can eat. Other options include 12/12, 20/4, every-other-day fasting (also called alternate-day fasting), 5/2 (five days of regular eating and two days of restricting calories), and eating one meal a day (OMAD) for one or more days a week. Intermittent fasting can help keep your brain healthy and may protect against brain-related diseases.

  According to Mark Mattson, PhD, a neuroscientist and adjunct professor at Johns Hopkins University School of Medicine, IF reduces inflammation and oxidative stress in the brain. I interviewed him for my podcast (*Menopause Reimagined*, episode #97), and he explained how this way of eating boosts the production of a protein called brain-derived neurotrophic factor (BDNF), which is key for memory and learning. This protein also helps grow new nerve cells and protects old ones from aging. Plus, IF boosts the number of mitochondria in your brain, which are like tiny power plants inside your cells. I found IF worked great when I was in perimenopause, and I did 16/8 for years. However, now that I'm in menopause, I still like to fast, but for a shorter period of time. Always do what feels right for you.

- **Take omega-3 fatty acids.** Fish oil and other sources of omega-3 fatty acids, in particular docosahexaenoic acid (DHA) and eicosapentaenoic acid (EPA), can help the glymphatic system do an even better job at cleaning out waste from the brain.

Studies show that people with higher levels of omega-3 tend to have better brain function, improved memory and learning capabilities, and a lower risk of getting Alzheimer's. Omega-3 fatty acids have strong anti-inflammatory benefits and can help to reduce inflammation in the brain (also known as neuro-inflammation).

- **Limit alcohol.** High consumption of alcohol has been linked to brain inflammation and disrupts the function of the glymphatic system, so be mindful of how much alcohol you consume.

- **Reduce exposure to toxicants.** While you can't control every-thing around you, there are some steps you can take to minimize your exposure to harmful chemicals, like choosing nontoxic household, cosmetic, and personal care products whenever possible. Be mindful about using synthetic fertilizers and pest control in your yard, and use them only when necessary. Buy organic foods when your budget allows. Minimize exposure to smoke and air pollution. Drink filtered water. And consider switching from plastic food containers to glass or stainless steel.

- **Stay hydrated.** The more hydrated you are, the better your cir-culation is, and the more easily blood can flow to your brain.

- **Stay regular.** Going to the bathroom every day helps your body clear out waste, making it easier for your glymphatic system to do its job.

Why Your Sleep Becomes Challenging in Perimenopause and Menopause

Estrogen influences how well we sleep. It helps us fall asleep faster, wake up less during the night, and get more overall sleep. Since estrogen levels change throughout the menstrual cycle, women's sleep patterns can also shift depending on the time of the month. Estrogen helps to make neurotransmitters that promote sleep, like serotonin and melatonin. It also helps to regulate body tempera-ture, so when levels fall, our body temperature can fluctuate. This can trigger night sweats, which make your sleep lighter and more interrupted.

Progesterone helps with sleep as it boosts the effects of the neurotransmitter GABA in the brain. GABA helps to calm the central nervous system so we feel less anxious and stressed. When progesterone lowers, the quality of sleep is affected, making it harder to fall and stay asleep.

The Study of Women's Health Across the Nation (SWAN) showed that beginning in perimenopause, women start to see a decrease in the quality and length of sleep, and it continues into menopause. And our published Morphus research shows that 66 percent of women in perimenopause and menopause have problems with sleep, and it's more prevalent for women in menopause than perimenopause.

Estrogen and progesterone help to regulate our circadian rhythm, so when they drop, our body's natural patterns of telling us when it's time to go to sleep and wake up can get thrown off. This can lead to trouble falling asleep and staying asleep, which in turn affects the quality of our sleep.

Also, melatonin levels start to gradually decline around ages thirty-five to forty. This is one reason we get less deep sleep, and more fragmented sleep, the older we get.

Repeatedly waking up during the night can mess with the different stages of sleep. Even if you spend enough total hours in bed, all the tossing, turning, and waking up can mean that you're not getting enough deep and REM sleep, leaving you feeling exhausted the next day.

Our published Morphus sleep research showed that the main factors contributing to sleep disturbances during this time include:

- **Waking up between 2 a.m. and 4 a.m.**

- **Bathroom visits**

- **Night sweats**

- Anxiety / racing mind / adrenaline rushes / racing heart / stress / heart palpitations

- Insomnia

- Pain / cramps, muscle aches / muscle spasms / charley horse, restless legs

- Sleep apnea (diagnosed or suspected)

- Medications

I bolded the three main reasons because I want to discuss them in a little more detail.

Waking up between 2 a.m. and 4 a.m.: Cortisol naturally starts to rise around 2 a.m. to 3 a.m., so if you're already stressed and have higher-than-normal cortisol levels, this surge can wake you up and keep you awake for hours, often just until it's time for your alarm to go off. Research shows that the brain functions differently at night, especially after midnight. It tends to focus more on negative thoughts and emotions, like worrying about money, health, or relationships, making it harder to fall back asleep.

Can you relate? Do you find that everything feels like a bigger deal in the middle of the night, but once you wake up, it often doesn't seem nearly as overwhelming? I know I do. I share my trick for minimizing this rumination later in the chapter.

Frequent bathroom trips, also referred to as nocturia: Frequent urination was reported by 36 percent of our respondents. It can be caused by a number of different reasons:

1. Drinking liquids too close to bedtime can cause your bladder to fill during the night.

2. As I discussed in Chapter 3, GSM, or genitourinary syndrome of menopause, can play a major role. As your estrogen levels decrease, the tissues of the bladder, urethra, and vaginal walls can become thinner, drier, and less elastic. This makes the urinary tract more sensitive and less able to hold urine for long stretches of time. The bladder may feel fuller faster (even when

it isn't), and urinary tract infections (UTIs) become more common, increasing both how often and how urgent you need to pee.

3. If you have a weaker bladder, as a result of pregnancy, aging, lower estrogen, or a health condition, it may have less capacity to hold urine for longer periods of time.

4. Taking diuretics before bed (including certain dietary supplements) increases urine production. Other medications can also affect the way your bladder functions or the amount of urine you produce.

5. Vasopressin, an antidiuretic hormone, decreases as you age. Reduced levels of this hormone mean the body doesn't retain fluid as well, leading to more trips to the bathroom.

6. Fluctuating blood sugar levels and diabetes can lead to increased urine production and frequent nighttime bathroom trips.

7. Sleep disorders such as insomnia, sleep apnea, or restless legs syndrome can interrupt your sleep cycle, and these interruptions often happen to coincide with the need to pee.

Night sweats: Our Morphus Signs and Symptoms research shows that 56 percent of women going through menopause and almost 53 percent of women in perimenopause have them. A woman from our sleep survey told us that her "night sweats are unbearable. They can be off/on all night long." Another said, "The hot flashes at night are my worst sleep disruption right now. I consider myself lucky to get three to four hours in a row a night."

Grace Pien, MD, MSCE, an assistant professor of medicine at the Johns Hopkins Sleep Disorders Center and a key researcher in the Penn Ovarian Aging Study analysis "Predictors of Sleep Quality in Women in the Menopausal Transition," led research suggesting that women going through perimenopause who have symptoms like depression or hot flashes are much more likely to have trouble sleeping. According to Dr. Pien, it's not the sweating itself that wakes women up. Instead, it's changes in the brain that make women wake up before they have night sweats.

Sleep Apnea

Sleep apnea is a condition where you stop breathing on and off during the night. The most common type, called obstructive sleep apnea (OSA), happens when the muscles in your upper throat relax too much, blocking or closing your airway. This blockage lowers oxygen in your blood and causes loud snoring as the air tries to get through the narrowed space. As a result, you may wake up gasping for air and feel super tired and unfocused the next day.

Sleep apnea can range from mild to severe. While it's more common in men, a woman's risk increases as she goes into menopause. As estrogen and progesterone levels lower, your airway is more likely to close up while you're sleeping, and your body may not control your breathing as well, which increases the risk of sleep apnea. Weight gain, especially visceral fat around the belly and the neck, also increases the risk.

If you snore, it doesn't always mean you have sleep apnea. However, many people with sleep apnea snore loudly and frequently, sometimes with pauses in breathing or gasps during the night.

Sleep apnea can be missed in women because the symptoms overlap with common menopause symptoms like fatigue, brain fog, or sleep problems.

It's important to be checked for sleep apnea once you're in menopause, as it's linked to metabolic dysfunction-associated steatotic liver disease (MASLD), or fatty liver. OSA can worsen MASLD. See Chapter 4 for a refresher on fatty liver.

If OSA isn't treated, it can lead to type 2 diabetes, heart disease, and high blood pressure. Women may not realize they have it because their symptoms can look different from men's. If you snore, wake up exhausted, have insomnia, feel depressed, have hypothyroidism, or suspect you might have it, speak to your doctor about doing a sleep study. While getting tested at a sleep clinic is often recommended, there are also home tests available, which are less expensive and more convenient. You can also check your oxygen levels using a pulse oximeter finger monitor or a blood oxygen saturation monitor. Many wearable devices, like smartwatches and fitness trackers, also have that capability. While these may provide you with some preliminary data, always speak to your doctor about getting properly tested to confirm a diagnosis.

Catching sleep apnea early and treating it (e.g., with a CPAP machine, which stands for "continuous positive airway pressure") protects your heart, brain, and liver. Plus, you'll feel much better and have more energy.

Strategies for Improving Sleep

Solving your sleep issues is like doing a puzzle: You have to figure out how all the pieces fit together. But where do you start? For simplicity, follow the *R.E.S.T.* Protocol, which I developed along with my team at Morphus:

Routine: Your sleep routine

Environment: Sleep hygiene

Support: Sleep support and aids

Technology: Helpful sleep tools and technology

Let's look at each one.

R: Routine

Do you end your day by watching a movie or show? Scrolling on your phone? Reading a book? Meditating or journaling? Taking a bath? Or maybe you prefer listening to a podcast. While having an evening wind-down routine sounds like a great idea, the reality is many of us are busy with work or work-related events, sports, driving kids around to their activities, taking a night school class, or meeting up with friends. And when the weekend rolls around, we tend to stay up later and sleep in the next day.

What does your current sleep routine look like?

A sleep routine refers to the activities, habits, or rituals you do every night before bed. Depending on what your routine is, some of your nightly activities may be telling your body it's time to rest, while others may be encouraging you to stay awake a little bit longer.

Your body likes to be on a schedule. It thrives on routine. Here are some tips for helping you get a good night's sleep:

- **Be consistent:** Going to bed and waking up at the same time every day, even on the weekends (I know, sorry!), tells your body what to expect, so you're more likely to have a good night's sleep.

- **Try calming wind-down activities:** Listen to calming music, take a bath, look at pictures of nature or from a happy occasion, meditate, or read a book. If you find that reading on your phone or tablet keeps you up, read a physical book.

- **Develop presleep rituals:** Every ritual, like putting on your PJs, brushing your teeth, taking a warm bath, or light stretching, tells your brain and body that sleep time is approaching. Do these rituals in the same order each night to reinforce this message.

- **Practice gratitude and end your day with positive thoughts:** Research shows that people who are grateful and practice gratitude have better-quality sleep, longer sleep, and fall asleep faster than those who don't. Gratitude also helps you shift into a positive mindset before bed, which sets the tone for peaceful sleep.

  Dr. Wayne Dyer said your last thought before you fall asleep can stay in your subconscious mind for up to four hours. If it's negative, that's four hours of negativity. If it's positive, that's four hours of positive programming. Combining gratitude with positive thoughts before bed creates a powerful bedtime routine that supports both your mental and physical health.

- **Journal:** One way to help you end your day on a positive note is to journal. Release any negative or ruminating thoughts or concerns onto a piece of paper or your device and let them go so they no longer keep you awake at night.

- **Say mantras:** Another option is to say mantras, affirmations, or prayers before you fall asleep. Here's one you can try from Frederick Dodson, success coach and author of more than fifty books, including *Parallel Universes of Self.* Whisper it out loud and repeat it anywhere from one to three times (no more) before falling asleep. Address your higher power (Universe, higher self, inner strength, inner wisdom, intuition, Source, Nature, God, or whatever feels right for you) and say:

    "[Higher Power], thank you for showing me that this issue is already solved."

    You can also add to it by inserting whatever it is you want to create. For example, *"[Higher Power], thank you for showing me that [insert your own thing] is already solved."*

- **Go to bed earlier:** For many people, going to bed between 10 and 11 p.m. works well with their circadian rhythms. If you go to bed too late, you may cut into the window when your body gets most of its deep, restorative sleep, which can leave you feeling groggy the next day. As a bonus, research shows that people tend to be more productive and more alert when they go to bed earlier rather than later, even when they get the same amount of sleep. I find I'm in a better mood the next day when I go to bed before 11 p.m.

Morning Routine

Your morning routine influences how well you sleep at night. Here are some tips to keep in mind:

- **Get some sun.** Good sleep habits don't just happen before you go to bed; rather, they start first thing in the morning and continue throughout the day. Morning sunlight is really important for sleep, as it helps to reset your circadian rhythm by telling your brain when it's time to wake up and when it's time to go to sleep. When you're exposed to natural light in the morning, it helps to give you more energy and makes you more alert by keeping melatonin production low. Melatonin naturally increases as the sun sets, helping your body prepare for sleep. When you can, go outside for at least twenty to thirty minutes in the morning to help reset your internal clock, and aim to do so within an hour or two of waking up.

- **Ease into your morning gently.** A calm start helps your body handle stress. Since we're more sensitive to stress in perimenopause and menopause, easing into the day can support your mood and help you manage and recover from stress more easily. Instead of setting a loud alarm, wake up to soft music that starts about ten to fifteen minutes before you need to get up.

- **Make mornings easier.** Prepare your clothes, lunch, snacks, and whatever else you need for the day the night before. This will make your morning routine smoother, which helps to minimize stress and ease your mind.

E: Environment—Sleep Hygiene

Our environment, or sleep hygiene, involves creating a calming space that supports healthy sleep habits. According to the Sleep Foundation, practicing good sleep hygiene can support longer and better-quality sleep.

Here are some ways to introduce sleep hygiene:

- **Sleep in a dark room.** Research published in the *Proceedings of the National Academy of Sciences* shows that sleeping in a room that's moderately lit (100 lux) versus a dimly lit room (less than 3 lux) *for just one night* can have a negative impact on your heart and insulin levels. To put that into context, direct sunlight on a typical day emits between 100,000 and 330,000 lux, an overcast day provides about 1,000 lux, and sunrise or sunset is around 400 lux. Moderate lighting can increase your insulin levels, raise your heart rate, and decrease heart rate variability (HRV), a measure of how well you handle stress. As I explained in Chapter 5, since insulin is a hormone that promotes fat storage, sleeping with the light on might contribute to weight gain.

  To improve your sleep, eliminate all light sources in your sleeping area. This includes ambient light from outside your windows (including streetlamps, Christmas lights, etc.), alarm clocks, cell phones, televisions, and other electronic devices. How?

» Use blackout blinds or curtains.

» Wear a sleep mask.

» Don't fall asleep in front of the TV.

» Turn off your bedside lamp or night-light before going to sleep.

» Cover any lights that you can't turn off, such as a clock or electrical outlet.

» If you wake up during the night to pee, don't turn on the lights. If you need light to see, use a dim light or a motion sensor.

» Even very low exposure from a night-light (around 5 to 10 lux) can disrupt your sleep by increasing lighter stages of sleep and reducing deep sleep. If you need to use one, choose one that emits red or warm amber light instead of bright white or blue, since these colors are less disruptive to the circadian rhythms.

• **Control the temperature.** Your body temperature naturally cools down when you sleep and starts to rise again before you wake up. The ideal temperature of your room should be between 65–68 degrees Fahrenheit (18–22 degrees Celsius). If your room is too hot, it's hard for your body to cool itself down, which can trigger night sweats or make them worse. If your room is too cold, you might have trouble falling asleep, or you may be woken up during the night.

So what can you do?

» Change your covers according to the seasons (heavier blankets in the winter, lighter ones in the spring and summer).

» Use cooling sheets and blankets.

» Wear light, breathable PJs (or nothing at all).

» Keep a fan close to your side of the bed or install a ceiling fan (if possible, avoid blowing air directly on you).

» Place cooling packs on the back of your neck, chest, inner thighs, or on the bottoms of your feet.

» If your room is too cold, use extra blankets and sleep with socks on.

- **Make sure your room is quiet.** If that isn't possible, wear earplugs (if you're able to). If you're a light sleeper, earplugs are great at blocking out any noise that may wake you up, such as snoring, horns, traffic, pet collars, kids, airplanes, et cetera.

- **Limit technology before bed.** Putting away your phone and other devices like tablets and laptops and turning off your TV at least half an hour to an hour before bed can help you sleep better. Screens, including TV screens, as well as LED lights and energy-efficient fluorescent light bulbs, can emit blue light, which suppresses and delays the production of melatonin, making it harder to fall asleep. Because it's similar to daylight, blue light tricks your body into thinking it's still daytime.

  Avoid exposure to blue light about thirty to sixty minutes before bed, but if you absolutely must use a device close to bedtime:

  » Try wearing blue light–blocking glasses. While the research is inconsistent, these glasses may help some people fall asleep faster and improve the quality of their sleep, especially when combined with other good sleep habits.

  » Put filters on your screens. Use Night Shift if you have Apple products, and Night Light or a blue light filter if you have Android products. Or download f.lux (justgetflux.com), free software that changes the color tone of your screen to adapt to the time of day you're using it.

  » Set a timer for the TV to turn itself off at a specific time if you tend to fall asleep in front of the television, or turn it off as soon as you feel yourself nodding off.

» Don't check your email or scroll on social media. Getting an upsetting email from a colleague, friend, or family member or a request from your boss right before bed will likely leave you tossing and turning while you figure out how to address it. You might even wake up in the middle of the night from the stress it caused you, ruining a good night's sleep (and probably ruining how you feel the next day too). And scrolling on social media before bed can be mentally stimulating, which in turn can make it harder to fall asleep. Social media platforms are designed to make us lose track of time, so what might start as a quick peek can easily turn into hours of scrolling, pushing your bedtime later and later.

- **Unplug.** Turning off your phone when you go to sleep is important, as notifications, vibrations, and even knowing your phone is next to you can disrupt deep sleep.

  Also, some research shows that even weak electromagnetic fields (EMFs) can interfere with sleep quality, and may decrease the production of melatonin. Consider turning off your router, unplugging your devices, or putting them on airplane mode before going to sleep. Another option is to keep your electronics away from your bed and pillow. If you need to keep your phone on for safety reasons, keep it three feet away from your head, or put it in another room where you can still hear it ring or ding.

- **Use essential oils.** Lavender oil can induce a sense of calm and improve the quality of your sleep. A small 2021 double-blind, randomized trial involving thirty-five menopausal women with insomnia found that inhaling lavender helped them fall asleep faster, improved their quality of sleep, and reduced menopausal symptoms like anxiety, depression, and hot flashes.

  Place a few drops on a cotton ball and inhale or diffuse it, or put some on a sachet and place it next to your pillow or on your pillowcase. You can also put a few drops on your wrists, then rub them together and inhale. Always test a small area first before applying essential oils directly on your skin to make sure they don't irritate you. Dilute essential oils with a carrier oil like almond or jojoba.

- **Try cognitive behavioral therapy for insomnia (CBT I).** Research shows that CBT I can be an effective treatment for sleep disorders, including insomnia. It helps you recognize and change worried or negative thoughts and beliefs that contribute to your lack of sleep. It also teaches you new sleep habits and helps you avoid behaviors that keep you up at night. Many people see an improvement after two to six sessions. CBT I has also been shown to help reduce stress, anxiety, hot flashes, and night sweats in menopausal women with insomnia. Look for a licensed therapist, menopause specialist, or a structured online program that specializes in CBT I for sleep and other menopause symptoms. One way I use CBT in my own life is to manage middle of the night rumination. If I wake up and feel ruminating thoughts coming on, I remind myself that this isn't the time to solve problems, and I'll deal with whatever comes up in the morning. It can take some practice, but it works!

- **Check your mattress and pillows.** Are you happy with your mattress and pillows? If you are, you're four times more likely to say you sleep well compared to those who aren't (48% vs. 11%), according to a 2022 report. This makes sense because worn-down mattresses and pillows may not provide you with the support your back and neck need, so you won't have as good of a sleep.

  » Depending on the type of mattress you have, consider changing it every seven to ten years. Latex and foam can last ten to fifteen years, and organic mattresses may last up to twenty years.

  » Rotate your mattress clockwise according to what the manufacturer recommends so you don't sleep on one section for too long, possibly wearing it down depending on the type of mattress you have.

» Invest in a good pillow: Years ago, I was getting terrible back and neck pain. My sister-in-law told me about a water pillow that she loves, so I tried it, and I've never looked back. The Sleep Foundation recommends changing your pillows every year or two.

» Pay attention to the smells and chemicals that come from beds, mattress covers, and pillows. They can affect sleep, memory, lungs, allergies, and hormones. Most mattresses and mattress covers are made from polyurethane foam, a petroleum-based material that releases volatile organic compounds (VOCs) that can affect indoor air quality over time.

When buying a mattress, look for brands that sell organic, natural latex, cotton, or wool materials. Also, choose brands that have third-party certifications that limit certain chemicals and VOC emissions, and whenever possible, avoid blended or synthetic latex, which typically off-gases more than natural latex.

Note: This applies to air mattresses as well. You may notice a strong chemical smell when you open the box. Allow the mattress to air out in a well-ventilated space (preferably outside or in your garage, basement, or storage unit) until the odor is gone before using it.

Tip: Look for a mattress cover made from organic cotton or wool. Placing it over your mattress can help reduce direct contact with treated materials and may limit your exposure to fumes.

S: Support—Sleep Aids

While sleep hygiene and environment can help with a lot of things, sometimes we need a little extra support.

Nutrition: As a nutritionist, I always try to emphasize the importance of a whole foods diet that is rich in nutrients. And here's why it's especially important when it comes to promoting sleep: A 2021 study in the *Western Journal of Nursing Research* found that what women eat may influence how much sleep they get across different stages of menopause. For example, women in perimenopause who ate more protein, healthy carbs, and certain vitamins and minerals (B1, folate, choline, phosphorus, sodium, potassium, and selenium) were more likely to get at least five hours of sleep a night. And women in menopause who cut down on sugar and had proper levels of phosphorus and zinc were more likely to sleep longer.

Dietary supplements: Supplements can be a game changer when it comes to falling asleep, staying asleep, getting more deep sleep, and waking up rested. However, *what*, *when*, and *how much* you take can make a difference.

Here are some of my favorite well-researched, science-backed supplement ingredients that support better sleep:

- **Magnesium bisglycinate or glycinate:** This chelated form of magnesium is one of my main go-tos when it comes to supporting sleep. When magnesium is combined with glycine, an amino acid that promotes relaxation, it can help you fall asleep and improve the quality of your sleep. Magnesium bisglycinate is easily absorbed, which makes it great for boosting your magnesium levels. This form is well tolerated and gentle on your stomach. Aim for 320–350 mg, about thirty to forty minutes before your head hits the pillow.

   Note: If you feel nauseous after taking magnesium, try taking it with food. Speak to your doctor if you have kidney issues or you're on medications such as bisphosphonates or antibiotics since magnesium can interfere with how they work.

- **Melatonin:** Your body naturally produces melatonin as a signal that it's time to go to sleep. As you age, you tend to make less of it. During perimenopause, lower or disrupted melatonin levels are often linked to sleep issues. Once you go into menopause, your nighttime melatonin levels are lower, and you may not produce it as steadily or for as long as you used to. These changes, as well as shifts in other hormones, can lead to sleep issues.

   A 2021 review of twenty-four studies published in the *Journal of Pineal Research* found that in perimenopausal and (post)meno-pausal women, supplementing with melatonin may improve overall sleep quality, and often helps women with existing sleep problems get into a deeper sleep. Adults aged fifty-five and older who took prolonged- or sustained-release melatonin also saw improvements in sleep quality and alertness the next morning without any withdrawal effects once they stopped taking it.

In addition to sleep, melatonin may help support bone density in perimenopausal and menopausal women. Early research in small clinical trials also suggests melatonin could play a role in brain, heart, liver, and metabolic health (including diabetes) and may offer support for vasomotor symptoms (like hot flashes and night sweats), but these areas need more research. Melatonin is also being studied for conditions like Alzheimer's, Parkinson's, IBS, and obesity, but the research is still in the early stages.

Melatonin also acts as a natural antioxidant that helps protect cells and may help support a healthy immune system.

Melatonin has only a few minor side effects. Most side effects, like morning grogginess and fatigue, can likely be prevented, or easily managed, by taking a dose that's right for you and timing it to coincide with your body's natural sleep cycle. Despite the rumors, there's no evidence that taking melatonin as a supplement is addictive or causes your body to stop making it.

I recommend starting with a dose of 1.5–3 mg, thirty to forty minutes before bed. If you need more, you can work your way up slowly, as some women need higher (or lower) doses than others. We're all different, so listen to your body. If you're new to taking melatonin and feel groggy when you wake up, either lower the dose or stay at that dose until your body acclimates. It can take a couple of weeks for the grogginess to dissipate.

Note: Before trying melatonin, speak to your doctor if you're taking medication(s) in case there are any contraindications. Certain medications can lower or suppress melatonin levels in your body. According to Dr. Carrie Jones, ND, FABNE, MPH, a functional medicine health and hormone doctor, these include hydrocortisone; prednisone; NSAIDs like ibuprofen, naproxen, and diclofenac; beta blockers; and in some cases anti-depressants like fluoxetine (Prozac). She recommends speaking to your doctor if you're taking any of these prescriptions.

Tip: Don't take melatonin with alcohol, since drinking can make it less effective and throw off your sleep.

- **Vitamin D:** Low levels of vitamin D are associated with several sleep problems, including not sleeping enough and having trouble falling asleep. Vitamin D may influence melatonin and serotonin, both important for maintaining a healthy sleep cycle. A 2023 study found that bringing vitamin D levels back into a normal range is linked to higher nighttime melatonin and better sleep. Vitamin D also helps to reduce inflammation, support mood, and reduce pain, all of which can impact the quality of your sleep. Getting some vitamin D by exposing yourself to natural light first thing in the morning can help regulate your circadian rhythm. You can also take a vitamin D supplement.

  Note: Some people find that taking vitamin D before bed negatively affects their sleep. If that's the case for you, take it earlier in the day.

- **L-theanine:** This naturally occurring amino acid, found in green tea, helps you relax by stimulating alpha waves in the brain. Research shows that L-theanine calms the nervous system, helping you get a better-quality sleep. It may also help to reduce PMS symptoms. Dosage is anywhere from 50 to 200 mg a day, thirty to forty minutes before bed. Its effects are typically felt for up to six hours. Look for the trademark Suntheanine® on the label, as it's well researched and has fifty clinical studies and virtually no side effects.

- **Lactium® casein hydrolysate:** With nine clinical studies conducted on more than five hundred people, this ingredient helps your body manage stress by increasing gamma-aminobutyric acid, or GABA, a key brain chemical that helps to lower stress and regulate the nervous system so you feel calm and relaxed. As a result, you get both the optimal amount of sleep you need and better-quality sleep. Lactium® is nonaddictive, even at high dosages, and has no reported side effects in experimental or human clinical studies.

Note: Lactium® is derived from dairy. However, the final product doesn't contain any casein or lactose. Always consult your healthcare professional if you have a dairy allergy or sensitivity.

- **Valerian root (*Valeriana officinalis*):** This ancient herb has been used for centuries. Many studies have shown valerian root is effective for promoting sleep and reducing anxiety.

- **Lemon balm:** Also known as *Melissa officinalis*, this herb from the mint family has calming properties. In a double-blind, placebo-controlled study, lemon balm reduced depression, anxiety, and stress, and improved sleep quality in those taking the herb for eight weeks when compared to a placebo. It has also been shown to help reduce pain. You can take it as a supplement or drink it as tea.

   Note: Lemon balm can interact with thyroid medications, so speak to your doctor before taking it if you have thyroid issues.

- **Chamomile (*Matricaria chamomilla*):** This popular herb has been shown to improve sleep quality in a number of studies. Although many people enjoy it as a tea before bedtime, chamomile is also available as an extract and in capsules.

- **Passionflower:** Research suggests this herb, also known as *Passiflora incarnata*, can ease anxiety and might also help with menopausal symptoms like hot flashes, mood swings, and sleep issues. It's available as a supplement or tea.

- **5-HTP:** Tryptophan is the amino acid in turkey known for making you sleepy after a Thanksgiving meal, but it's found in many other foods as well. It converts into 5-HTP, which then transforms into serotonin, a neurotransmitter that supports sleep, behavior, and mood. Serotonin is converted into melatonin, and supplementing with 5-HTP may help to boost melatonin levels. A 2021 single-blind, twelve-week randomized control trial with twenty adults in their sixties found that 5-HTP helped them fall asleep faster, though the effect only lasted about eight weeks. 5-HTP supplements come from a plant called *Griffonia simplicifolia* and are sold alone or combined with melatonin, GABA, or other sleep-supporting ingredients.

Note: Speak to your doctor before taking supplements with 5-HTP if you're on medications, including antidepressants, or if you're pregnant or breastfeeding.

- **Iron:** If you're experiencing tingling, crawling, pulling, or uncomfortable sensations in your legs, this may be due to a condition called restless legs syndrome, or RLS. You usually feel it in the evening or at night, or while you're relaxing, and it tends to get worse when you're lying down. This condition is more common in women than men and tends to increase with age. If restless legs are keeping you up, ask your doctor to check your iron. Low ferritin is common in RLS, and supplements can help if you're deficient. You can also try supplementing with magnesium. In addition to supplements, try moving, stretching, and massaging your limbs to help alleviate your symptoms.

  Note: Ask your doctor to check your iron levels before taking an iron supplement. This is especially important if you're in menopause.

Note: Always take sleep supplements according to the directions on the label and discuss possible interactions with your doctor or healthcare provider.

Move more. Regular exercise helps improve sleep, and getting a good night's sleep provides energy and motivation for exercise. Research shows that exercise increases deep sleep and improves sleep quality. Thirty minutes, five days a week may be enough to see immediate results.

Stress and sleep are tightly linked, so when you don't get enough sleep, you're tired and more vulnerable to stress. Regular exercise is a great way to break this cycle, as it relieves stress and improves sleep. It also gives your mind a break from stressful thoughts. Plus, research shows that exercise not only lowers stress but also helps you build resilience to handle it better.

Exercise can also help improve symptoms of sleep apnea, and a randomized controlled trial found that practicing tai chi improved sleep by about as much as a commonly used prescription medication in older adults with insomnia.

When you exercise can make a difference too. The National Heart, Lung, and Blood Institute says daytime exercise positively impacts sleep at night, especially if you exercise outdoors in natural light. Keep in mind that exercising later in the day can be too stimulating for some people, as it raises heart rate, body temperature, endorphins, and adrenaline, all of which can make it harder to fall asleep. At the end of the day (yeah, I know), it really depends on you and how your body responds. If exercise is too stimulating for you at night, do it earlier in the day, or try light exercise like yoga, walking, or stretching before bed. Do what's best for you, and exercise whenever you can fit it into your schedule.

Manage stress. Since stress is the number one reason we're waking up during the night now that we're in perimenopause and menopause, what can you do when you're staring at the ceiling at 3 a.m., knowing that the next day will be disastrous if you don't get some sleep? In addition to the stress-relieving tips I shared in Chapter 6, like deep-breathing exercises and taking a warm bath before bed (the combination of the drop in body temperature after getting out of the warm water and the cooler air lets your body know it's time for sleep), try these relaxing tips:

- **Write it down.** If you have a "brilliant idea" in the middle of the night and you don't want to forget it in the morning, write it down. Keep a notebook and pen next to your bed to record your genius thoughts.

- **Listen to calming music or sounds.** Try a white noise machine, soft music, guided meditation, poetry, an audiobook, or a soothing podcast. Another option is to listen to a sound bath on your phone or online. Sound baths work on three levels—sound, vibration, and frequency—to quickly relax your body and mind. Search "sound baths" on YouTube for different options.

> As we go into perimenopause and menopause, a drop in progesterone is linked to more disrupted sleep. Research suggests that oral micronized progesterone at bedtime can help with falling asleep and staying asleep. Progesterone has a calming and soothing effect on the body and mind. It works with GABA, a brain chemical, which helps you feel calmer, sleep better, and feel less anxious. Research shows that in menopausal women, micronized progesterone may help reduce hot flashes and night sweats. Speak to your doctor or healthcare provider for more information.

T: Technology—Helpful Sleep Tools

We live in a world of technology where we can track, measure, and even improve many parts of our lives, including sleep. Examples of sleep technology and tools include wearables that track your heart rate and sleep cycles, apps that help you relax, and smart lights that adapt to your biological clocks. Here are some tools that can help improve your sleep now that you're in perimenopause and menopause:

Cool your bed. You can look into a cooling system that goes on or near your bed. There are different choices available. I own a BedJet and really like it. I put it at the end of my bed, and it blows air under my blanket, which helps to keep me cool while I sleep. There is also the option of temperature-controlled mattresses, which allow you to adjust the temperature. If you sleep with a partner, many smart mattresses allow you to set the temperature according to each of your preferences.

Wear a continuous glucose monitor (CGM). If you think that blood sugar fluctuations might be the reason you're waking up during the night, speak to your doctor about trying a CGM. Wearing one for a short period of time can help you understand what your blood sugar levels are and whether they're a culprit in your sleepless nights. Since both high and low blood sugar can disturb your sleep, maintaining balanced blood sugar levels is important when it comes to sleeping through the night.

Check your sleep DNA. Platforms like the DNA Company, 3X4 Genetics, LoveMyHealth, as well as SelfDecode and GeneRX (which can import your existing 23andMe health data if you have it), offer genomic testing that can reveal what kind of sleep and bedroom environment you need based on your genetics and provide health tips that match your unique genetic makeup. Check out the Resources section at www.nourishingmenopausebook.com for more information.

Try meditation and breathing apps. There are some great meditation and calming apps available for your smartphone. Search "meditation apps," "sound bath," or "deep breathing" in the app store or on YouTube.

Wear a sleep tracker. These devices are typically worn on the wrist, finger, ankle, shirt collar, or forehead, although some are designed to be placed on your night table and pointed at your chest so they can monitor you during the night.

I use a ring to track my sleep. It gives me my overall sleep score and tells me how much total sleep I get, and it breaks it down by sleep cycles (light, deep, and REM). It also shows me how long it takes me to fall asleep, what my resting heart rate is, how often I wake up during the night, excessive movements (meaning did I toss and turn all night or did I get a restful sleep?), how much time I spent sleeping versus lying awake in bed, average HRV, what time I fell asleep and woke up, blood oxygen levels, body temperature, exercise including number of steps, breathing regularity, and daily stress levels.

Some rings measure data that can help you spot the signs of perimenopause. They track patterns such as changes in body temperature, poor sleep, changes in HRV, and irregular cycles. Over time, this information can highlight trends, which become even more useful when you add your own notes and observations.

Add weights. Weighted blankets can help improve the quality of your sleep by lowering stress levels. They're like a hug for your nervous system, helping to calm and relax you. A 2020 Swedish study found that adults with insomnia, along with anxiety, depression, ADHD, or bipolar disorder, slept better using a weighted blanket than a lighter one.

Still Can't Sleep?

Try the following:

Take a nap: Short daytime naps can recharge your energy and may even be linked to better brain health. A large study found that people with a natural tendency to nap may have brains that look up to six years younger than those who don't. Aim for a twenty-to-thirty-minute power nap, and avoid napping after 3 p.m. if you have trouble falling asleep at night.

Check your blood pressure: If you have unexplained high blood pressure, a lack of sleep could be one reason for it. Speak to your doctor or healthcare provider about treatment options, including a sleep apnea test.

Keep your tootsies warm: Warming up your feet before bed, like by wearing socks, using a hot water bottle, or putting them into a warm bath or shower, tells your brain it's time to sleep. A small 2018 study found that people who wore socks to bed fell asleep faster, slept longer, and woke up less during the night than those who didn't. The sample size was small, but other research supports this idea as well.

Breathe through your nose: Are you a nose or mouth breather? Breathing through your nose while you're sleeping (rather than through your mouth) can improve sleep quality. Nose breathing increases nitric oxide (NO), which helps open up your airways and improve oxygen flow so you feel calmer and more relaxed, which may help you sleep more soundly. NO may also support cognition and mental focus. One way to encourage nose breathing while you sleep is to try mouth taping. However, keep in mind that taping your mouth shut at night isn't for everyone; this is especially true if you have allergies, sleep apnea, sinus issues, a deviated septum, or trouble breathing through your nose. Not being able to talk or open your mouth can also be triggering for some people. If you aren't sure if it's right for you, speak to your doctor or healthcare provider about this option before trying it.

Limit caffeine: Caffeine is stimulating, so you may have a harder time falling asleep after consuming food and beverages that contain it (such as caffeinated coffee and tea, energy drinks, and chocolate). Caffeine can disrupt your sleep by blocking a chemical in your brain called adenosine. Adenosine makes you feel drowsy and tells your body it's time to go to sleep, so when it's blocked, your body doesn't get the signal that it's time to wind down. Caffeine can also push back the release of melatonin, which can affect how long it takes you to fall asleep and stay asleep. Research shows that even a moderate amount of caffeine consumed within six hours of going to bed has a significant impact on sleep. It's also a diuretic, so it can cause you to wake up to pee during the night.

My coauthor of *Unjunk Your Junk Food* (and coffee lover), Lisa Tsakos, has trouble falling asleep and gets relentless night sweats if she has a second cup of coffee in the morning, which was her norm before menopause. Sticking to one cup a day has made all the difference for her. Even though it's so far away from bedtime, the additional caffeine negatively affects her body.

Also, chocolate can be stimulating because it contains theobromine, a caffeine-like compound that gives it its bitter taste. Personally, if I eat chocolate too close to bed, it triggers major night sweats for me.

Avoid alcohol at least three hours before bed: If you like to unwind with a glass of wine in the evening, keep in mind that although alcohol might help you doze off quicker, it could disrupt your sleep later in the night. Once your body processes the alcohol, you're likely to wake up, and you may find it hard to fall back asleep. Drinking alcohol before bed affects deep sleep, so you get less of it, as well as REM sleep, so you may have more intense or vivid dreams.

Alcohol can raise cortisol levels once your body starts metabolizing it, which can cause you to wake up during the night. And it can raise blood sugar levels, leading to overnight bathroom trips as your body tries to regulate the spike.

It can also trigger or worsen hot flashes and night sweats. I can't even have a sip of wine anymore without it triggering an immediate flash.

Alcohol is metabolized by the liver, and as we age and go into perimenopause and menopause, our bodies become more sensitive to it, so we tend to feel its effects even more intensely.

Drink less before bed: Alcohol aside, drinking too much of any fluid within a few hours of bedtime may wake you up to use the bathroom one or more times during the night. A cup of chamomile tea just before bed can be very relaxing, but if you find it results in too many overnight bathroom visits, try drinking it earlier in the day.

Quit smoking: Smoking is stimulating, so it can lead to lighter and less restorative sleep.

Don't eat too close to bed: Finish your last meal at least three to four hours before your head hits the pillow. This gives your body enough time to digest your food rather than doing it overnight, when it should be resting and repairing. Also, for some people, lying down too soon after eating can cause gastroesophageal reflux disease (GERD), indigestion, or gas, so you may find it hard to fall asleep if you're feeling full or bloated.

Another reason you may want to avoid eating a heavy meal before bed is that some people get nightmares when they go to sleep on a full stomach. Certain foods, like spicy and junk foods, increase your chances of having them, possibly because they can upset your stomach, raise your body temperature, and make your brain more active when eaten too close to bedtime.

Going to bed hungry can have the opposite effect. It can disrupt your sleep by raising cortisol levels, especially if your blood sugar level drops too low in the middle of the night. If this happens, you might wake up even hungrier and have trouble going back to sleep. Some people find that having a light protein or low-glycemic snack about thirty to sixty minutes before bed can help. Try these snack suggestions: a tablespoon of nut butter or nuts (cashews, almonds, walnuts, and pistachios), half a cup of plain Greek yogurt sprinkled with cinnamon, a celery stick with cream cheese, turkey breast (turkey is known for inducing sleep), a small apple, or a cube of cheese.

Try Emotional Freedom Technique: EFT, also known as tapping, helps to calm the nervous system by gently tapping on specific acupressure points, which can make it easier to fall asleep. For more information and guided EFT sessions, check out Nick Ortner's website, www.thetappingsolution.com.

WAKING UP IN THE MIDDLE OF THE NIGHT

Many of us feel anxious or worried when we don't sleep straight through the night. I totally get it. I used to feel that way, too, until I learned that it's normal to wake up between sleep cycles. It's called "Middle Sleep." I first heard the term from Dr. Ellen Vora several years ago at a conference. The key, though, is falling back to sleep within a reasonable amount of time so you still get enough sleep.

One thing I learned from my sleep trackers is that you can wake up in the middle of the night and *still* have a great night's sleep. Both can be true at the same time.

When assessing the quality of your sleep, consider several factors: the time you went to bed, how long you slept before waking up, the amount of deep sleep you got, and how much total sleep you had. If you wake up tired, that could mean your sleep wasn't the best. But if you wake up feeling energetic and alert, even if you didn't sleep a full seven to eight hours, you likely got a decent amount of deep, restorative sleep.

If you wake up during the night but have a hard time falling back to sleep, here are some tips you can try tonight that work for me, in addition to what I've already shared:

- Before your mind starts to wander, repeat these four sentences over and over again until you fall back asleep. Trust me when I tell you, it works!

I am sorry.

Please forgive me.

Thank you.

I love you.

  It's called Ho'oponopono, and it's a powerful Hawaiian spiritual healing method and practice created by Morrnah Nalamaku Simeona, a Hawaiian Kahuna. I learned about it when I read the book *Zero Limits* by Dr. Hew Len and Joe Vitale. I loved the book and highly recommend it. To learn more, visit: https://hooponoponomiracle.com. You can also listen to Ho'oponopono meditations on YouTube.

- Try not to look at your phone or clock. Worrying about how much time you have left to sleep before your alarm goes off will wake up your brain and stress you out even more. It can also open the door for intrusive or ruminating thoughts to creep in.

- Count sheep. Or dogs. Or butterflies. The point is to do something that doesn't require much mental stimulation so you can block out the stressful ideas and racing thoughts that could otherwise keep you awake.

I hope you feel more confident about being able to tackle sleep now that you're in perimenopause and menopause. And while it may feel unpredictable, it's not entirely out of your control. The most important thing is to pay attention to your body, your habits, and your needs, and to create a sleep routine that works for you and your schedule. Rest is essential now and is one of the main foundations of how to nourish yourself. Another equally important foundation is nutrition, so next we'll look at how to fuel your body with the building blocks it needs.

8

The Building Blocks of Nutrition: Macros

If there's one thing I've learned from my personal journey through perimenopause and then menopause, it's that no two women are the same. My journey is unique to me, and yours is to you.

There is, however, one thing we *all* have in common at this stage: a need for nutrient-rich, nourishing whole foods. There's a good chance that how you ate and the lifestyle choices you made before you got to this stage may no longer serve you now that your needs have changed. Changes in hormones, body shape, stress levels, and mood mean taking a fresh look at your dietary habits to meet your body's changing demands.

Making nutrition a priority will help you manage your symptoms better, and you'll feel emotionally and physically stronger. It's really important to be mindful of what you're putting *into* and *onto* your body, because once you're in menopause, you're in it for the rest of your life. Be discerning. Ask questions. Experiment and see how you feel. What you choose to eat and drink affects everything from your symptoms, mood, energy, and stress levels to the quality of your sleep. Choosing foods that are rich in nutrients sets you up for success to power through your day.

But with all the food advice bombarding us 24/7, how do we even start to make smarter eating choices? Have any of these thoughts crossed your mind: *What* should *and* shouldn't *I be eating now? What diet* should *I be following? What time of day* should *I be eating? And how much* should *I be eating at each meal or in a day?*

That's a whole bunch of "shoulds," and it can feel like a lot, even for someone like me who has spent over two decades learning about our food system and nutrition. In this chapter and the next three, I'll share what I've learned from over twenty years as a nutritionist and twenty-six years working in health and wellness with the goal of helping you manage your symptoms and feel your best.

As you read through the next several chapters, keep in mind that there are no strict rules, as I don't endorse the "all or nothing" mind-set. My intention is to share insights and information you can adapt easily, so choose what resonates with you and find ways to weave it into your life in a way and pace that feels right for your body. That might mean making one small change at a time, adopting the 80/20 rule (eat whole, unprocessed foods at least 80 percent of the time), or jumping in fully. The most important thing is to take action.

Food Basics

Get this: According to the U.S. government's Dietary Guidelines for Americans report (2020 to 2025), about "60% of adults have one or more diet-related chronic diseases."

You read that right: *diet-related* chronic diseases.

In other words, the chronic diseases they're referring to, like heart disease, type 2 diabetes, obesity, liver disease, and some types of cancer, can often be reduced or prevented by making healthier food choices.

Since these diseases become more common as we age, and go into perimenopause and menopause, doing what we can to lower the risks only has an upside.

In this chapter, and the next two, I'll take you through the essentials of food. You'll learn about macronutrients, micronutrients (vitamins and minerals), and antioxidants.

Let's start with macronutrients.

The Big Three

When it comes to nutrition, it's important to identify and consume the right amounts of macronutrients; these are nutrients that we need in large amounts for energy, growth, and overall body function. I'll refer to them as the "Big Three." They are protein, fat, and carbohydrates.

Each of these has specific roles and functions in the body that involve:

1. How we digest food and absorb nutrients,

2. Body composition (what your body is made of, beyond just weight),

3. The strength of our immune system,

4. Hormone production, and

5. Energy, growth, healing, and more.

Macronutrients provide our bodies with calories, or energy. This is why we need them in relatively large amounts. Each macronutrient has a different number of calories per gram:

1. Protein has 4 calories per gram.

2. Fat has 9 calories per gram.

3. Carbohydrates have 4 calories per gram.

As an example, if a food label lists 10 grams of carbohydrates, 0 grams of protein, and 0 grams of fat per serving, that food contains 40 calories, all from carbohydrates.

Most foods contain two or all three macronutrients in different ratios.

Fruits are mainly made up of carbohydrates. For example, a banana is made up of mostly carbohydrates, with only tiny amounts of protein and fat. An avocado is made up of mostly fat, with a smaller amount of carbohydrates, and some protein, so it's considered a fat-based food. A grilled, skinless chicken breast is mainly protein, with some fat, and zero carbohydrates, so it's considered a protein-based food.

Knowing the breakdown of what you're eating can help you pick foods that better support your body's needs during perimenopause and menopause.

Let's start with protein.

Protein

Proteins are the "building blocks" of the body. They help to keep it strong, support muscle and tissue repair, and help it work properly.

Proteins are pretty much everywhere in your body. They build your muscles, tissues, organs, and even your hair, skin, and nails. They also help make brain chemicals and enzymes that support digestion and mood, and they help fix damaged cells.

Proteins are made from twenty different amino acids. Nine are called "essential" because your body can't make them, so you need to get them from food. The other eleven are "nonessential" because your body can usually make them on its own. However, during perimenopause and menopause, and also when you're stressed or sick, your body might not make enough of some of the nonessential ones, and your body's need for certain amino acids increases, so you may need to get more from your diet. You can also get amino acids from supplements.

It's important to get enough protein during any period of physical change (puberty, pregnancy, perimenopause, and menopause) since your body uses it to fix and grow tissues, support muscle growth, and fight off infections. Our body can't store extra protein the way it stores carbohydrates (as glycogen) and fat (as body fat), so we need to get it from food on a regular basis.

In addition to what I've already mentioned, protein helps to:

- Keep your muscles, bones, and immune system strong,

- Support metabolism and weight management,

- Keep your blood sugar levels steady, and

- Lower the risk of frailty by improving muscle mass and strength.

As we age, our bodies don't use protein as well as they used to. Hormonal shifts, slower digestion, muscle loss, and changes in how our bodies respond to insulin all make it harder to build and maintain muscle. For all these reasons and more, getting enough protein now is really important.

Protein mainly comes from animal (meat, fish, eggs, dairy) and plant-based sources (legumes, nuts and seeds, whole grains, and vegetables). Fruits contain a little bit as well, but they're not considered a major source.

Protein is so critical in perimenopause and menopause that it's one of the seven key principles of my B.A.L.A.N.C.E. Blueprint™, outlined in Chapter 11.

Fat

The second component of the Big Three is fat.

There are different types of fat, and each one affects the body differently. Some increase the risk for disease, while others help protect against it.

The Role of Dietary Fats

Dietary fats (fats that come from food sources) are a concentrated source of energy. Think of them like logs in a fireplace. Just like logs keep the fire going for long periods of time and provide a steady source of heat or energy, fats do the same for your body.

Fat supports everything from making and protecting cells to helping your body absorb fat-soluble vitamins (A, D, E, and K) in the small intestines. It also helps your body make important hormones. Cholesterol, a type of fat, is used to produce hormones like estrogen, progesterone, testosterone, and adrenal hormones like cortisol. Since hormone levels fluctuate and then fall in perimenopause and menopause, it's important to prioritize good-quality fats to support hormone production, along with heart health, metabolism, and joint health.

Unsaturated Versus Saturated Fats

There are two main categories of fat: *unsaturated* and *saturated*. Unsaturated fats stay liquid at room temperature, and saturated fats are typically solid at room temperature.

The two main types of unsaturated fats are *monounsaturated* and *polyunsaturated*.

Get ready, because a lot of acronyms are coming your way!

MONOUNSATURATED FATS (MUFAs)

MUFAs have been shown to lower LDL cholesterol, raise HDL cholesterol, help with weight management, improve insulin sensitivity, improve blood sugar control, and lower inflammation. MUFAs are a great choice for a heart-healthy diet and lowering the risk of heart disease, especially when they replace unhealthy fats like trans fats.

MUFAs are found in many plant-based foods, and one of the most popular sources is olive oil. They're also found in olives, nuts (almonds, cashews, hazelnuts, pecans, pistachios, and macadamia), pumpkin and sesame seeds, avocados, and avocado, canola, and peanut oils.

POLYUNSATURATED FATS (PUFAs)

There are two main types of polyunsaturated fatty acids: *omega-3* and *omega-6*. These are known as *essential* fatty acids (EFAs) because your body can't make them on its own, so you need to get them from food or supplements. EFAs keep your heart, brain, and immune system healthy.

PUFAs are more sensitive to heat than saturated and monounsaturated fats, and can be damaged by heavy processing, so you'll want to avoid cooking them at high temperatures, especially unrefined PUFA-rich oils (like flaxseed oil and walnut oil).

OMEGA-3

Omega-3s are very popular, and for good reason! They've been shown to support brain health, and are linked to better memory, focus, and reaction time. The brain, whose dry weight is about 60 percent fat, relies on omega-3s, especially DHA, for thinking, memory, and overall function. They've also been shown to help with heart health, mood and depression, and joint pain and stiffness (linked to conditions like arthritis), all key areas to support as we go into perimenopause and menopause.

There's a lot of research on omega-3s. A large meta-analysis reported that omega-3 fats may help lower the risk of heart disease and the chances of dying from it. Another review found that there's "clear evidence from multiple studies that higher doses of omega-3s (2,000 to 4,000 mg/day of EPA + DHA) appear to be safe and reduce cardiovascular disease (CVD) events in multiple CVD populations." Research also suggests that omega-3s can help keep the gut lining healthy and make your stools a bit softer and easier to pass.

There are three kinds of omega-3s:

1. *Alpha-linolenic acid (ALA):* ALA is found in many plant-based foods, like flaxseeds, chia seeds, and their oils. While it has cardiovascular and anti-inflammatory benefits, ALA doesn't convert well into EPA and DHA (conversion is less than 10% for EPA and anywhere from 0.05% to 5% for DHA).

2. *Eicosapentaenoic acid (EPA):* EPA helps to lower inflammation, making it especially helpful for heart health and inflammation-related conditions like arthritis.

3. *Docosahexaenoic acid (DHA):* DHA is important for brain, skin, heart, and eye health. DHA makes up nearly 90 percent of the omega-3s found in the brain and about 10–20 percent of the brain's total fat content.

There isn't a specific recommended dietary allowance (RDA, or how much you should get in total every day, from food and supplements combined) for omega-3s. Recommended doses vary anywhere from 250 to 4,000 mg a day of EPA and DHA depending on your specific health needs. Many experts suggest aiming for somewhere between 1,000 and 3,000 mg a day if you don't have any health issues. I find taking 2,500 to 3,000 mg a day helps with dry eyes, dry skin, and itchy ears. To put that dose into perspective, the European Food Safety Authority (EFSA) says that taking up to about 5,000 mg (5 grams) of combined EPA and DHA from supplements is safe for adults.

While omega-3s have a mild blood-thinning effect, research shows that for most people taking standard doses, the effect is minimal. However, always speak to your doctor if you have a bleeding disorder or you're on blood-thinning medication to ensure they don't interact.

OMEGA-3s AND DRYNESS

As you saw in Chapter 2, dryness is very common in peri-menopause and menopause. It can show up as itchy ears; dry or watery eyes; dry skin, scalp, or mouth; and even vaginal dryness. When estrogen levels drop, it becomes harder for our skin to stay moisturized and produce enough natural oils. Omega-3 fatty acids, especially EPA and DHA, also have many advantages for the skin. They may help:

- Reduce water loss, helping to keep your skin hydrated,

- Reduce the severity of acne,

- Reduce redness and calm inflamed, itchy skin, and

- Protect your skin from the sun's UV rays.

Foods high in omega-3 fats include cold-water fish (salmon, herring, mackerel, anchovies, trout, and sardines), walnuts, and seeds (ground flaxseeds, chia, and hemp). Two servings of fatty fish a week is usually enough to meet the minimum omega-3 requirements.

If these foods aren't a regular part of your diet, or you want higher doses, you can also get omega-3s from supplements like fish oil or vegan options like algae oil, which is the best vegan source of DHA and EPA. When choosing an omega-3 supplement, look for one in a triglyceride form. It's easier to digest and absorb than an ethyl ester form, and it's more stable and less prone to oxidation, so you minimize the chances of getting fish burps. In addition, make sure the brand filters out heavy metals like mercury and contaminants like PCBs (look for products that are third-party tested). The oil should taste fresh (you can bite into softgels to check) and should come in a dark bottle, as light exposure can degrade the quality of the oil, causing it to go rancid. Store the bottle in the fridge to keep it as fresh as possible.

OMEGA-6

Omega-6 fatty acids support brain and bone health, strengthen your immune system, and help build cells. Your body uses them to make hormones that affect blood clotting, inflammation, and blood pressure.

Omega-6 fatty acids are found in many nuts (pine, almonds, cashews, and walnuts), legumes such as soybeans and tofu, peanuts and peanut butter, seeds (hemp, sunflower, and sesame), and animal foods such as chicken, pork, turkey, and eggs. Seed oils, such as soybean, canola, corn, sunflower, cottonseed, safflower, grapeseed, and rice bran oils, as well as ultra-processed packaged foods, are the most common food sources of omega-6 fatty acids and make up the largest share of omega-6 in our diet.

But before adding these to your grocery list, one issue with omega-6 oils is that most of us already get too much from our diet. To put it into perspective, our ancestors consumed omega-6 and omega-3 in a 1:1 or 4:1 ratio, but our Western diet provides a lot more omega-6s than omega-3s, and some experts estimate today's ratio is closer to 10:1 or 20:1. This imbalance matters because getting too much omega-6 without enough omega-3 may contribute to chronic inflammation, so it's important to be mindful of how much omega-6 you eat and to aim for a more balanced intake.

SATURATED FAT

Saturated fat is usually solid at room temperature. It's most often found in animal and animal-sourced products like meat, lard, tallow, ghee, egg yolks, cheese, whole milk, and butter. It's also found in tropical oils like coconut, palm, and cocoa butter.

Chicken, turkey, and other poultry, as well as fish, contain some saturated fat, but they typically have less than red meat.

Saturated fat has been a source of debate for many years, linking it to one of the main causes of heart disease. However, in 2010, studies started questioning this theory. While the debate continues, newer research shows mixed findings on the connection. (In fact, many experts have turned the blame to refined ultra-processed carbs and seed oils instead.) Until there's a definitive conclusion, foods high in saturated fats should be eaten in moderation. I interviewed Dr. Jonny Bowden regarding fats, oils, and cholesterol on my podcast, *Menopause Reimagined*, a couple of times. Look for episodes #40 and #58.

TRANS FATS

Trans fats, or trans-fatty acids, are another type of fat, and we want to avoid them at all costs. Experts now agree that trans fats are linked to heart and blood vessel disease, cancer, and diabetes.

While trans fats have been banned in many countries, they may still appear in some foods, so it's important to read labels carefully. You may find trans fats in vegetable shortening and any foods that contain it, like pie crusts and other baked goods. They are also used in peanut butter, crackers, popcorn, ice cream, cakes and cookies, granola bars, frozen pizza, baby food, and more. You can spot artificial trans fats on an ingredient label by looking for the terms *partially hydrogenated oils* and *vegetable shortening*.

Carbohydrates

Ah, carbohydrates. Should we eat them? Cut them out completely? The answer lies somewhere in between.

Carbohydrates, or carbs, are one of the body's main sources of energy, along with protein and fat. However, the body prefers carbs for quick energy since they're the easiest to convert.

Carbs are found in fruits, vegetables, whole grains, and legumes, and there are small amounts in nuts and seeds, as well as dairy products. They're also in starchy vegetables (like potatoes, corn, peas, and winter squash), nonstarchy vegetables (like broccoli, carrots, and leafy greens), processed foods like bread and pasta, breakfast cereals, baked goods (cookies and donuts), soft drinks, and many snack foods (chips and popcorn). They're also in condiments and sauces (like ketchup and barbecue sauce), candy, desserts, rice, energy and sports drinks, and even alcoholic beverages like beer.

When you eat carbs, your body converts them into glucose. As discussed in Chapter 5, the glucose goes into your bloodstream, where it's brought to every part of your body, including your brain, muscles, and even your toes!

Your body needs carbs; that's why they're part of the Big Three. But the type matters. Complex carbs like whole grains, legumes (including beans), and vegetables are high in fiber, so they slow down digestion and help keep blood sugar levels balanced. As a result, you have steady, longer-lasting energy. On the other hand, refined carbs such as cookies and donuts cause your blood sugar to spike quickly, giving you a quick burst of energy, only to crash soon after. The less processed the carbs, the more gradual the rise in blood sugar tends to be, which helps to avoid the quick spikes and crashes.

Carbs are important for women in perimenopause and menopause. They provide steady energy, support healthy thyroid function, help your endocrine (hormonal) system run more smoothly, influence the quality of your sleep, and fuel the brain.

The key, however, is not to overdo it. Even though carbohydrates are a main source of energy, too many refined ultra-processed high-carb foods, like bread, cake, and sugary snacks, can affect your blood sugar and insulin levels. And as estrogen levels fluctuate in perimenopause and fall in menopause, your digestion can also be affected, changing your metabolism and making it harder for your body to handle carbs the way you used to. When this happens, it can contribute to weight gain, especially around your belly, mood swings, energy crashes, and an increased risk of insulin resistance, type 2 diabetes, and cardiovascular disease. Choosing complex carbs with more fiber can improve digestion, keep you full longer, and may help you cut down on snacking.

Here are some additional tips for choosing carbs:

- **Choose whole and ancient grains whenever possible.** In addition to whole wheat and brown rice, experiment with ancient grains like quinoa, millet, farro, teff, amaranth, sorghum, and spelt, as they're less processed and contain fiber, protein, vitamins, and minerals.

- **Prioritize vegetables and low-glycemic fruits.** Whole veggies and fruits contain fiber, antioxidants, vitamins, minerals, and certain enzymes that help digestion and support the growth of beneficial bacteria in our gut (refer to Chapter 4 on why this is important).

THERE ARE THREE MAIN TYPES OF CARBOHYDRATES: SUGARS, STARCHES, AND FIBER.

Sugars (monosaccharides and disaccharides): Also known as simple sugars, or simple carbohydrates, these are the types of carbs to be the most mindful of, as they spike our blood sugar quickly, especially when they're coming from ultra-processed foods and sugary drinks.

Simple sugars are common in processed foods with added sugar. Natural sugars are also simple sugars, but they're found in whole foods like unsweetened dairy products, fruit, and in smaller amounts in many vegetables. The big difference is that whole foods also contain fiber, water, and nutrients that help to slow down how quickly we absorb the sugar, helping to keep our blood sugar levels more stable.

In the United States, you'll see simple sugars listed on product labels in two ways: "Total Sugars," which includes both naturally occurring and added sugars, and "Added Sugars," which only shows the sugars added during processing (listed in grams and % Daily Value). In Canada, they're listed as "Sugars/Sucres," which includes both naturally occurring and added sugars without separating them.

Complex carbohydrates (polysaccharides): Complex carbs include starches and fiber. Unlike simple sugars, whole food sources of complex carbs often contain fiber, so they slow digestion and prevent quick blood sugar spikes.

Starch: Starch is the main type of complex carbohydrate. The body converts starches into glucose, which is then used for energy. Foods that contain starch include whole grains, pasta, rice, potatoes, peas, and corn. However, not all complex carbohydrates affect blood sugar the same way. For example, refined starches, like white bread, rice, and pasta, have less fiber, so they raise blood sugar levels faster than whole-grain starches.

Fiber: Fiber is another type of complex carbohydrate, but your digestive system can't fully break it down. Think of it as the body's broom, sweeping through your colon to keep digestion moving smoothly. Because of that, it helps with intestinal health, helps lower cholesterol levels, helps you feel full, and helps stabilize blood sugar levels. Fiber is found in plant-based foods such as vegetables, fruits, nuts, seeds, legumes, beans, peas, lentils, tubers (sweet potatoes, tigernuts), and whole grains. You can also take it as a supplement. When choosing a fiber supplement, look for one that contains soluble fiber and has a short, simple ingredient list. Many fiber products contain unnecessary additives such as food coloring (Blue 1, Red 40, and Yellow 6), artificial flavors, artificial sweeteners (aspartame and acesulfame potassium), seed oils (sunflower oil and corn oil), and added sugars (sucrose and maltodextrin).

Even though starch and fiber often come together in the same meal, they're doing different, but equally important, jobs for your health. Fiber keeps your digestive system moving, while starch gives you the energy to power through your day.

I go into more detail about fiber in Chapter 11.

By choosing the most beneficial types and portions of carbohydrates, you may start to notice positive changes in your symptoms, like higher energy levels, more stable moods (fewer ups and downs), better focus and concentration, improved digestion, better weight management, more balanced blood sugar and insulin levels, and fewer cravings.

Choosing Carbs Wisely

Healthy carb options include minimally processed foods that have a low glycemic index (GI). The glycemic index measures how quickly foods raise your blood sugar (glucose) levels after you eat them using a scale ranging from 0 to 100. Keep in mind that the GI value is calculated based on 50 grams of carbohydrates from a single food, so it doesn't always reflect how an actual portion would affect blood sugar levels.

Low-GI foods, for the most part, take longer to digest, which leads to a slower rise in blood sugar, helping to keep your energy levels steady. The GI index is helpful when making food choices, but the total number of grams of carbohydrates may have a bigger impact than GI on your blood sugar levels, so it's important to consider both factors when selecting foods.

Here's a quick list of some lower-glycemic carbs: apples, blackberries, blueberries, grapefruit, oranges, pears, strawberries, black-eyed peas, chickpeas, green beans, kidney beans, lentils, hummus, asparagus, broccoli, cucumber, leafy greens, lettuce, tomatoes, onions, zucchini, almonds, chia seeds, sunflower seeds, walnuts, soy (tofu, edamame; organic, non-GMO), ancient grains (quinoa, buckwheat), wild rice, and unsweetened plant-based milks like almond and coconut.

Another factor to consider is the glycemic load, which measures the amount of carbohydrates and the GI in a typical serving.

Blood Sugar-Friendly Tip: Looking for ways to reduce your intake of carbohydrates? Swap wheat flour for almond, cashew, and coconut flours.

You can read more about the glycemic load and glycemic index at https://glycemicindex.com/.

Your perimenopausal and menopausal body and mind depend on more than the Big Three macronutrients to keep you in optimal physical and mental health. They also need micronutrients, vitamins, minerals, antioxidants, and fiber. I'll go into those in the following chapters.

9

The Building Blocks of Nutrition: Minerals

A central theme of this book is to choose nourishing, whole, unprocessed foods as much as possible.

But *why*?

Unfortunately, many of the macro- and micronutrients are lost or greatly reduced when foods are processed and packaged (which is why they're often added back in during processing, a step called fortification). Fortified foods have added vitamins and minerals to make them more nutritious, but in many cases, your body doesn't always absorb them as well as the naturally occurring nutrients found in whole foods.

All vitamins and minerals are important for optimal health, but at this stage, when hormones are changing, some are more critical than others due to an increased risk of certain conditions like cardiovascular disease, osteoporosis, and metabolic diseases. Ensuring we get enough of them can help offset the potential risks and support our changing bodies' needs.

I'll take you through them one by one.

Mighty Minerals

Minerals help your body function. Your body can't make minerals, so you need to get them from food. Plants absorb minerals from the soil, and then animals and humans eat those plants or plant-eating animals.

During perimenopause, certain minerals help to support your body as it adjusts to your changing hormones. Getting enough magnesium, calcium, zinc, selenium, and iron may help ease symptoms such as poor sleep, mood changes, heavy periods, and fatigue. This is especially true if you're low in any of them.

Once you're in menopause, minerals continue to support your body. For example, calcium and magnesium help to maintain strong bones and healthy nerves, and selenium and zinc support your thyroid and immune system.

Calcium

What's the first thing that comes to mind when you hear the word *calcium*? Probably "bone health," and for good reason. Calcium is the most abundant mineral in the body, and almost all of it (99%) is stored in the bones and teeth.

In addition to bone health, calcium is important for teeth, muscle function, releasing hormones into the blood, heart rhythm, muscle contractions, and blood pressure regulation.

Throughout our lives, our bones are constantly being broken down and rebuilt, but around the time we go into menopause, we start to lose bone faster than we build it. According to the Bone Health & Osteoporosis Foundation (BHOF), women can lose about 1–2 percent of their bone density each year around the time they go into menopause, and some women may lose up to 20 percent in the first five to seven years (post)menopause, when bone loss happens the fastest.

So what's happening during late perimenopause and menopause that causes our bones to break down?

Estrogen helps keep bones strong by balancing the amount of bone the body breaks down with the amount it builds back up. However, when estrogen levels fall, it makes bone density loss more likely, and lower bone density raises the risk of osteoporosis.

According to the North American Menopause Society's 2021 Osteoporosis Position Statement, calcium and vitamin D are important for women in perimenopause and menopause to keep their bones healthy, but they aren't enough on their own to increase bone mass density (BMD) or treat osteoporosis. They work best as part of a bigger plan that includes exercise and strength training, fall prevention, and, when needed, treatments like hormone therapy (HT) or other osteoporosis medications. Speak to your healthcare professional if you're at risk.

The Menopause Society and the National Academies of Sciences, Engineering, and Medicine (NASEM) advise that women fifty and under aim for 1,000 mg of calcium a day, and women fifty-one and older aim for 1,200 mg a day from food and supplements combined. They also recommend a target of 600 IU of vitamin D a day if you're between the ages of fifty and seventy, and 800 IU a day if you're seventy-one or older, and The Menopause Society adopts these targets in its osteoporosis statement. The Endocrine Society recommends (post)menopausal women get 800 IU a day, regardless of age, for bone health.

The best way to get calcium is from food. Rich sources include dairy products, like cottage cheese, Greek yogurt, and cheese (parmesan has the most calcium), canned salmon and sardines with bones, (organic, non-GMO) tofu, seeds (chia, sesame), dark leafy greens (collard greens, spinach, bok choy, and kale), broccoli, beans and lentils, almonds, some brands of almond milk, and foods fortified with calcium.

If you aren't getting enough calcium from your daily diet, you can consider taking a calcium supplement. However, I want you to be aware: a 2021 meta-analysis of thirteen double-blind, placebo-controlled randomized controlled trials (RCTs) with 28,935 participants suggested that taking around 1,000 mg of calcium alone, without vitamin D, was linked to a 15 percent increased risk of cardiovascular disease (CVD) and a 16 percent increased risk of coronary heart disease (CHD) in healthy (post)menopausal women. Unfortunately, the type of calcium wasn't always mentioned. If you've been advised to take a calcium supplement, speak with your doctor or healthcare provider about which type and dose are appropriate for you.

For best absorption, take a calcium supplement in divided doses.

In addition to calcium and vitamin D, bone health also depends on phosphorus, magnesium, zinc, manganese, boron, vitamins K2-MK4 and K2-MK7, potassium, copper, iron, vitamin C, B vitamins, and, of course, lifestyle habits such as getting enough protein and including weight-bearing and resistance exercises, safe sun exposure (for vitamin D), and supporting gut health.

If you're open to exploring the option of hormone therapy for bone health and the prevention of osteoporosis, speak to someone who's up to date on the latest research. You can find a knowledgeable doctor or healthcare practitioner who understands hormones for women in perimenopause and menopause at menopause.org and www.wakeherup.co.

Magnesium

Magnesium is the second-most-abundant mineral inside our cells (after potassium) and the fourth most abundant in our body overall. It's responsible for over three hundred to six hundred enzymatic processes, and every cell needs it to function properly. About 99 percent of magnesium is stored in muscles (25–30%), bones (50–60%), and other soft tissues. Less than 1 percent is found in the blood.

Magnesium plays a big role in how the body uses the Big Three— protein, fats, and carbohydrates—for energy and overall health. It also helps your body make protein, a process known as protein synthesis, so it's a good idea to include magnesium-rich veggies like leafy greens, artichokes, and cruciferous vegetables (broccoli, cauliflower, bok choy, Brussels sprouts, etc.), to support this process.

One of magnesium's jobs is to help activate and metabolize vitamin D, and your body needs the active form of vitamin D to absorb calcium. Without enough magnesium, vitamin D may not fully switch on, so your body may have a harder time absorbing calcium, even if you get plenty of vitamin D. In other words, vitamin D can't do its job as well without magnesium helping to activate it.

Magnesium is critical for women's health in general, and especially now.

As I mentioned in the calcium section, as we go into menopause, our bodies break down bone faster than we build it, so we're more prone to bone loss. Studies have shown that perimenopausal and menopausal women with osteoporosis have low levels of magnesium. Making sure you get enough magnesium supports bone density and bone quality, and is important for hormones that help to build bones. Magnesium works with vitamin D to help move calcium into the bones, instead of depositing it in soft tissues like arteries where too much calcium can calcify and contribute to heart disease. It also helps to reduce inflammation and oxidative stress, which can weaken bones.

Magnesium has a calming effect on the nervous system, so it's amazing for helping us cope better with stress and anxiety. It can improve the quality of our sleep, help regulate mood, and provide relief from muscle (including menstrual) cramps, spasms, and tension, which can become more frequent during this stage of life. It's also been shown to improve energy levels, and some small studies suggest it may reduce the frequency and intensity of hot flashes and night sweats, but more research is needed in this area.

And if all that isn't enough, it can also help ease premenstrual syndrome (PMS) symptoms, headaches, and migraines; regulate blood sugar levels; improve insulin sensitivity; and support cardiovascular health, including modest reductions in blood pressure.

How Much Magnesium Do You Really Need?

The recommended dietary allowance (RDA) for women thirty-one and older is 320 mg a day in both the United States and Canada. However, on average, women consume around 228 mg a day.

The typical Western diet generally provides enough magnesium to prevent *severe* deficiency but not necessarily enough to protect us from heart disease, bone loss, and other long-term health risks. It's estimated that a significant portion of the population, half or more, is deficient, and 50 to 75 percent may not be getting enough magnesium from diet alone on a daily basis. This is especially true for women.

Research shows that many of us would benefit from increasing our magnesium intake by about 300 mg a day on top of our regular diet to reach a range that's beneficial for longevity and overall health.

Here are some signs that your body might need more magnesium: fatigue or low energy, anxiousness or feeling on edge, heart palpitations, constipation, brain fog, weakness, muscle spasms or twitches (including eyes and lips), nausea, sleep disturbances, loss of appetite, mood swings, leg cramps, restless legs, headaches, migraines, tingling in your hands and feet, PMS, and painful menstrual cramps.

Research has linked low magnesium levels to several chronic conditions such as type 2 diabetes, low-grade inflammation, anxiety, and depression. It also plays an important role in blood sugar regulation.

A deficiency in magnesium can also raise the risk of serious heart problems such as high blood pressure, irregular heart rhythms, hardening and stiffening of the arteries, heart failure, blood clots, and, in some cases, the heart stopping suddenly.

But here's the thing: If you're thinking, *No problem, I'll get a blood test to check my levels*, it's not that simple, unfortunately. Since the majority of the body's magnesium is stored in bone, muscle, and soft tissues, with less than 1 percent in blood, you might still be deficient *even if* your test results come back "normal." Your body does a great job at keeping magnesium levels in your bloodstream steady, so if the levels start to drop, it'll pull magnesium from your bones, muscles, and other soft tissues to top it up, potentially masking the issue. Therefore, a standard serum (blood) magnesium test isn't the most accurate way to assess your overall magnesium levels. One option is to ask for a red blood cell (RBC) magnesium test. It looks at the amount of magnesium inside cells, which gives a little bit more information, but it's still not a perfect test. Truthfully, you can often tell if you need more magnesium by the symptoms you're exhibiting (which I listed earlier).

So why are so many of us deficient in magnesium?

Unfortunately, there are many reasons, including environmental, dietary, health-related, and lifestyle factors.

The overuse of chemical fertilizers, improper farming practices, and deforestation have depleted the amount of nutrients, including minerals, in the soil.

Many of us don't get enough magnesium from our diet, and most ultra-processed foods are high in compounds that leach magnesium from the body. Also, refined foods are stripped of minerals, including magnesium, when processed.

As we saw in Chapter 4, our digestive system can change now that we're in perimenopause and menopause, affecting how we absorb nutrients. And certain health-related causes, like some digestive issues (e.g., celiac or Crohn's disease, IBS, chronic loose stools) or kidney conditions, make it harder for our body to absorb or retain it. Research also shows that people with type 2 diabetes often have lower magnesium levels, and a magnesium deficiency itself may increase the risk of developing insulin resistance. Therefore, supplementing with magnesium may help you become more insulin sensitive, especially if you have prediabetes or type 2 diabetes and your magnesium intake is on the low side.

Stress, alcohol, and certain medications, such as proton pump inhibitors (PPIs), diuretics, anti-inflammatories, and certain hormone therapies (oral contraceptives), can deplete magnesium from the body.

It's unlikely you'd consume too much magnesium from food alone, since your body naturally gets rid of any excess through urine.

Good food sources of magnesium include green leafy vegetables (collard greens, kale, spinach, mustard greens), legumes and beans (black beans, kidney beans, navy beans, lima beans, peanuts, lentils), whole grains (brown rice, oatmeal), avocados, dark chocolate, nuts (almonds, cashews), seeds (sesame, sunflower, chia, flaxseeds), and fruits and vegetables such as bananas, blackberries, and avocados. Magnesium is found in smaller amounts in animal protein (beef, chicken, halibut, and salmon). A helpful rule of thumb is to look for foods high in dietary fiber, as they often contain magnesium. If you aren't getting enough in your diet, consider taking a supplement. As I mentioned previously, my all-around favorite option is magnesium bisglycinate.

Phosphorus

Phosphorus (as phosphate) helps your body produce energy and helps your hormones work properly. It's also a powerhouse mineral for building and protecting strong bones.

When estrogen fluctuates during perimenopause and drops in menopause, your body may not use or process minerals like phosphorus, calcium, and magnesium the same way it did before, so keeping them in a healthy range helps to support stronger bones.

Unlike magnesium, a phosphorus deficiency is rare. Most of us meet our daily needs without any issues. The RDA is 700 mg, and you can get it from meat, fish, dairy products, eggs, nuts, seeds, beans, and whole grains.

Note: Watch out for ultra-processed foods and drinks like frozen dinners, soda, processed meats, and fast foods. Many of these contain high amounts of phosphorus because of added phosphate preservatives, and they can increase how much you're ingesting on a daily basis. Higher amounts can throw off the balance of other minerals like magnesium and calcium, potentially leading to bone health issues.

Iron

In general, women in pre- and perimenopause tend to have lower levels of iron because of their monthly cycles (we lose iron through blood). It's estimated we lose between 15 and 30 mg every time we get our period. Vegetarians and vegans can have lower levels of iron (and other nutrients like B12), as it's harder to absorb it from plant-based foods. People with inflammatory bowel conditions such as celiac, Crohn's, and ulcerative colitis may also have a hard time absorbing iron because of gut inflammation, even if they're getting enough.

Optimal Iron Levels and Testing

The RDA for iron for premenopausal and perimenopausal women is 18 mg per day, and 8 mg per day for menopausal women.

Many symptoms of low or high iron overlap with those of perimenopause and menopause, including fatigue, hair loss, brain fog, heart palpitations, and joint pain, so I encourage you to ask your doctor or healthcare provider to check your ferritin level at least once a year.

Blood tests measuring ferritin are commonly used to diagnose iron deficiency anemia and iron overload disorders like hemochromatosis. If ferritin levels are low, it may mean you're deficient in iron. If they're high, it may mean you have too much iron, but high ferritin doesn't always mean you have iron overload. Ferritin levels can also increase because of inflammation, infection, liver disease, autoimmune conditions, or metabolic issues, so doctors may want to check other markers like serum iron, transferrin saturation, and total iron-binding capacity (TIBC) to get a full picture of your iron levels.

"Normal" ferritin levels for adult women can vary quite a bit (from very low to very high), but many experts agree that an "optimal" range often falls somewhere between 50 and 100 ng/mL (μg/L). Experts such as Christy Sutton, DC, author of *The Iron Curse*, prefer to see ferritin levels below 100. Dr. Thomas Perls, MD, MPH, and founder and director of the New England Centenarian Study, has also noted that lower ferritin levels are associated with greater longevity, as long as you don't have any symptoms. You can listen to my interviews with both Christy Sutton and Thomas Perls on my podcast, *Menopause Reimagined*, episodes #71 and #67, respectively.

Iron Deficiency

In perimenopause, your periods can get longer, shorter, lighter, or heavier, and many women have excessive bleeding, commonly referred to as flooding. Or you may also skip periods altogether. Heavier or longer-lasting periods can slowly drain iron stores over time and lead to low levels or iron-deficiency anemia. My good friend had an ablation, a medical procedure that removes or destroys the uterine lining to reduce or stop bleeding, because her perimenopause periods were super heavy and would last for weeks at a time without reprieve. She'd bleed through her pads so quickly that she'd have to change them hourly. Another friend of mine chose to have a hysterectomy because of the flooding. If you're experiencing any type of heavy bleeding, please speak to your doctor.

The more common signs of low iron levels include fatigue and exhaustion, brain fog, memory loss, lack of focus, irritability, mood changes, frequent headaches, heart palpitations, dizziness or light-headedness, shortness of breath, very pale skin, brittle nails, hair loss, cracks on the side of your mouth, and a dry or burning mouth or tongue.

Other possible signs are tinnitus (ringing in the ears), restless legs, muscle weakness, and cold hands and feet.

Another reason you may want to check your ferritin level is if you have low thyroid hormone levels (hypothyroidism). The thyroid needs iron to produce hormones (T3 and T4), so low ferritin can make it harder to balance your thyroid.

If your iron is low, here are some tips to increase your levels:

- **Reach for iron-rich foods.** Sources of well-absorbed iron (heme iron) include meat, fish and shellfish (clams, mussels, and oysters), chicken, turkey, and organ meats. Plant-based sources of nonheme iron, which isn't absorbed as well as heme iron, include quinoa, beans, legumes, brown rice, broccoli, nuts and seeds (pumpkin and sesame), dark chocolate, and enriched foods like some unsweetened fortified plant-milks, and protein powders and bars. Pair nonheme iron–rich foods with vitamin C foods (citrus, strawberries, kiwi, bell peppers, tomatoes) or, if needed, a vitamin C supplement, to help with absorption.

  Be mindful of eating nonheme iron–rich foods with "antinutrients," meaning nutrients that can decrease its absorption. These include oxalates (found in spinach, beet greens, and chard), phytates (found in whole grains, legumes, nuts, and seeds), and tannins (found in tea [caffeinated], coffee, and legumes like lentils and chickpeas). This doesn't mean you shouldn't eat them; just space them out (wait about an hour before or after eating nonheme iron–rich foods), and either cook, soak, sprout, or ferment them to lower their antinutrient activity.

- **Check your vitamin B12 levels.** Even if you get enough iron, your body still needs B12 to make healthy red blood cells. Low B12 can cause anemia, too, and it's possible to be low in both at the same time.

- **Cook with cast-iron pans.** Cooking with cast-iron cookware can increase the iron content of foods, especially if they're acidic and left to simmer, boil, or stew in liquid for more than thirty minutes. Shorter cooking methods like frying, sautéing, or searing for less than ten minutes won't transfer as much iron as would slow, wet cooking. You can also try an iron cooking tool, like the Lucky Iron Fish or Leaf, which adds 6 to 8 mg of iron to any liquid you add it to.

- **Consider iron medications or supplements.** Talk to your doctor, pharmacist, or healthcare practitioner about nonconstipating options. If you take an iron supplement, you may want to look into a chelated form like iron bisglycinate, which is often easier on the stomach, or heme iron polypeptide, which comes from animal sources and is usually well absorbed.

High Iron

If you're in menopause, be mindful of how much iron you're getting from food and supplements, because once you stop having periods, the risk of being iron deficient drops. When iron builds up over time, it can increase oxidation in the body. Think of it like rust on metal that slowly wears on your tissues and organs. This kind of stress can lead to inflammation and long-term health issues, which is why once you stop menstruating, it's really important to continue testing your levels at least once a year.

Classic symptoms of iron overload include feeling weak or having unexplained fatigue; skin changes like hyperpigmentation, darkening, or bronzing; and joint stiffness or pain. Other possible symptoms include inflammation, joint and muscle aches (due to iron deposits in the tissues), and abdominal pain if the liver is affected. Liver problems (such as fatty liver or cirrhosis) are also a possible sign. Over time, too much iron can lead to serious health issues like diabetes and liver damage. If iron builds up in the heart, it can increase the risk of cardiovascular disease. It can also weaken the immune system, making you more prone to infections.

A 2023 study of 12.1 million Canadian women found that premenopausal women had lower average iron levels than (post)-menopausal women. Too much iron was rare before menopause (2.7%) and much more common after (21%).

If your ferritin level is high, here are some steps you can take to lower it:

- Be mindful when cooking with cast-iron pans because they can leach iron into your food.

- Read the ingredients on supplements, including multivitamins, to see if they contain iron.

- Donate blood.

- Eat less red meat (once a week or once a month depending on your levels).

- Avoid alcohol, smoking, and ultra-processed sugar, as they put extra stress on your liver, which is already strained if you have iron overload and, as you saw in Chapter 3, during perimenopause and menopause.

- Drink green tea with meals that contain iron to lower absorption, because its tannins can block the absorption of nonheme iron.

- Check if you have hereditary hemochromatosis (a condition that causes high iron levels).

Iodine

Iodine helps to keep your thyroid working properly. The thyroid gland controls your metabolism, energy levels, mood, and how clearly you can think, all things that can be affected during perimenopause and menopause.

If iodine levels are too low, your thyroid can't make enough hormones (T4 and T3), which may cause or worsen hypothyroidism, and lead to symptoms like a sluggish metabolism, cold hands and feet, low libido, depression, and low energy levels. Low iodine can also cause the thyroid to enlarge, creating what's known as a goiter. Because thyroid hormones play a big role in memory and focus, getting enough iodine is important for brain health.

But how much is ideal? The RDA for iodine for adults, including women in perimenopause and menopause, is 150 mcg a day. If you're pregnant, the RDA is 220 mcg, and it's 290 mcg if you're breastfeeding.

However, if you have a thyroid condition, you'll want to be *very mindful* of how much iodine you're getting from food and supplements combined. According to Danielle Meitiv, MS, a functional health coach, "Hypothyroidism is especially common in women, and the risk increases during hormonal transitions like perimenopause and menopause. Estrogen and progesterone influence thyroid hormone activity, so declining sex hormones can unmask or worsen underlying thyroid dysfunction. Studies suggest that 10–25 percent of women in midlife may have overt or subclinical hypothyroidism, though many go undiagnosed because symptoms like fatigue or brain fog are often attributed to menopause alone. Autoimmune thyroiditis (Hashimoto's) is a leading cause and is common in women during these transitional years."

Dr. Izabella Wentz, PharmD, FASCP, the best-selling author of several books, including *The New York Times* bestseller *Hashimoto's Thyroiditis: Lifestyle Interventions for Finding and Treating the Root Cause*, says that too much iodine can be an issue, as high levels can stress the thyroid and lead to thyroid "dysfunction." Too much iodine may worsen or trigger conditions like hypothyroidism, hyperthyroidism, or Hashimoto's. Dr. Wentz recommends that most people (whether they're deficient or have an excess) should keep iodine intake to around or under 150 to 200 mcg a day from all sources and warns against taking supplements that contain more than 500 mcg a day without medical supervision (including thyroid formulas). Food sources like seaweed and their extracts (kelp, dulse, and hijiki) can contain high levels of iodine per serving, so consume them in moderation. She recommends looking for hidden sources of iodine in supplements, medications, skin care, and personal care products (e.g., topical antiseptics and seaweed- or kelp-based creams, masks, shampoos, and lotions).

Other less potent food sources of iodine include seafood (such as cod, shrimp, and tuna), egg yolks, and dairy products like milk, yogurt, cheddar cheese, and cottage cheese. If you use table salt, iodine is found in iodized salt, but to be honest, I don't recommend using that type of salt. Instead, consider Himalayan pink salt, gray sea salt, or Celtic salt, since these salts only have negligible amounts of iodine.

Unfortunately, testing iodine levels isn't widely accessible or recommended. The preferred option is a twenty-four-hour urinary iodine concentration (UIC) test. However, if you suspect you have high levels and need a faster answer, you can ask for a blood test, but it's less reliable. You can also check your thyroid hormones (TSH, free T4, and free T3) and do a review of your diet (do you eat a lot of sushi? Enriched breads?) and supplements. If your iodine intake is high, it's important to make sure you're getting enough selenium, as it helps to protect the thyroid. As always, consult your doctor.

Selenium

The thyroid has the highest concentration of selenium of any organ per gram of tissue, and this trace mineral is essential for thyroid function. Selenium helps to keep your heart healthy and your immune system strong. It supports your liver, too, by helping to process and clear metabolized hormones and other substances you no longer need.

A study from New Zealand found that many (post)menopausal women were getting less selenium than what's recommended due to low levels in the soil, so it's important to pay attention to how much of this mineral we're getting now.

If you're low in selenium, you may have a hard time losing weight and notice thinning or brittle hair. Low selenium levels may affect your brain, possibly contributing to irritability and depression. All of these are common during perimenopause and menopause. Autoimmune thyroid diseases like Hashimoto's and Graves' have also been associated with low selenium levels.

You can check selenium levels with a serum blood test, where the typical reference ranges are between 70 and 150 µg/L depending on the lab. Some specialty labs also offer RBC selenium testing, which shows your levels over several months.

The RDA for adult women is 55 µg, or micrograms (mcg). However, 200 mcg is often used in research and in certain clinical settings.

Food sources of selenium include Brazil nuts, shellfish, canned sardines with the bones, pork, beef liver, eggs, barley, baked beans, and brown rice. You can also take it as a supplement. Take it with vitamin E for added antioxidant support since they work together as a team to protect your cells.

Chromium

This trace mineral helps your body process fat, protein, and carbohydrates, and improves how your body responds to insulin, which is why it may help if you have insulin resistance or type 2 diabetes.

Low chromium has been linked to higher levels of blood sugar and, in some cases, higher triglycerides and cholesterol levels, especially in people with metabolic issues. Early research shows that it may also play a role in mood, memory, and concentration.

Since we're more susceptible to all the above now that we're in perimenopause and menopause because of changing hormone levels, getting enough chromium may help offset some of these metabolic changes.

Chromium is found in many foods, including meat, whole grains, fruits, vegetables, and spices like basil and garlic, but the amount can vary a lot depending on the mineral content of the soil, how it's grown, and how the foods are processed, which is true for most minerals.

There isn't an official RDA for chromium. Instead, there's something called an adequate intake (AI) level, an estimate of how much chromium is assumed to meet our nutritional needs. The AI for chromium for women in the United States and Canada is 25 mcg for ages nineteen to fifty and 20 mcg for ages fifty-one and older.

Potassium

This important mineral is also an electrolyte, which means it helps your heart beat regularly and supports nerve signals that make your muscles contract. It also helps with balancing fluids, blood pressure, blood sugar, and other aspects of heart health. Other minerals that are also electrolytes are calcium, magnesium, and sodium.

Eighty percent of the body's potassium is stored in muscle, and 20 percent in bones, where it works with magnesium, calcium, and phosphorus to support bone density. Eating foods rich in potassium may help prevent bone loss, making it particularly important for those of us who are already in menopause.

Hormonal changes around menopause can affect how our bodies handle fluids and electrolytes like sodium and potassium, so our kidneys might hold on to a little more sodium and water, which can cause mild water retention and symptoms like bloating, swelling, and blood pressure changes. Also, hot flashes and night sweats can make us slightly dehydrated, which may temporarily affect fluid and electrolyte balance. Low potassium levels can trigger or worsen symptoms such as fatigue, constipation, bloating, swelling, high blood pressure, heart palpitations, and muscle cramps and twitches. Studies also show that people who don't get enough potassium or have low amounts may develop kidney stones and often have higher fasting blood sugar levels, insulin resistance, and an increased chance of developing type 2 diabetes.

Although there's no RDA for potassium, the AI recommendation is 4,700 mg. Unfortunately, most of us only get about 2,250 mg a day, which is less than half the recommended amount. In fact, a women's health study with over ninety thousand (post)menopausal women found that only about 3 percent were getting the AI recommendation, so this is another mineral worth paying attention to in order to meet the daily suggested intake.

Some experts recommend aiming for a 2:1 ratio of potassium to sodium, meaning potassium intake should be about twice as high as sodium. A higher potassium-to-sodium ratio has been shown to lower blood pressure and reduce the risk of cardiovascular events (like heart attacks and strokes). It helps by relaxing blood vessel walls and eliminating sodium through the urine.

Research published in 2022 in the journal *Hypertension* found that (post)menopausal women with high blood pressure who took a potassium supplement excreted more sodium than before they took it. This is important because getting rid of extra sodium helps to regulate blood pressure and may lower the risk of cardiovascular disease, which becomes more common in perimenopause and menopause.

Food sources include veggies (spinach, mushrooms, zucchini, Brussels sprouts, and acorn squash), fruits (berries, kiwi, and bananas), avocados, nuts (almonds and walnuts), seeds (pumpkin), legumes (lentils and beans), dairy (Greek yogurt and cottage cheese), eggs, and animal protein (chicken, salmon, pork, and beef).

You can also take it as a supplement.

You can check your potassium levels with a serum potassium blood test. Results of 3.5 to 5.0 mmol/L are considered normal.

Sodium

Sodium is a mineral and an electrolyte that helps control fluid levels in your body and allows your nerves and muscles, including your heart, to function properly. Sodium works with other electrolytes like chloride and potassium to do its job.

Sodium is well-known for its connection to high blood pressure. Research shows a clear relationship between the amount of sodium consumed and high blood pressure. In some populations where people eat very low-sodium diets, they don't experience the same increase in blood pressure with age. A study in the *Journal of the American Medical Association* (*JAMA*) found that reducing your intake of sodium from food and beverages significantly lowered blood pressure in middle-aged and older adults within just one week.

Shifts in estrogen and progesterone during perimenopause and menopause can change how your body handles fluids. As a result, you might notice you hold on to water easier, feel more bloated, have a puffy face, or have swelling in your hands, feet, or belly. Because your body may be more sensitive to sodium at this stage, salty foods can make bloating, heaviness, swelling, and puffiness feel even worse.

Another reason to be mindful of how much sodium you're ingesting is bone health. A 2017 study published in *Osteoporosis International* found that consuming 2,000 mg of sodium per day, or more, was associated with lower bone mineral density and a higher risk of osteoporosis in (post)menopausal women.

The current recommendation for sodium intake for the general population is a maximum of 2,300 mg a day, and closer to 1,500 mg if you have heart disease or high blood pressure. However, most of us are getting closer to 3,500 mg a day. One level teaspoon of salt (~5 g) contains about 2,200 to 2,300 mg of sodium.

When we think about sodium, we usually equate it with table salt, but that's only one of many sources of sodium in our diet. About 80 percent of the sodium we consume comes from processed, packaged, and restaurant foods, not the saltshaker. It's often added in large amounts to enhance the flavor of foods or act as a preservative. Be mindful of these high-sodium foods at the grocery store: deli meats and hot dogs, pizza, snack foods (like potato chips), tomato sauces, salad dressings, condiments, frozen or ready-to-eat appetizers, cured and pickled foods, baked goods (bread, muffins, cookies, and crackers), and prepared soups and entrées, such as frozen fries and lasagna.

While getting *too much* processed *sodium* can be detrimental to your health, *not getting enough* of the *right type of salt* can be as well. According to Ben Azadi, functional diagnostic nutrition (FDN) practitioner and author of *Metabolic Freedom*, not all salt is created equal. "The highly processed, iodized white table salt found in most households and packaged foods is stripped of its natural minerals and often contains anti-caking agents like sodium aluminosilicate and sodium ferrocyanide (yep, that's a cyanide compound!). On the other hand, unrefined, mineral-rich salts, like Himalayan pink salt and Celtic gray salt, contain trace amounts of essential electrolytes such as magnesium, potassium, and calcium, which help maintain proper fluid balance, muscle function, and even healthy blood pressure levels." Another unrefined salt to check out is Himalayan black salt, as it contains a little bit less sodium than white table salt and provides small amounts of antioxidants.

Over the years, studies have found that some people are more salt sensitive than others, which may explain why results of sodium intake and hypertension have been inconsistent.

Ben says that when it comes to women in perimenopause and menopause who are already more prone to specific symptoms, getting enough real, unrefined salt may help to reduce fatigue, brain fog, dizziness, muscle cramps, and irregular heartbeat. This is because natural, unrefined salt plays an essential role in hydration, electrolyte balance, and even blood pressure regulation.

My perspective? Consume sodium in moderation and choose unrefined varieties as opposed to bleached white table salt.

You can measure sodium through a twenty-four-hour urine test to assess how much you're consuming since we pee out 90–95 percent of sodium within approximately one day.

Zinc

Probably best known for its role in immune health, this trace mineral is found in nearly every cell of the body. It's involved in many processes, including wound healing, digestion, taste and smell, hair and skin health, eye health, bone health, and hormones (including metabolizing thyroid hormones and helping the pancreas make and store insulin).

Seventy percent of zinc is found in muscles and bones. Your body doesn't store it in large amounts, so you need to get it from food on a regular basis.

As we age, we can become deficient in zinc due to absorption problems and certain medications. Genetics can also play a role. We lose zinc when we pee, poop, sweat, and menstruate. During perimenopause and menopause, hormonal and metabolic changes in the body can make it easier to lose more zinc than we take in.

Some studies on postmenopausal women show that those who get less zinc tend to lose more bone than those who get enough. In one study, adding zinc with calcium and copper slowed bone loss in women whose dietary zinc intake was low. Some research suggests that very low intake of zinc-rich foods (below recommended levels) is linked to lower bone density. And another study on (post)menopausal women found that taking a higher dose of 50 mg of zinc a day for eight weeks was linked to higher vitamin D levels and lower leptin (which in this case likely means the body is responding better to it), a hormone tied to weight and metabolism (see Chapter 5). Early research is looking at how zinc may help support mood, including anxiety and depression, and neurodegenerative disorders like dementia and Alzheimer's.

Low levels of zinc have also been linked to hypothyroidism, as well as hair loss, one of its well-known side effects.

The RDA for zinc is 8 mg for adult women. The tolerable upper-intake limit (UL) is 40 mg a day.

You can meet this daily amount by eating zinc-rich foods like oysters (by far the highest source), sardines, beef, pork, turkey, egg yolks, nuts and seeds (especially pumpkin seeds), oatmeal, quinoa, soybeans (organic, non-GMO), chickpeas, and lentils.

Zinc from animal foods is absorbed more easily than plant-based foods. If you're vegetarian or vegan, be mindful that legumes, grains, and nuts and seeds contain phytates, which can block the absorption of zinc. Lower phytate plant foods like cashews, quinoa, mushrooms, spinach, kale, and broccoli are good options. To improve absorption, soak, sprout, or ferment grains, legumes, and seeds to lower phytates, and pair them with protein or vitamin C–rich foods. And if you take calcium or iron supplements, take them separately from zinc-rich foods since they compete for absorption.

You can also take zinc as a supplement, but be mindful about taking too much for too long (over 40 mg a day), as it can throw off the balance of other minerals, especially copper. Check the label to see if the supplement also has iron, as it can interfere with the absorption of zinc (however, this isn't the case with food).

Note: Toxicity has been shown at extremely high levels of 1–2 grams taken at once.

Copper

This trace mineral helps the body with a number of important tasks, including collagen production. Collagen is the most abundant protein in the body (about 30% of total protein) and is important for skin, bones, and connective tissues. As estrogen levels drop, collagen loss speeds up as well, which can contribute to thinner, looser skin, painful and less flexible joints, and bone loss.

Copper is needed for the body to use and transport iron, and it helps with the production of brain chemicals that regulate mood and help keep blood vessels and the heart healthy, which is especially important in menopause, when the risk of heart disease increases.

You can get copper from seafood, particularly oysters, crab, and lobster, as well as organ meats such as liver, as they're among the richest food sources. Nuts, seeds, legumes, whole grains, dark chocolate, and certain fruits and vegetables also contain copper, though in smaller amounts. Including a variety of these foods in your diet helps ensure you get enough.

Both zinc and copper play a role when it comes to hair health.

Zinc can help with growth and repair, and copper can help make melanin, the pigment that gives hair its color. When these minerals are out of balance, low copper can lead to premature graying, while a zinc deficiency is linked to hair loss.

Word of Caution: Excess Copper

Copper and zinc have an inverse relationship as they compete for absorption in the intestines. This means that if one goes high, the other goes low, possibly leading to a deficiency. Too much copper can be an issue because it can interfere with the absorption of zinc, and vice versa.

My friend EJ had a copper IUD inserted after she had her kids. Unfortunately, it was left there for much longer than it was supposed to be (approximately eight years), and it started to break down in her body. She got really sick, but nobody could figure out why. She did her own research and discovered that her symptoms were consistent with copper toxicity, and the source was her IUD. She insisted it be removed, and once it was out, she started to feel much better. If you have an IUD, whether for contraception or to help manage heavy bleeding during perimenopause, please make sure you're on top of your regular checkups.

Symptoms of excess copper levels include stomach pain, yellowing of the skin or eyes, loss of appetite, extreme thirst, headaches, anxiety, nausea, vomiting, depression, sudden mood changes, diarrhea, and dizziness.

If you have high copper levels, be mindful of copper cookware and pipes, and use a water filter if your water contains high levels.

Manganese

Manganese supports important changes during midlife. Research suggests that our levels may drop once we go into menopause, possibly due to changing hormones and higher iron stores once our periods stop, since manganese and iron seem to have an inverse relationship.

Manganese helps to build bone and connective tissue (e.g., cartilage) and may help protect you from bone loss when combined with other nutrients like calcium, zinc, copper, and vitamin D. Some studies link it to better metabolic health, including a lower risk of type 2 diabetes in (post)menopausal women. It's also an antioxidant, so it helps protect cells from damage as we age through an enzyme called superoxide dismutase (SOD). Research on manganese and its effects, particularly on menopause and bone health, is limited, so it's best to think of manganese as one piece of your larger mineral puzzle.

The AI is 1.8 mg a day for adult women. The tolerable upper intake level is 11 mg/day from all sources.

It's best to get manganese through a whole foods diet or a multi-mineral formula (not to be confused with a multivitamin) rather than taking it on its own, unless specifically recommended by your healthcare practitioner.

High-manganese foods include mussels, clams, oysters, steel-cut oats, brown rice, quinoa and other whole grains, tea, hazelnuts, pecans, walnuts, spinach, kale, legumes, and berries.

As you saw, some nutrients are harder to test than others, so I recommend checking out the Nutrient Zoomer by Vibrant Wellness. They have a wide range of tests you can ask your healthcare provider about including vitamins, minerals, amino acids, fatty acids, antioxidants, hormones, gut and heart health, autoimmune, environmental toxins, infections, and more!

We hear so much about nutrition and the foods that nourish our bodies. Understanding what these foods are made up of and how they affect us now that our bodies are changing, or have changed, can help you understand why it's important to make sure you get enough macro- and micronutrients. They give us energy; affect our sleep, mood, cognitive function, and bone and muscle strength; and impact hormones. Think of them as the foundation for nutrition, the bricks that hold the house together.

In the next chapter, I'll talk about vitamins and antioxidants and their importance for overall health in perimenopause and menopause and how they complement these essential nutrients to keep you feeling your best.

10.

The Building Blocks of Nutrition: Vitamins and Antioxidants

Minerals help to keep your body strong and balanced, and vitamins bring their own important benefits too. Vitamins help your body do its daily jobs, from converting food into energy to keeping your cells working properly. Understanding vitamins and how they impact you during perimenopause and menopause can help support your energy, mood, skin, muscles, sleep, brain function, stress levels, and immune health.

There are thirteen essential vitamins, and they're grouped into two categories: fat-soluble (vitamins A, D, E, and K) and water-soluble (vitamin C and the B vitamins).

- The four fat-soluble vitamins are A, D, E, and K, and they're stored in the liver, muscles, and fatty tissue. They're absorbed more easily when eaten with fat, and most foods that contain them naturally have some fat in them. If you're taking them as a supplement, it's best to take them with food that contains fat.

- The water-soluble vitamins include vitamin C and all eight B vitamins (collectively known as the B complex vitamins). For the most part, your body doesn't store large amounts of these vitamins, and whatever you don't need is flushed out through urine. Because they're not stored in your body, you have to consume them on a regular basis to keep your levels steady. The major exception is vitamin B12, which your liver can store for several years.

Here are important vitamins for this stage of life, and why:

Vitamin A: Did your mother or grandmother make you take cod liver oil as a kid? If you answered yes, the reason was because it contains vitamin A! It's a fat-soluble vitamin that's important for your immune system, vision, lungs, heart, and many other organs.

Vitamin A comes from both animal and plant-based foods. Animal sources like liver, eggs, and dairy provide preformed vitamin A (retinol), the active form your body can use right away, while plant foods like carrots, red and orange peppers, cantaloupe, sweet potatoes, and leafy greens (spinach, kale, and collard greens) supply provitamin A carotenoids, including beta-carotene, which your body has to convert into vitamin A.

Retinol promotes healthy cell turnover and overall skin health. It also plays an important role in eye health. As we age, we may notice changes in how well we see, especially when there isn't a lot of light. Vitamin A supports the formation of rhodopsin, a pigment that helps with night vision. Beta-carotene acts as an antioxidant in the body, which helps to protect our cells from oxidative stress.

The recommended daily allowance (RDA) for women ages nineteen to sixty-four is 700 micrograms (2,333 IU). A severe deficiency can lead to night blindness and eventually loss of vision.

Vitamin C: Also known as ascorbic acid, this powerful antioxidant helps protect cells from damage caused by free radicals, which are unstable molecules that can harm your cells and contribute to aging. I talk more about free radicals in the next section on antioxidants. Vitamin C helps the immune system work the way it should, which is especially important when we're stressed or going through hormonal shifts during perimenopause and menopause.

One of its main roles is producing collagen, a protein that helps keep skin firm, elastic, and glowing. As estrogen levels decrease during menopause, skin can lose elasticity, leading to more wrinkles and sagging skin. While vitamin C won't reverse the aging process, it may help reduce the appearance of some of these visible changes.

When you consume foods with vitamin C, your body uses it to help with the absorption of nonheme iron from plant-based sources. This is important for women of all ages, as low iron levels can lead to fatigue and anemia. As I mentioned in Chapter 9, having optimal iron levels is important for energy and a healthy immune system.

Symptoms of low or deficient levels of vitamin C include sensitive or bleeding gums due to the breakdown of collagen in connective tissue, irritability, bruising, fatigue, skin changes, and rough, bumpy skin.

The RDA for vitamin C is 75 mg per day for adult women nineteen and older, although experts feel this amount is too low and believe the intake should be closer to 200 mg a day. The tolerable upper intake is 2,000 mg/day.

Your body can't make or store very much vitamin C, so you need to get it from external sources. To make sure you're getting enough, eat a whole foods diet rich in colorful fruits and vegetables. Some excellent sources include kiwi, strawberries, citrus fruits, bell peppers, broccoli, Brussels sprouts, cauliflower, spinach, kale, tomatoes, and herbs like parsley and thyme. Three to five servings of raw fruits and vegetables a day can provide 200 mg or more of vitamin C.

Note: Storing food for too long and cooking it at high temperatures can lower vitamin C levels because it dissolves in water and breaks down when exposed to heat. Steaming your food, rather than boiling it, is a good option to help preserve it.

You can also take vitamin C as a supplement. It's best to take it in smaller doses throughout the day because your body absorbs less when you take a large dose all at once. Absorption is about 70–90 percent when you take a moderate amount (30–180 mg a day) but drops to less than 50 percent if you take more than 1,000 mg all at once. High-dose supplements of vitamin C are available, although more isn't necessarily better because the excess is excreted through urine. However, there are times when taking more may be helpful, like when you're stressed, feeling under the weather, or managing a specific medical condition. Speak to your doctor if you have kidney issues or hemochromatosis before taking higher amounts.

Vitamin D: Nicknamed the "sunshine vitamin," vitamin D is made by our body when our skin is directly exposed to UVB sunlight without sunscreen. However, many factors can affect your vitamin D levels, including where you live (the climate), time of day, time of year, lack of sunlight, aging, darker skin, poor nutrition, medical conditions, genetics, medications, obesity, and health conditions that affect metabolism and absorption, each of which can reduce the body's ability to produce or utilize vitamin D effectively. Interestingly, women, and people with insulin resistance, high blood pressure, obesity, high cholesterol, or kidney disease, are more likely to have low vitamin D levels.

Vitamin D is especially important for women in perimenopause and menopause. It supports bone health by helping the body absorb calcium and phosphorus, keeping bones and muscles strong, and lowering the risk of fractures and falls. However, it's important to note that vitamin D does not treat osteoporosis.

Vitamin D is really important for supporting a healthy immune system. Lower estrogen can affect how your immune system functions, which may change how your body responds to inflammation and infections. It may also help lower the risk of developing type 2 diabetes, although research is still evolving.

And bringing vitamin D levels into a healthy range may help improve mood and reduce fatigue in people who have low levels. A couple of years ago, my husband, who is usually Mr. Chill, started acting strange. He was always in a bad mood, which was so out of character for him, and he'd overreact to things that normally wouldn't bother him. I recommended he ask his doctor for a blood test to check his hormone levels because I thought maybe he was in andropause, or male menopause (yes, it's a thing!). He ended up finding out he was deficient in vitamin D, so he started supplementing with it, and within days (I'm not even exaggerating), his mood and energy levels were so much better, and after a few weeks he was back to his usual self.

When you're low in vitamin D, which about 50 percent of adults are, you may feel exhausted, achy, or stiff. You might notice joint or muscle pain, muscle weakness, sleep issues, sadness, irritability, or even hair loss. Chronically low levels have also been linked to weaker muscle strength. Another important thing to note is that if you have ongoing bone pain, it may be a sign you're deficient, so please ask your doctor for a blood test (I mention which test to ask for in a bit).

The RDA for vitamin D for women ages fifty-one to seventy is 600 IU, and for women seventy-one and older, it is 800 IU. According to the National Institutes of Health (NIH), most adults need 600–800 IU per day, but taking up to 4,000 IU is generally considered safe for most people. However, some experts and organizations believe many adults should be getting closer to between 2,000 and 5,000 IU a day.

Dr. Michael Holick, a leading vitamin D researcher with more than 600 peer-reviewed papers and over 150,000 citations in the fields of calcium, vitamin D, and bone metabolism, says that optimizing vitamin D levels may be linked with a lower risk of many health issues, including chronic inflammation, autoimmune conditions, and type 2 diabetes.

The Vitamin D Society recommends maintaining blood levels between 40 and 60 ng/mL (100 and 150 nmol/L), with the ideal being around 50 ng/mL (125 nmol/L). Some researchers say that this range is similar to levels seen in our hunter-gatherer ancestors who lived near the equator.

In my opinion, annual vitamin D testing should be mandatory for every woman in perimenopause and menopause (thirty-five and older). It's important to know what your levels are so you can supplement accordingly, if need be. Ask your doctor for a 25-hydroxyvitamin D or 25(OH)D blood test.

Dr. Holick's research shows that when you take a vitamin D supplement, the vitamin D in your bloodstream rises and then starts to fall within approximately seventy-two hours (three days), which is why taking it consistently helps to keep your levels steady in the long run. Most studies show that both forms of vitamin D, D3 (cholecalciferol) and D2 (ergocalciferol), increase blood levels. However, D3 is generally more potent and lasts longer in the body. It's also the form our bodies naturally make from sunlight. The form you take it in, meaning whether you take it as an oil, liquid, tablet, or capsule, matters less than dose and consistency, as they're all pretty well absorbed and converted into 25-hydroxyvitamin D, or 25(OH)D, in the body.

Low levels of magnesium can affect how your body activates and uses vitamin D. This is another reason it's important to ensure you're getting enough magnesium on a consistent basis. Speak to your doctor about checking your vitamin D levels at least once a year to ensure they're in the optimal range.

You may have heard that you should always take vitamin D with vitamin K2 to support bone and heart health. You actually don't! According to Dr. Holick, vitamin D works perfectly well on its own to support bone health. He also points out that the data supporting the combination for heart health is weak at best.

Some emerging research suggests vitamin K2, particularly in the MK7 form, may offer *additional support* for bone health in some people. For example, vitamin K may help switch on proteins that help build bone, but results are mixed. And since vitamin D helps your body absorb calcium, vitamin K may help guide calcium into the bones and teeth rather than soft tissues like the arteries. However, it's important to note that large studies *have not* found that taking vitamin D supplements on its own increases the risk of heart disease.

Other research has looked into whether taking vitamin D together with vitamin K2 MK7 (menaquinone-7) may be more effective at slowing bone loss in menopausal women than taking either one alone. Early studies have also looked at the potential benefits of the combination for cardiovascular health, but findings are mixed.

Researchers often use the MK7 form because it's well absorbed and stays active in the body longer.

Vitamin K also has its own important health benefits, which I'll discuss after the next section.

Food sources of vitamin D include salmon, mackerel, herring, cod liver oil, fortified cow's milk, fortified orange juice, plant-based beverages, and mushrooms exposed to sunlight. As you can see, this isn't a very long list, and since it's really hard to reach the recommended minimum of 600 IUs a day from food alone, you may want to consider supplementing if you need to increase your levels.

Vitamin E: This vitamin is also an antioxidant with powerful health benefits that help to counteract oxidative stress, fighting the signs of aging both inside and out.

Food sources include nuts, seeds, avocados, olive oil, sunflower seeds, spinach, broccoli, and whole grains.

It's important to know that not all forms of vitamin E are the same when taken as a supplement. While alpha-tocopherol is the most researched form, tocotrienol, a unique type of vitamin E, may act as a more powerful antioxidant. Research shows that tocotrienol (specifically delta and gamma types) may help lower LDL cholesterol and triglycerides, regulate blood sugar, lower blood pressure, improve brain health and memory, decrease fat in the liver, speed up wound healing, support weight loss, and help reduce bone loss. It may even promote hair growth due to its anti-inflammatory benefits.

Tocotrienol can be sourced from palm[*] and rice,[**] but the highest concentration of gamma and delta[***] comes from annatto, a natural food coloring and flavoring agent made from the seeds of the achiote tree. To date, there have been more than twenty human clinical studies done on annatto tocotrienol, and the suggested dose is 125–300 mg a day.

Since tocotrienol is fat-soluble, take it with a meal for better absorption. If you're already taking a vitamin E supplement that contains alpha-tocopherol, take it at least six hours apart from tocotrienol, as tocopherol can interfere with the absorption of tocotrienol. I interviewed Dr. Barrie Tan, the man who discovered tocotrienol, on my podcast, *Menopause Reimagined*, episode #78.

Vitamin K: This fat-soluble vitamin has gained a lot of popularity because of its role in blood clotting, brain, and bone health.

It exists in two main forms: phylloquinone (K1) and menaqui-

---

[*] 75% as tocotrienol and 25% as tocopherol.
[**] 50% as tocotrienol and 50% as tocopherol.
[***] 100% as tocotrienol and 0% as tocopherol.

nones (K2). K2 has several subtypes, with the most studied being MK4 and MK7. Vitamin K1 primarily supports blood clotting, works quickly, and is cleared relatively fast from the body. Vitamin K2, on the other hand, lasts longer in the body and has been studied for its potential role in supporting bone health in (post)menopausal women.

Adequate intake for vitamin K1 is 90 mcg for adult women. There currently isn't an official Adequate Intake for K2, but a common range found in supplements is between 90 and 120 mcg. These amounts are generally considered safe and are based on doses often used in research.

Note: If you're on blood thinners, be mindful of how much vitamin K you're getting, including both K1 and K2. Speak to your doctor before taking supplements that contain vitamin K or making major changes to your diet.

Phylloquinone (K1) is found in greens such as mustard, spinach, and Swiss chard; cruciferous vegetables like kale, cabbage, and Brussels sprouts; and herbs including parsley, basil, and cilantro. Menaquinones (K2, especially MK7) are found in fermented foods like natto and some cheeses, particularly aged or fermented varieties like gouda, Brie, and edam. MK4 is found in animal products (eggs, dairy, and meat), and it's naturally made in your body from K1.

Because vitamin K is a fat-soluble vitamin, it's best absorbed when eaten with food that contains fat. You can also take it as a supplement.

B Vitamins: B vitamins support our entire nervous system, and we use more of them during times of stress. Because most of us are under more stress and have less resilience than we used to, keeping B vitamin levels steady is crucial for energy, mood, focus, and handling stress.

Vitamins B1 (thiamine), B2 (riboflavin), and B3 (niacin) help your body turn food into energy and may help fight fatigue. B5 (pantothenic acid) helps your body make energy and cope better with stress, and B7 (biotin) supports healthy hair and skin. Pyridoxine, or B6, is important for mood because it helps make brain chemicals like gamma-aminobutyric acid (GABA) and serotonin. Folate, or B9, helps your body make DNA and red blood cells, and supports

WORDS OF CAUTION

Folic Acid vs. Folate: Best known for preventing neural tube defects during pregnancy, folic acid is a common ingredient in multivitamins and other prenatal supplements. Women in perimenopause and menopause may be taking it for heart, brain, and bone health. About 30–40 percent of the population has a variation in the MTHFR gene that can make it harder to convert folic acid (the synthetic form) into methylfolate, the active form your body uses. Folate found naturally in food is generally well absorbed and used by the body. If you know you carry this gene (confirmed with genetic testing), talk with a practitioner before supplementing with folic acid, since they may recommend products with 5-MTHF (5 methyltetrahydrofolate) or folinic acid instead.

B12: Methylcobalamin is the natural, active form of B12 that your body can use right away, and may be a better choice for people with certain absorption problems or methylation issues. Cyanocobalamin is a synthetic form that needs to be converted in the body, but most people can handle the conversion without a problem.

B6: Although B6 is water soluble like other B vitamins, too much can build up in the body with long-term use or high-dose supplements and cause nerve damage in the arms and legs that may not be reversible (called peripheral neuropathy). The form of B6 to be most mindful of is pyridoxine HCl, which is the type that's most often linked to this risk. If you have symptoms like tingling, burning, numbness, electric shocks, pain in your hands or feet, nausea, tinnitus, or burning skin, ask your doctor to check your B6 levels.

heart health. This type of B vitamin is especially important if you have an MTHFR gene variant, which can affect how your body uses folate (you can find out if you have it by getting genetic testing). B12 is important for brain function and energy, but it becomes harder to absorb from food after the age of fifty because of lower stomach acid and other digestive changes.

Many signs of low B vitamins can look similar to perimenopause and menopause symptoms, including:

- Irritability or mood changes (often B1, B6, B9/folate, or B12)

- Fatigue or tiredness (B1, B5, B9/folate, or B12)

- Tingling, numbness, or pins and needles in hands and feet (B1, B6, B9/folate, or B12)

- Burning feet (mainly B5, but also B1 or B6)

- Thinning hair and brittle nails (B7/biotin, sometimes B9/folate)

- Memory problems, poor concentration, or confusion (B12, B9/folate, B1, or B6)

- Digestive upset like nausea or poor appetite (B3, B9/folate, or B12)

- Dry or irritated eyes (most commonly B2)

- Skin rashes or rough, scaly skin (B2, B3, B6, and more rarely B7/biotin)

- Muscle weakness or unsteady movement (B1, B6, B12, or B5)

- Headaches, heart palpitations, or shortness of breath (most often B9/folate or B12)

Other symptoms include cracks in the corners of your mouth (B2 or B6) or a sore, swollen, or red tongue (B2, B9/folate, B12, or B6).

The Bs work best as a team and are commonly found together

in foods like whole grains, nuts and seeds, legumes, eggs, dairy, meat, and dark leafy green vegetables. Vitamin B12 is the exception, as it's only found in animal foods, so if you're vegan or vegetarian, you may need to supplement with it. Ask your doctor to check your levels with a blood test.

You can also take B vitamins in supplement form. Look for a balanced B-complex formula. I take them a few times a week, or during high stress periods when I feel I need the extra support.

Almighty Antioxidants

You're probably familiar with the term *antioxidants*, but what are they exactly, and how do they work in the body?

Think of antioxidants as your body's cleanup crew, neutralizing unstable molecules, called free radicals, that can damage cells and are believed to be a major factor in aging and many degenerative diseases. This kind of damage is known as oxidative stress, and if oxidative stress is too high for too long, it can lead to inflammation, heart disease, and certain types of cancer.

Free radicals are produced during normal body processes like metabolism, but many lifestyle and environmental exposures create them too. Physical and emotional stress, alcohol, pesticides, certain food additives, high blood sugar, air pollution, cigarette smoke, and infections all add to the overall load your body has to manage.

As you enter perimenopause and menopause, hormonal changes can increase oxidative stress, which may trigger or worsen symptoms like fatigue, inflammation, hot flashes, mood swings, depression, and anxiety. Over time, it can raise the risk of long-term issues like cardiovascular disease and osteoporosis.

Antioxidants help to support your body during these changes by reducing free radicals and oxidative stress.

You can get antioxidants from many foods. To make sure you're getting enough, focus on a diet rich in plant-based foods. Fruits and vegetables are some of the best sources. The top choices in these categories include cruciferous veggies (broccoli, cauliflower, cabbage, Brussels sprouts, arugula, kale, bok choy, turnip, and collard greens), berries (all kinds), carrots, spinach, sweet potatoes, purple potatoes, red cabbage, artichokes, green tea, asparagus, avocados, beets, squash, herbs and spices (like turmeric, ginger, clove, oregano, rosemary, cumin, parsley, and cinnamon), and dark chocolate (without added sugar).

Some standout antioxidants that are especially helpful during perimenopause and menopause include:

- **Oleocanthal:** Found mostly in high-quality extra virgin olive oil, oleocanthal has strong anti-inflammatory and antioxidant properties, and may help lessen joint discomfort and support heart health. Both animal and early human studies suggest that olive oil may help protect the brain and possibly lower the risk of neurodegenerative diseases like Alzheimer's and Parkinson's, but more research on humans is needed.

- **Phenolic compounds:** These plant chemicals are known for their antioxidant and anti-inflammatory properties. More than eight thousand phenolic compounds have been identified in different plant species, with flavonoids being the largest and most studied group. Phenolic compounds may help women in perimenopause and menopause by lowering oxidative stress and inflammation, and may also support heart, bone, and brain health.

  In a large ten-year observational study of women aged thirty-six to eighty, those who ate the most flavonoid-rich foods had a lower risk of developing depression. The strongest mood benefits were seen in women over fifty who ate the most flavonoid foods, compared to those who ate the least.

  Examples of phenolic compounds include quercetin (apples, onions), catechins (tea, berries, cocoa), resveratrol (grapes, peanuts, berries), coumaric acid (berries, spices), caffeic acid (coffee, apples, pears, artichokes), lignans (flaxseeds, sesame seeds), proanthocyanidins (cranberries, cocoa, apples, cinnamon), and anthocyanins (berries).

- **Carotenoids:** Carotenoids are potent antioxidants found in colorful fruits and veggies. There are more than six hundred different types of these plant pigments, and they too help to reduce oxidative stress and inflammation in the body. The most common carotenoids include beta-carotene, lutein, lycopene, and zeaxanthin. Food sources include carrots, dark leafy greens, egg yolks, tomatoes, pink grapefruit, red and orange peppers, butternut squash, spinach, and kale.

Antioxidants often work best together as part of a varied diet, along with other nutrients and plant chemicals (polyphenols) found in foods. For example:

» **Strawberries:** The antioxidants responsible for their bright red color are called anthocyanins. When combined with vitamin C, this powerful duo supports immunity and reduces oxidative stress.

» **Tomatoes:** The combination of lycopene, an antioxidant in tomatoes, and other antioxidants like beta-carotene (carrots, orange peppers) helps to support heart health and may reduce the risk of certain cancers.

» **Green tea:** Catechins, a type of polyphenol with strong antioxidant properties, contribute to this tea's amazing health benefits. Drinking green tea with vitamin C foods (like a slice of lemon) enhances its antioxidant effects. A 2025 review of clinical trials found that catechins found in green tea, including EGCG, may help support healthy aging, heart health, and overall wellness.

Caution: Drinking green tea on an empty stomach can cause nausea. This happens to me, so I wanted to share these tips. The tannins and caffeine in tea made from the *Camellia sinensis* plant (like green, black, oolong, and white tea) can make your stomach produce more acid and irritate its lining. If this happens to you, try steeping it for less time, drinking decaf, or eating something right before or while drinking it. This usually isn't an issue with herbal teas since most are caffeine-free and lower in tannins.

» **Curcumin:** Turmeric has incredible antioxidant and anti-inflammatory properties. Curcumin, its active ingredient, is best absorbed when combined with black pepper, which contains piperine, a compound that can increase absorption by up to 2,000 percent!

Tip: Spices are packed with antioxidants, and studies show that some spices, gram for gram, have antioxidant power up to ten times higher than many fruits and vegetables! Spices that have the highest amounts of antioxidants are cloves, cinnamon, turmeric, ginger, oregano, thyme, rosemary, sumac, and sage. Adding a variety of spices and herbs to your diet can substantially raise your antioxidant intake.

Additional Nutrients for Women in Perimenopause and Menopause

Black Seed Oil (*Nigella Sativa*)

Black seed oil (BSO), also known as black cumin, has been used for thousands of years by many cultures. It's been studied for a variety of health conditions that often show up during perimenopause and menopause, including digestive, respiratory, immune, memory, and cardiometabolic concerns. I talked about cardiometabolic health in Chapter 5, and it covers the heart, blood vessels, and metabolic factors like blood sugar control, insulin sensitivity, obesity, fatty liver, inflammation, blood pressure, cholesterol, and triglycerides. In smaller studies, BSO has also been shown to have promising effects for arthritis and joint pain, as well as Hashimoto's thyroiditis.

Studies in menopausal women suggest that taking BSO may improve total cholesterol, triglycerides, LDL, HDL, and blood sugar control. A small 2025 pilot study published in *Nutrients* found that taking 800 mg of BSO a day for eight weeks was associated with lower blood pressure, fewer hot flashes and night sweats, and some weight loss.

A BSO supplement should:

- Be cold-pressed, meaning the oil is extracted without using heat (which damages its effectiveness)

- Be standardized to 3 percent for thymoquinone, the main active ingredient, to ensure consistent strength and effectiveness

- Contain less than 1.25 percent free fatty acids. Free fatty acids can go rancid, which compromises the thymoquinone and makes it less effective. The balance between thymoquinone and free fatty acids is critical for optimal results, making it easier for the body to absorb.

Look for a branded BSO like ThymoQuin®, which will have all the above qualities. That way you know you're getting a high-quality product with maximum benefits.

The suggested dose is 500 mg a day taken on an empty stomach. If you can't take it on an empty stomach, then take it with a small amount of food.

EstroG-100®

A good friend of mine introduced me to this ingredient when I was suffering from hot flashes and night sweats. He told me there was good human research on how it helps with different perimenopause and menopause symptoms, including vasomotor symptoms (hot flashes and night sweats), vaginal dryness, fatigue, sleep quality, nervousness, joint pain and inflammation, libido, moods and emotions (sadness), vertigo, paresthesia (pins and needles), and abnormal skin sensations like crawling skin. It's made from a combination of three herbs, *Cynanchum wilfordii*, *Angelica gigas*, and *Phlomis umbrosa*, and studies have shown it doesn't bind to estrogen receptors, so it's nonestrogenic.

The daily dosage is 514 mg, and it can be taken all at once or in divided doses.

Reasons to Consider Taking Supplements in Perimenopause and Menopause

Food should always be your first go-to, as you can't out-supplement poor nutrition. The word *supplement* means something that *adds* to your main routine, not something that *replaces* it. Supplements can help you reach your daily nutrient goals or give you an extra boost, but they can't, and shouldn't, replace real food, unless a doctor or healthcare professional tells you otherwise. Everyone's body is different, so please always consult your primary care physician before taking anything new.

I believe there's a time and place for supplements once you're in perimenopause and menopause. Here are some important reasons to consider adding them to your routine:

- **Digestive changes:** Reduced stomach acid, chronic or new food sensitivities, and inflammation can all interfere with how well your body breaks down and absorbs nutrients.

- **Nutrient intake:** You may not be eating enough to meet your body's needs, or you might be eating too many ultra-processed foods that lack key vitamins, minerals, and antioxidants.

- **Vitamin D levels:** If you don't get much sunlight, your body may produce less vitamin D.

- **Smoking:** Smoking can deplete important nutrients such as vitamins C and E, antioxidants, and several B vitamins.

- **Medications:** Certain prescription medications can block the absorption of or deplete nutrients, including vitamins and minerals.

- **Symptom support:** If you want to manage perimenopause and menopause symptoms without medications or hormone therapy, supplements can play a role. You can also take them alongside hormone therapy when appropriate, provided there are no interactions. Always work with your healthcare provider to discuss what's right for you.

By keeping these factors in mind, supplements can help cover nutrition gaps and provide additional options to manage your symptoms.

These last few chapters covered the building blocks of nutrition, providing a foundation for fueling and defending our cells from daily wear and tear as we enter perimenopause and menopause. Next, we'll put it all together with a simple eating plan.

11.

Eating Your Way Through Perimenopause and Menopause

By this stage of life, most of us realize there are things we can't control, but we also know there's a lot we can. The choices we make about what we put in and on our bodies are more important now than ever, from the food we eat to the products we use every day. Those daily decisions can make a powerful difference in how we feel and our long-term health.

As your body transitions, so do your nutritional needs. The focus now is less about calories and more about the quality of the foods you're eating and how they make you feel. Do they support

Now that you're in perimenopause or menopause, extreme dieting, severely restricting calories, and exercising to exhaustion can take a real toll on your body, raising cortisol levels, slowing your metabolism, and causing you to store more fat, especially around your midsection. Your body needs enough food to keep your bones and muscles strong and your energy stable. Your brain alone uses about 20–25 percent of the calories you eat every day, and it needs proper nourishment to think clearly. Focus on nourishing your body with enough whole, nutritious foods, managing stress, making sleep a priority, building and keeping your muscles strong, and exercising with intention.

your energy, mood, and hormones? Or do they make you feel anxious, inflamed, and exhausted? Reading food labels, understanding ingredients, and choosing foods that nourish your body and mind give you back a sense of control and confidence to thrive in this next chapter of your life.

Up until this point, I've shared *why* and *how* your body is changing in perimenopause and menopause and what's driving those changes. Now, I want to put it all together to give you clear, actionable steps that make a real difference in your day-to-day life, steps that help you feel like yourself again while also honoring the strong, new version of you that's emerging.

I created the acronym B.A.L.A.N.C.E. to make the basic nutrition principles I recommend easier to remember. These are the principles that help you get started and stay consistent in the long run. Balance is exactly what we need most right now.

Here's what B.A.L.A.N.C.E. stands for:

B: Balance blood sugar levels

A: Add more fiber

L: Load up on protein

A: Add good-quality fats

N: Nurture digestion

C: Choose more plants

E: Ensure you're hydrated

Let's dive into each of these principles:

Principle #1: Balance Blood Sugar Levels

If there was one thing I could tell my younger self, I'd say to do whatever I could to support my blood sugar and insulin levels. It's been a central theme in the book so far because it drives so many of the symptoms and changes we're dealing with. That's why I made it the first principle.

When your blood sugar levels are steady, your energy and mood are too. It makes it easier for key hormones like estrogen, progesterone, cortisol, and insulin to do their jobs, and it improves sleep. It also supports brain and metabolic health, lowering the risk of cardiovascular disease, type 2 diabetes, and chronic inflammation.

As we learned in Chapter 5, when your blood sugar levels are stable, your body runs more smoothly. It uses carbohydrates for longer-lasting energy and keeps insulin more balanced.

But if your blood sugar is high, low, or constantly fluctuating, it can lead to metabolic issues like insulin resistance, which we're more prone to now. It can cause weight gain, especially around the belly, make it harder to lose weight, make you feel hungrier, and cause cravings. As time goes on, it can increase inflammation and mood swings, and affect the way your hormones, brain, organs, and body function, including your liver, pancreas, kidneys, teeth and gums, immune and nervous systems, heart, feet, and eyes.

I previously explained why it's harder to keep your blood sugar regulated now that you're in perimenopause and menopause, and how both chronically high and unstable blood sugar levels can raise your risk for serious conditions like type 2 diabetes, dementia, and cardiovascular disease.

This is why doing your best to manage your blood sugar levels is important for long-term health.

It's never too early or late to start. Being mindful of what you're eating and drinking, how much you're moving and exercising, and how you're handling stress are all important factors when it comes to balancing blood sugar.

Supporting Healthy Blood Sugar Levels

I went into detail about blood sugar support, management, and insulin resistance in Chapter 5, and in this chapter I'll share even more actionable steps.

Since nutrition plays an important role when it comes to balancing blood sugar levels, let's start with that:

- **Never eat carbs alone; always pair them with some protein and fat.** When you eat or drink carbs by themselves, they can cause your blood sugar to spike quickly and then crash. Eat

WHAT ABOUT LOW-CARB DIETS?

A low-carb diet may seem like a quick fix for balancing blood sugar, but it's far from the whole answer. Many women in perimenopause and menopause do well with some fiber-rich, whole food carbohydrates rather than cutting them out completely. While cutting out carbs can lower blood sugar in the short term, especially if you're insulin resistant or have type 2 diabetes, having a healthy metabolism isn't about avoiding them altogether; it's about helping your body switch between burning sugar and fat for energy, a process called *metabolic flexibility*. Long-term metabolic flexibility comes from a balanced approach that includes both carbs and fat.

A low-carb diet doesn't solve the underlying issues with *how* your body processes glucose, which are often at the heart of blood sugar imbalances. Here's the thing: Your brain, muscles (during exercise), and certain tissues depend on glucose to function properly. When you don't eat enough carbs, your body turns to a process called gluconeogenesis, which means "making new glucose." It does this by converting amino acids (from protein in foods or muscle tissue) and glycerol (from fat) into glucose. Making it this way is more work for your body, so eating an extremely low-carb diet for a long time can be more demanding than simply getting some glucose from carbs.

When you're stressed (whether it's physical, emotional, or metabolic stress, like not eating enough or eating very low carb),

sweet potatoes with chicken, berries with slivered almonds and Greek yogurt, and apple slices with nut butter.

- **Drink vinegar before carbs.** Before eating a meal rich in carbohydrates, drink a glass of water (8–10 ounces) with 1 tablespoon of vinegar (any type is fine: apple cider, wine, or rice). The acetic acid in vinegar (and in pickled foods) slows down the digestion of carbohydrates and reduces the rate at which sugar enters your

your body releases cortisol. Cortisol tells your body it needs fuel or glucose *now* to handle that stress. If there isn't enough glucose available because you skipped a meal, cut carbs too low, or your glycogen stores are already depleted, your body starts pulling glycogen from the liver. If your glycogen stores are also too low, it will start burning fat for immediate energy, but as we saw in Chapter 6, chronically high cortisol levels encourage your body to hold on to belly fat, so this becomes counterproductive. As time goes on, your body may also break down muscle tissue, especially if you're following a long-term ultra-low-carb diet.

Now you might be wondering: Can my body use fat to make energy? That's a great question, and yes, it can! It does that through a process called ketogenesis, where your body turns fat into ketones (you might already be familiar with this term if you've tried a keto diet). However, some parts of your body, like your brain and red blood cells, still need glucose to function properly. That's why following a low-carb diet for too long at this stage of life may cause your body to start breaking down muscle to make glucose for energy, especially if you're not eating enough protein or calories.

So choose complex carbohydrates like sweet potatoes and squash instead of simple carbs like white bread and white rice, as they'll take longer to digest and provide steadier support for energy and blood sugar.

bloodstream. Doing this could lower your blood sugar after a meal, in some cases by around 20–30 percent. Another option is to add a tablespoon or two of vinegar into your homemade salad dressing and eat the salad as an appetizer.

- **Cool your starches.** After cooking starchy foods (like potatoes, rice, pasta, or bread), let them cool in the refrigerator for at least twenty-four hours before eating or reheating them. The cooling process changes some of the starch into a type called "resistant starch" (through a process called starch retrogradation), which is harder for your body to digest. Instead of being fully broken down in the small intestine, it moves through to your large intestine, where it feeds the healthy bacteria in your gut. Those healthy bacteria then produce postbiotics like short-chain fatty acids (including butyrate) that support gut health (see Chapter 4). An easy way to remember this hack is to think of it as "cook-cool-eat-or-reheat." Choose sweet potatoes, purple potatoes, or smaller potatoes over larger white ones (like russet), as they won't raise your blood sugar as quickly, and boiling them instead of baking them will also help lower the impact on blood sugar.

- **Add cinnamon.** Research from 2025 shows that taking two capsules of cinnamon (1,000 mg/day) helped to lower fasting glucose, especially in people with type 2 diabetes. While there is some evidence that dietary cinnamon (specifically Ceylon) may improve blood sugar levels in some people, it isn't conclusive. However, it shouldn't stop you from adding cinnamon to your food and beverages. Sprinkle it into your smoothies, coffee, and tea, on top of hot cereal or yogurt, or mix some with nuts and seeds. I love it on sliced or baked apples (yum!).

- **Eat in an orderly fashion.** The order in which you eat your food, called food sequencing, may help. Starting with fiber-rich veggies, then eating quality fats, then protein, and saving your carbs for last can help with digestion and keep your blood sugar more stable. What would this look like? Eat your salad or veggies first, tossed with your favorite dressing. Next, eat your protein (chicken, meat, fish, or organic tofu), and finish with your carbs (brown rice, sweet potato, squash, or quinoa).

Principle #2: Add More Fiber

How much fiber do you get a day?

Take a guess.

On average, we eat about 12–15 grams of fiber a day, which is about half of the 25–30 grams recommended by many health experts, including me.

Getting enough fiber is important at every stage of life, but it becomes especially important for supporting healthy hormone levels during perimenopause and menopause, because fiber helps your body process and clear estrogen it no longer needs. I explained this in Chapter 4.

The liver helps break down estrogen into a form your body can clear, which supports hormonal balance and may ease estrogen-related symptoms such as bloating, constipation, and sore breasts.

Here's how fiber can help:

- Fiber is another way to help support healthy blood sugar levels and lower your risk of type 2 diabetes. Soluble fiber, in particular, slows down the absorption of glucose (sugar) in your bloodstream, preventing spikes after you eat carbs. This helps to stabilize your blood sugar levels.

- Fiber can help with weight management. It adds bulk to your stomach, making you feel fuller faster, curbing your hunger and appetite. There's research linking increased dietary fiber to ideal body weight and better weight management, including a lower risk of obesity.

- Fiber helps keep you regular. This is really important, because fiber binds to broken-down (metabolized) estrogen in the gut and helps to remove it through your stool. Without enough fiber and regular bowel movements, that estrogen can be reabsorbed instead of being cleared from the body, potentially leading to symptoms like PMS or heavy periods if you're in pre- or perimenopause, as well as other estrogen-related symptoms such as bloating, breast swelling or tenderness, and water retention.

- In addition to estrogen, soluble fiber binds to and removes (via your stool) cholesterol (which tends to rise during menopause), as well as bile acids. It also feeds your gut bacteria and helps your body remove waste by forming a gel-like substance that softens and bulks stool, making it easier to pass through your colon.

- Fiber helps reduce the risk of cardiovascular disease and bowel diseases, such as irritable bowel syndrome, diverticulosis, diverticulitis, hemorrhoids, and polyps. It has also been shown to lower the risk of many types of cancer, including ovarian, colon, and breast. A meta-analysis and systematic review of twenty studies found that eating high amounts of fiber may be associated with a lower chance of getting breast cancer. This was true for both soluble and insoluble fiber and for women across the years leading up to and including menopause.

- Dietary fiber from a variety of plant foods supports a healthy gut microbiome. The more diverse your gut microbiome is, the better your overall physical and mental health tends to be.

- Finally, fiber has been shown to reduce inflammation and can reduce the risk of some diseases or slow down their progression. The good bacteria in your gut help break down the fiber you eat into short-chain fatty acids (SCFAs) that can fight off inflammation and help prevent long-term health issues.

The two forms of fiber are *soluble* and *insoluble*. Plant foods in their natural form typically have both types.

Soluble fiber: This type of fiber helps with blood sugar control and lowers cholesterol. Soluble fiber dissolves in water. Think of it as a sponge, soaking up cholesterol and helping your body clear and regulate certain hormones. Soluble fiber feeds the good bacteria in your gut, helping them produce short-chain fatty acids (butyrate, propionate, and acetate), which support gut health and reduce inflammation.

Insoluble fiber: Think of this type of fiber as "roughage." Picture it as a broom that sweeps debris and waste products through the colon, pushing them out of the body. It gives bulk to your stools, making them larger and softer. Whole grains, nuts, seeds, and the skins of fruits and vegetables are good sources.

We need to get both types of fiber every single day.

Note: Animal products, such as meat, fish, poultry, eggs, and dairy, as well as refined grains used in white rice and white pasta, contain little or no fiber.

Now, let's circle back to my question at the beginning of this section: *How much fiber do you get a day?* Are you reaching the recommended goal of 25–30 grams? If not, track your fiber intake.

Fiber is found in whole plant foods like fruits, veggies, nuts and seeds, legumes, and whole grains. Examples include:

Insoluble Fiber Sources (Mostly)	*Soluble Fiber Sources (Mostly)*
• Bran	• Steel-cut oats (unsweetened)
• The skin of raw fruits: e.g., apples, pears, peaches, and plums	• Legumes: e.g., dried beans and lentils
• Berries*	• The flesh of apples, pears, and peaches
• Green leafy vegetables: e.g., kale, spinach, cabbage, and collard greens	• Citrus, especially the pith (white part inside the peel)
• Vegetables, especially broccoli, cauliflower, Brussels sprouts, green beans, and zucchini (with the skin)	• Berries
• Whole grains: e.g., whole wheat, bulgur, brown rice, oats, quinoa, hulled barley, rye, millet, and whole-grain cereals	• Vegetables, especially carrots (with their peels), winter squash (butternut, acorn, and kabocha), sweet potatoes, asparagus, artichokes, okra, Brussels sprouts, beets, turnips, onions, and garlic
• Seeds: flaxseeds (whole), chia, pumpkin, basil, sunflower, and sesame seeds	• Seeds: e.g., flaxseed (ground), chia, basil, and hemp hearts
• Nuts: e.g., almonds (with skin), walnuts, pecans, and pistachios	• Pectin-rich foods, including citrus, apples, plums, berries, cooked carrots, tomato skins, and sweet potato peels
	• Avocado

Note: Most whole plant foods contain both soluble and insoluble fiber. These lists highlight foods that tend to provide more of one type than the other.

* Seeds contribute insoluble fiber, while the flesh contributes soluble fiber.

Tips to maximize fiber:

- Whenever possible, eat fruits and vegetables with their skins or peels on. That's where most of the fiber is found, as well as extra nutrients and antioxidants. Be sure to wash them before eating, even if they're organic.

- Eat vegetables and fruits (including the membranes, pith, and pulp) whole for maximum fiber content.

- Cook certain vegetables like carrots, sweet potatoes, or okra to soften fiber to make them easier for your gut to digest.

- Seeds are a great source of fiber. A tablespoon of chia seeds has 5 grams of fiber, and a tablespoon of basil seeds has 7.5 grams of fiber. Soaking them for 10–15 minutes helps to activate and enhance their soluble fiber benefits.

Adding More Fiber to Your Diet

Here are some tips on how to add more fiber to your diet:

1. Grind 1–2 tablespoons of ground flaxseeds into your yogurt, salad, or smoothies.

2. Add 1–2 tablespoons of basil or chia seeds to water, iced tea, smoothies, or yogurt.

3. Try to include some veggies whenever you can. Even a few carrot sticks count!

4. Choose 100 percent whole-grain products. Try new grains such as farro, purple rice, and millet (my fave!) to mix things up.

5. If you can tolerate beans and legumes, add them to salads, chili, and soups. Make bean spreads and dips and enjoy them with raw veggies.

6. Read labels and choose foods and beverages that have 4 or more grams of fiber per serving.

7. Consider a soluble fiber supplement (refer to Chapter 8 for what to look for).

8. If need be, try spreading out your fiber throughout the day instead of getting it all in at once, as it makes it easier on your digestion and helps to keep things moving smoothly.

9. And be sure to drink lots of water when increasing your fiber intake to help things move along your colon.

Principle #3: Load Up on Protein

As you read in Chapter 8, protein is a building block of the body, and it's important for different structures and functions, including muscles, bones, skin, hair, nails, tissues, organs, metabolism, and the immune system. And as we go into perimenopause and menopause, we need to make sure we're getting enough of it! Protein supports your bones and muscles, builds and repairs tissues, helps with energy and hormone production (some hormones are made of proteins), keeps skin firm by supporting collagen, helps keep blood sugar steady, and supports brain health. In short, getting enough protein becomes even more important for feeling strong, stable, and energized during this time of our lives.

How Much Protein Do You Need in Perimenopause and Menopause?

This is a great question, and one you'll get many different answers for depending on what your goal is. What we do know from current research is that women over forty need more protein than women under forty, and women in perimenopause and menopause need more protein than women in premenopause to support muscle, metabolism, and overall health. Getting enough protein helps keep your muscles and bones strong, helps stabilize blood sugar and insulin levels, supports steady energy, may help with mood and focus, supports your metabolism and immune system, and helps manage weight by keeping hunger and cravings under control.

Depending on who you ask or where you look, you'll find rec-ommendations for protein intake ranging anywhere from 0.8 to

2 grams of protein per kilogram of body weight per day, with many experts suggesting between 1.0 and 1.6 grams per kilogram.

A study in *Frontiers in Nutrition* (May 2024) suggested that older adults (sixty and over) would benefit from getting around 30 grams of protein at each meal, starting with the first meal of the day, to build and maintain muscle.

After reviewing the research, speaking to other nutrition and fitness experts, and taking my personal experience into account, I believe an appropriate and fair starting point for calculating daily protein needs for women in perimenopause and menopause is around 1.2 to 1.4 grams per kilogram of body weight (about 0.5 to 0.6 grams of protein per pound of body weight).

To keep it simple, for most women:

- If you're under 140 pounds, aim for a *minimum* of 60–75 grams of protein a day. This works out to 20–25 grams at each meal, assuming you're eating three meals a day.

- If you're over 140 pounds, aim for a *minimum* of 75–90 grams. This works out to 25–30 grams at each meal, assuming you're eating three meals a day.

Now *adjust that amount according to your needs and lifestyle.* A few factors to consider when figuring out the right amount of protein for *your* body include:

- **Height, weight, activity level, and personal goals.**
    If you're sedentary, the baseline amount may be enough for you.
    If you're taller or have a larger frame, your protein needs will be higher.
    If you're active (e.g., lift weights, go for daily walks, do High Intensity Interval Training [HIIT] exercises, etc.), you'll need more protein to repair and rebuild muscle, support bone strength, and help reduce post-workout aches and pains.
    If you're an athlete, your protein needs will be significantly higher, closer to 1.4–2.2 grams per kilogram of body weight per

day (approximately 0.6 to 1 gram of protein per pound of body weight), depending on training volume and type, says Selene Yeager from Feisty Menopause. She suggests, in addition to getting 25–30 grams at meals, also including 15–20 grams at snack time.

While 25–30 grams of protein at each meal is a great general guideline for most women, you can calculate exactly how much you need by using this online calculator from Calculator.net (https://www.calculator.net/protein-calculator.html). You can also speak to a qualified healthcare or nutrition expert.

Other things to keep in mind about protein include:

- **Are you still hungry after a big meal?** If so, you may need more protein. This is a big one for me. I know if I've had enough protein (and food) by how snacky I am afterward. When I eat enough protein in one sitting, I'm satiated for hours and have fewer cravings for carbs. Make protein the center of each meal.

- **Symptoms:** Watch for signs of weakness, hair thinning or loss, dull or sagging skin, slow wound healing, frequent sores inside the nose or mouth, mood changes, and muscle wasting. All these may be associated with a low protein intake or not absorbing it properly.

- **Harder to digest:** Protein can be harder to digest as we age and go into perimenopause and menopause because our stomach acid production can decrease, making digestion more challenging. Be sure to revisit the digestion tips in Chapter 4, especially if you're experiencing bloating, gas, or heaviness after eating a meal high in protein. Supporting healthy digestion will help your body properly break it down and absorb it.

Tip: If you can't reach your daily target with food alone, try a high-quality protein powder.

Tip: Spread your protein out over the course of the day. This will help digestion, keep your energy levels up, and help you feel fuller longer.

Protein helps your body make and regulate hormones, like thyroid, insulin, glucagon, and many made by the adrenal glands. It also supports the processes that help keep sex hormones in balance and working properly.

Not getting enough protein may be associated with memory issues, mood changes like depression and anxiety, irritability and moodiness, a lack of motivation, and feeling more easily overwhelmed by stress. It can also leave you feeling drowsy or fatigued. Eventually, low protein intake can lead to sarcopenia, or muscle loss. In fact, a 2017 study found that (post)menopausal women who ate more protein and stayed active had more muscle than those who didn't.

Protein helps you feel full and satisfied after eating by stimulating the release of hormones such as glucagon-like peptide-1 (GLP-1), cholecystokinin (CCK), and peptide YY (PYY), which help to manage hunger and control cravings.

How to Identify Protein in Foods

You'll find the amount of protein *per serving* listed on the Nutrition Facts panel.

You can use the chart on the next page as a guide. It is a short reference list. For a more detailed list, visit www.nourishingmeno pausebook.com and click on the Resources tab.

Balance your protein choices with nutrient-rich foods such as vegetables, low-glycemic fruits, good-quality fats, complex carbohydrates, nuts, seeds, and legumes. Include probiotic-rich foods and omega-3 fatty acids.

Note: If you have kidney disease or are at risk for it, consult your doctor before increasing your protein intake.

Principle #4: Add Good-Quality Fats

Gen Xers, baby boomers, and older millennials grew up in the era of "low fat is better" and "fat makes us fat." This message is so ingrained in our brains that many of us still fear fat. So much has changed as far as that thinking goes, so I don't want you to shy away from eating it. Rather, pay attention to the *types* of fat you consume.

Food Source	Amount Protein (Approximate)
LEAN MEAT, POULTRY, AND EGGS	**PER 3-OUNCE SERVING (UNLESS OTHERWISE STATED)**
Skinless chicken breast	26 g
Yellowfin tuna	25 g
Lean ground beef	25 g
Turkey breast	24 g
Lean pork	22 g
Sockeye salmon	22 g
Rainbow trout	19 g
Eggs	6–8 g per large egg
DAIRY PRODUCTS	
Greek yogurt (plain, non-fat)	20 g (1 cup serving)
Cottage cheese	14 g (½ cup serving)
Parmesan cheese	10 g (1 ounce)
Milk (skim, 1%, 2%, whole)	8 g (1 cup)
Swiss cheese	7.6 g (1 ounce)
Mozzarella cheese (whole milk)	6.3 g (1 ounce)
LEGUMES AND OTHER PLANT-BASED FOODS	
Firm tofu	20 g (½ cup)
Hemp hearts	10 g (3 tablespoons)
Pumpkin seeds (hulled)	8–9 g (¼ cup)
Lentils (boiled)	9 g (½ cup)
Chickpeas (boiled)	7.5 g (½ cup)
Kidney beans (boiled)	7.5 g (½ cup)
Dry roasted chickpeas	7 g (⅓ cup)
Almonds (1 oz, approx. 23)	6–7 g (¼ cup)
Walnuts	4.5 g (¼ cup)
Quinoa	4 g (½ cup cooked)
Peanut butter	4 g (1 tablespoon)
Almond butter	3.4 g (1 tablespoon)
Avocado	2.7 g (1 avocado, medium)
Hummus	2 g (2 tablespoons)

Good-quality, or healthy, fats are essential for women in peri-menopause and menopause. Fats can help with the following symptoms:

- **Brain health and cognitive function.** About 60 percent of your brain is made up of fats (at dry weight, meaning when the water is removed). The type of fats you eat can have an impact on your mental health, moods, cognition, memory, and focus. To give you an example, a 2021 study in *Frontiers in Nutrition* showed that adults sixty and older who ate avocados performed better on certain memory and attention (cognitive) tests than those who didn't. See Chapter 8 for the fats to prioritize.

- **Lowering inflammation.** Monounsaturated fats (olive oil, olives, avocados, nuts, and seeds) and omega-3 fatty acids (fatty fish like salmon, walnuts, chia and hemp seeds, and algae oil) have anti-inflammatory properties. MUFAs help to calm inflammation and omega-3s are used to create anti-inflammatory compounds that help reduce inflammation.

- **Heart health.** Monounsaturated fats and omega-3 fatty acids can also help lower cholesterol and the risk of heart disease.

- **Bone health.** Some studies suggest that women who eat more monounsaturated fat–rich foods, like olive oil, have better bone mineral density, which may lower their risk of osteoporosis. Omega-3 fats may also help support stronger bones by stimulating the cells that build them (osteoblasts) and slowing the ones that break them down (osteoclasts).

- **Improved energy.** Considering that fatigue is the number one symptom (refer to Chapter 2), this is a huge bonus!

- **Satiety.** When we eat fat as part of a balanced meal, it helps us feel full and satisfied for longer periods of time.

- **Skin health.** Healthy fats help your skin feel soft and smooth, stay flexible and hydrated, and become less prone to inflammation.

How Much Fat Do You Need?

Ideally, dietary fats should make up 20–30 percent of your diet, with a focus on omega-3s, monounsaturated fats, and some saturated fats.

For example, for a 150-pound woman eating an 1,800-calorie-a-day diet, getting 30 percent of her calories from fat equals 540 calories, or about 60 grams. Here's what that could look like over the course of a day:

FOOD ITEM	SERVING SIZE	FAT (G)	PROTEIN (G)
Avocado Toast	1 slice whole grain bread, ¼ avocado	6 g	5 g
Salmon (wild, cooked)	100 g (about 3.5 oz)	9 g	25 g
Cheddar Cheese	1 oz (28 g)	9 g	7 g
Olive Oil (extra virgin)	1 tablespoon (15 ml)	14 g	0 g
Almonds (raw, ~10 nuts)	~12 g	7 g	2.5 g
Eggs (whole)	3 large (150 g total)	15 g	18 g
Total		**60 g**	**57.5 g**

Plant-Based Fats Only

FOOD ITEM	SERVING SIZE	FAT (G)	PROTEIN (G)
Avocado (½ medium)	75 g	12 g	1 g
Almond Butter	2 tablespoons (32 g)	18 g	7 g
Chia Seeds	1 tablespoon (14 g)	4.5 g	2.5 g
Tahini	1 tablespoon (15 g)	8 g	2.5 g
Olive Oil (extra virgin)	1 tablespoon (15 ml)	14 g	0 g
Dark Chocolate (85%)	1 small square (5 g)	2.5 to 3 g	0.5 g
Total		**59.5 g**	**13.5 g**

A 2024 study published in the *Journal of Nutrition* followed 1,024 older adults for nearly seven years (the average age was eighty-one) and found that eating at least one egg a week was associated with a 47 percent lower risk of developing Alzheimer's compared to those who rarely ate eggs. The researchers believe it's partly due to choline found in the yolks, a nutrient that supports brain health.

Principle #5: Nurture Digestion

In Chapter 4, I talked about how common digestive issues are at this stage of life, and how your gut microbes help break down and regulate estrogens (estrone, estradiol, and estriol). When your gut microbiome has a healthy mix of different types of bacteria, your body can use and clear these estrogens the way it's supposed to. Your gut microbes play a major role in keeping your hormones balanced and supporting your overall health.

In addition to what I shared in Chapter 4, here are other ways to nurture your digestion:

Monitor stimulants. Do you feel jittery or wired when you have sugar or caffeine? That's your nervous system kicking in. Both activate your nervous system, which can trigger or exacerbate stress and anxiety. And because your brain and gut are connected through the vagus nerve (the two-way highway), they can also mess with digestion and lead to gas, bloating, loose stools, and a sudden urge to *go*. These reactions can feel more intense during perimenopause and menopause because fluctuating hormones make the nervous system and gut more sensitive. Pay attention to how your body reacts to these stimulants and make adjustments accordingly. Caffeine, particularly in coffee, activates your body's gastrocolic response (it's what makes you have to *go* after eating). If you find your morning coffee is too harsh for you, try having half a cup instead, or switch to decaf or a coffee alternative like Teeccino, which has chicory root (inulin), a type of prebiotic fiber.

Herbal help. Herbal teas and supplements can soothe digestive symptoms. Ginger helps with nausea, peristalsis (gut contractions), and indigestion. Chamomile can help calm an upset stomach, and peppermint and fennel help to relax the muscles of the digestive tract, easing cramping and bloating. *Note:* Go easy with peppermint if you're prone to heartburn. You can eat these herbs, drink them as teas, or take them in supplement or tincture form.

Aloe vera juice can help with easing heartburn, as it helps to soothe the mucus membranes along the esophagus. A 2015 pilot study found that taking 10 ml of aloe vera as a supplement once a day (standardized to 5.0 mg polysaccharide per ml) reduced the frequency of GERD symptoms with few side effects. Check out Lily of the Desert for a whole line of digestive support products.

Manage stress. When you're stressed, your body naturally slows down digestion. Stress is a recurring theme throughout this book, as it impacts nearly every aspect of perimenopause and menopause for all the reasons I discussed in Chapters 2 and 6.

Stay well-hydrated. Drinking enough liquids on a daily basis helps you to better digest and absorb the nutrients from food. It also helps move fiber through your digestive tract so you can poop and pee out the waste. Not getting enough water may worsen symptoms like constipation, bloating, and gas. I talk more about hydration in Principle #7.

Principle #6: Choose More Plants

Nutrient-rich plant foods offer incredible health benefits for perimenopausal and menopausal women. From colorful fruits and veggies to hearty legumes, whole grains, nuts, and seeds, the options are endless. Plant foods can help support hormone health and overall well-being. Include these delicious foods in your meals:

- **Vegetables**
  - » *Leafy greens:* spinach, chard, collards, kale
  - » *Cruciferous:* broccoli, cauliflower, Brussels sprouts, cabbage, arugula, bok choy
  - » *Root veggies:* carrots, sweet potatoes, beets
  - » *Nightshades:* potatoes, tomatoes, bell peppers, eggplant
  - » *Alliums:* onions, garlic, leeks (also great prebiotics)
  - » *Fermented veggies:* sauerkraut, kimchi, pickles (naturally fermented)
  - » *Sprouts and microgreens*
  - » *Okra*
  - » *Gourds and squashes:* zucchini, yellow squash, butternut squash, acorn squash, spaghetti squash, pumpkin
  - » *Stalks and stems:* celery, fennel bulb, asparagus, kohlrabi, rhubarb

- **Fruits:** fresh or frozen for variety and convenience. More details on fruit coming up shortly.

- **Legumes:** beans, lentils, chickpeas, peas, soy (edamame, tempeh, tofu), peanuts, mung beans, adzuki beans, black-eyed peas, lupini beans

- **Whole grains:** quinoa, brown rice, oats, whole wheat, barley, millet, farro, amaranth, teff, buckwheat, bulgur, sorghum, freekeh, sprouted grains

- **Tubers:** tigernut, jicama (also a prebiotic), yucca, yacón, Jerusalem artichokes (very high in inulin)

- **Aquatic veggies:** lotus root, water chestnut

- **Nuts and seeds:** almonds, walnuts, pumpkin, flaxseeds, chia, basil, sunflower seeds, hemp, sesame (great for calcium), Brazil nuts (selenium), pistachios, macadamia nuts

- **Herbs, roots, and spices:** both fresh and dried, like rosemary, basil, parsley, turmeric, cinnamon, ginger, oregano, thyme, coriander, fennel, horseradish, wasabi

- **Sea greens and algae:** seaweed (nori, kelp, wakame, dulse), spirulina, chlorella, phytoplankton

- **Fungi:** all types of edible mushrooms

- **Healthy fats:** omega-3s (plant sources), monounsaturated fats (olive and avocado), coconut, and their oils

Plant foods can help support your body as it adapts to the hormonal changes of perimenopause and menopause. Fruits, veggies, nuts, and seeds are packed with nutrients that help to lower inflammation, regulate mood, improve energy, and support how your body responds to stress. Plant foods are also filling without being too high in calories. Fiber and healthy fats support gut and heart health and help to balance blood sugar and keep you full for longer. And eating a variety of plant foods helps to diversify your gut microbiome, including your estrobolome (Chapter 4). Since estrogen influences mood, weight, digestion, and even libido, feeding the beneficial microbes in your gut may have a positive ripple effect throughout your body.

Plant Goals

According to the American Gut Project and research at the University of California, San Diego, people who eat thirty or more different plant foods a week tend to have a wider variety of healthy gut microbes than those who eat ten or less. Having a broader range of gut bacteria can help support your immune system, skin health, blood sugar, and the absorption of nutrients. Refer to Chapter 4 in the section on *prebiotics*, *probiotics*, and *postbiotics*.

Starting today, set a goal to eat five *unique* plant foods every couple of days (including different-colored produce). Some days you'll hit your goal and some days you won't, and that's okay. The idea is to use what you already have, then switch things up when you're ready to replenish your stock. Most of us tend to eat the same things over and over (me included!), so do your best to change it up as much as you can by adding or swapping out two new plant-based items on your grocery list a week. Over time, those small changes will help you hit that weekly goal. I created a plant foods cheat sheet to use when planning or shopping for groceries. You can download it by going to www.nourishingmenopausebook.com under the Resources tab.

Whenever possible, and when your budget allows, choose organic, as certain pesticides can mimic or interfere with estrogen in the body and mess with hormones. One way to prioritize which produce to buy organic or not is by referring to the Environmental Working Group's Dirty Dozen™ and Clean Fifteen™ lists. They release revised lists every year. You can learn more at ewg.org.

A Note About Fruits: Nature's Candy

This question comes up often: *Should I or shouldn't I eat fruit?*

My answer is yes, in moderation.

Fruits are healthy, as they contain fiber, vitamins, minerals, and antioxidants like polyphenols (Chapter 10). However, they also contain natural sugars, so portion size and the type of fruit matter, especially when it comes to blood sugar.

That said, context matters. According to Nicole Avena, PhD, associate professor of neuroscience and author of *Sugarless: A 7-Step Plan to Uncover Hidden Sugars, Curb Your Cravings, and Conquer Your Addiction*, "Fruit offers sweetness wrapped in fiber, water, and micronutrients, a package our brains and bodies are designed to handle. The challenge today is that many ultra-processed foods mimic fruit's sweetness while stripping away everything protective, creating a level of reward our biology was never meant to manage."

Even with whole fruits, some affect blood sugar more than others, but how much will vary from person to person. Since there's a huge push toward personalized medicine, more and more companies are developing technology to help identify how specific foods affect blood sugar levels (and other metrics). One way to know how certain fruits affect *your* body is to wear a continuous glucose monitor (CGM) or use a blood sugar monitor glucose meter. If you have or suspect you have diabetes, please speak to your doctor about which technology is best for you. If you don't have access to a CGM or glucose monitor, you can use the glycemic index (GI) and glycemic load (GL) as a reference. Refer to Chapter 8 or search for low GI foods.

Limit fruit to one to three a day (about 200 g each), depending on the size and type of the fruit, how ripe it is, what you're eating it with, and your own blood sugar response.

One way to keep blood sugar in check is to eat fruits with other foods, for example, coupling them with a fat and protein like almond butter, cottage cheese, or Greek yogurt for a snack rather than after a large meal, which may cause gas and bloating.

Eat Your Berries

Berries are amazing for perimenopausal and menopausal women! Research shows that eating blueberries and strawberries may support better brain function and is linked with a lower risk of dementia later in life, thanks to antioxidants called anthocyanins. Anthocyanins are potent plant chemicals that give berries their deep colors. A 2020 review found that blueberries help to reduce inflammation and oxidative stress, and may improve blood sugar balance, which supports metabolic health, and may help lower the risk of developing type 2 diabetes. They also support heart health. Even a moderate amount, one-third of a cup a day, has been associated with a lower risk of disease.

A 2023 double-blind, placebo-controlled study showed that eating strawberries every day helps to lower blood pressure.

In addition to improving cognitive health, blueberries help to protect our skin and bones from damage by reducing inflammation. Eating a cup of blueberries a day has been shown to help keep skin more hydrated, protect the skin's natural barrier, and make skin feel smoother. Blueberries also have a positive effect on bone health by reducing resorption, the process where bone breaks down into the bloodstream, which helps slow bone loss in menopausal women. Another study found that eating ¾ to 1 cup of blueberries a day may help to slow bone loss in healthy menopausal women.

Raspberries and blackberries* share the title of *queen* when it

---

* Be mindful of blackberries if you are on a low-FODMAP diet, as they are high FODMAP (high in polyols), even in low amounts.

comes to blood sugar balance with their 8 grams of fiber per cup. In general, berries are excellent sources of anti-inflammatory antioxidants, vitamins, minerals, and fiber. Like blueberries and strawberries, they're linked with a lower risk of type 2 diabetes and metabolic syndrome.

Cruciferous Vegetables

Cruciferous vegetables are great to include in your diet during perimenopause and menopause thanks to compounds like indole-3-carbinol (I3C) and sulforaphane. I3C converts to 3,3' diindolylmethane (DIM) in the body, which may help your liver break down and clear estrogen more effectively. Sulforaphane is a powerful antioxidant that's been studied for its potential role in certain types of cancers, including breast cancer. Aim to eat an assortment of the following cruciferous veggies three to five times a week:

- Leafy greens: arugula, bok choy, collard greens, kale, mustard greens, watercress

- Cabbage: green, red, napa, savoy

- Broccoli, broccoli rabe (rapini), broccolini, broccoli sprouts, Chinese broccoli

- Cauliflower

- Brussels sprouts

- Root vegetables: radishes, daikon radish, turnips, rutabaga, wasabi

- Kohlrabi

- Horseradish

- Moringa

- Mustard seeds

- Sprouted radish seeds

Principle #7: Ensure You're Hydrated

When we're born, about 75 percent of our body weight is water. As adults, that drops to around 50–55 percent for women.

As we age, we're more prone to dehydration for the following reasons:

- We lose muscle and gain more fat (muscle holds more water than fat. In fact, it's about 70–75 percent water);

- Excessive sweating from vasomotor symptoms like hot flashes and night sweats;

- Urinary incontinence;

- Our sense of thirst changes, so we may not feel thirsty;

- We may not drink enough;

- Kidney function changes;

- Illnesses, which can lead to blood loss, vomiting, and diarrhea;

- Chronic conditions (e.g., diabetes); and

- Medications, including diuretics.

I can't stress enough the importance of staying hydrated once you go into perimenopause and menopause. Here are some reasons why:

- **Moisture:** Keeps the mucous membranes (eyes, ears, and nose), skin, scalp, and vagina moist.

- **Digestion:** Flushes waste from the body, helps break down nutrients including protein and carbs so we absorb them better, and makes saliva.

- **Regularity:** Helps soften stool and move waste through the colon so you can poop regularly and avoid constipation.

- **Energy:** Helps your cells work properly, so you feel more energized.

- **Body temperature:** Helps to cool the body and replace lost fluids from sweating.

- **Brain function and cognition:** Dehydration can trigger or exacerbate headaches, brain fog, poor concentration, and memory issues.

- **Moods:** Keeps your emotions more balanced. Even mild dehydration can make you feel tired, irritable, and anxious.

- **Heart health:** Helps with blood flow, which helps your heart work more efficiently.

- **Joint health:** Keeps your joints lubricated, reducing stiffness and pain.

- **Bone health:** Carries nutrients like magnesium and calcium to your bones.

- **Electrolyte balance:** Electrolytes like sodium, potassium, magnesium, and calcium help your muscles move and your nerves communicate. When you lose a lot of fluid through sweating, stress, and hormone shifts, these electrolytes can be depleted, which may lead to muscle cramps, fatigue, and dizziness.

DID YOU KNOW YOU CAN ACTUALLY DRINK *TOO MUCH* WATER?

If your pee looks totally clear, like plain water, you might be overdoing it. That can mean you're drinking more than you need to, which can dilute your blood and lower your sodium levels. Ideally, your urine should be pale yellow.

On the other hand, if your pee is dark yellow or amber, or has a strong smell, it could mean you need to drink more!

Note: If you're taking B vitamins, your urine might be bright or neon yellow because your body gets rid of what it doesn't need. The bright yellow is generally due to vitamin B2, or riboflavin.

- **Urinary health:** Flushes bacteria from the urinary tract and keeps your bladder healthy, which can lower your chances of getting a urinary tract infection (UTI).

How to Hydrate: What Should You Drink?

When it comes to staying hydrated, focus on both water and electrolyte-rich fluids:

- **Plain water:** If you don't like the taste of plain water (to be honest, I don't), try infusing it with sliced cucumbers or berries. My mother uses a water bottle that comes with a built-in infuser, and she finds it really helps her drink more water. You can also add mint chlorophyll to your water, as it's been shown to help with digestion. It also tastes great. Chlorophyll turns your water green, so it's a fun conversation starter!

- **Herbal tea:** Personally, I like to drink herbal tea (no sugar or caffeine).

  Just be mindful; if you're drinking tea all day long, some herbal teas have medicinal properties, so try not to overdo it on one particular type. Brew them lightly and remove the tea bag early so it doesn't steep for long, making your tea too strong. My personal go-to choices are Bigelow Tea's lemon ginger plus probiotics and their cold-water infusions.

- **Electrolytes:** These minerals are especially important if you're experiencing muscle cramps, increased sweating, or fatigue. Some of my favorite electrolyte-rich beverages include:

  » **Teas*:** Varieties that naturally support electrolyte balance include:
    - *Alfalfa leaf:* calcium, magnesium, and potassium
    - *Oatstraw:* magnesium, calcium, and silica
    - *Hibiscus:* potassium and vitamin C

---

* These teas offer light electrolyte support rather than high dose replacements. If you're looking for therapeutic doses, consider commercially prepared electrolyte drinks or powders.

      – *Moringa:* potassium, calcium, and magnesium

      – *Rooibos:* potassium, calcium, magnesium, and antioxidants

» **Homemade electrolyte drinks:**

      – Water with a pinch of sea salt, lemon, and a little bit of raw honey

      – Nettle tea (magnesium, calcium, potassium, iron) with a splash of lemon juice and a pinch of pink or gray salt

» **Bone broth:** contains sodium, potassium, and magnesium

» **Coconut water:** a natural source of potassium and magnesium (look for brands without added sugar)

Here are some other things to keep in mind when hydrating:

- Drink throughout the day rather than chugging your liquids all at once.

- Set reminders to drink, especially if your thirst cues are off.

- Listen to your body. If your mouth is dry, or you're tired or have a headache, try increasing your fluid intake.

- Drink a glass or two of water when you wake up to rehydrate after sleeping.

- Carry a water bottle or travel cup so you always have something to sip on (choose brands that can keep your liquids cold or hot for several hours).

- Add electrolyte powders if you sweat excessively or have a lot of cramping.

- Eat more soups and high-water-content fruits and veggies.

- Caffeine and alcohol can be dehydrating. Either limit them or balance them with extra water.

A Hormone-Supportive Diet: Estrogen, Progesterone, and Testosterone-Building Foods

Can foods boost sex hormones—estrogen, progesterone, and testosterone—the way menopause hormone therapy (MHT) does?

The short answer is not exactly.

Unlike MHT, which provides bioidentical or synthetic hormones to directly supplement falling or fluctuating levels, foods can't increase hormone levels the same way.

However, they can play a supporting role.

Food and beverages can give your body the nutrients it needs to make hormones, help your liver metabolize and clear them, reduce inflammation, and support overall hormone health during perimenopause and menopause.

Estrogen-Supporting Foods: Phytoestrogens

Phytoestrogens are natural compounds found in plant foods like soy, flaxseeds, and legumes that can mimic estrogen in the body, but in a much weaker way than estradiol (17-beta-estradiol, or E2), the primary form of estrogen in premenopausal women. Phytoestrogens share a similar structure with estradiol, so they can attach to estrogen receptors in the cells in your breasts, uterus, ovaries, bone, liver, and fat tissue, affecting how estrogen functions.

Research shows that phytoestrogens can have both estrogenic and anti-estrogenic effects, so they can either act like estrogen when your levels are low, like during menopause, or have a balancing effect if your levels are high, like in perimenopause.

This unique ability, and the research behind it, suggests that phytoestrogens may help ease symptoms like hot flashes, improve glucose and cholesterol levels, and support cardiovascular and bone health. They may also support gut health by helping to feed the good bacteria in your gut.

Phytoestrogens can play a supportive role in hormone health, making them a good addition to your perimenopause and menopause diet.

— PHYTOESTROGEN-RICH FOODS —

SEEDS

- Flaxseeds (very high in lignans)
- Sesame seeds
- Sunflower seeds
- Pumpkin seeds

NUTS

- Pistachios
- Almonds
- Cashews
- Walnuts
- Hazelnuts
- Peanuts

LEGUMES

- Soybeans (edamame, tofu, tempeh, soymilk)
- Chickpeas (including hummus)
- Lentils
- Kidney beans
- Pinto beans
- Lima beans
- Black-eyed peas
- Mung beans
- Split peas

FRUITS

- Dried fruits (dates, prunes, raisins, dried apricots)
- Pomegranates
- Berries (strawberries, raspberries, blueberries)
- Plums
- Peaches
- Cranberries
- Cherries

GRAINS

- Oats
- Barley
- Rye
- Wheat (whole grain, especially wheat germ)

VEGETABLES

- Alfalfa sprouts
- Onion
- Broccoli

- Cabbage
- Brussels sprouts
- Cauliflower
- Collard greens
- Carrots
- Garlic

HERBS & SPICES

- Rosemary
- Sage
- Fennel
- Anise
- Thyme
- Parsley
- Turmeric

OILS

- Flaxseed oil
- Sesame oil

BEVERAGES

- Soymilk
- Green tea
- Black tea
- Red wine

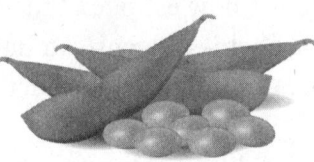

Foods rich in phytoestrogens are shown on the next page.

More than three hundred foods have an estrogenic effect, but the type and strength of phytoestrogens they contain can vary significantly. The most well-known and researched types of phytoestrogens are *isoflavones*, *lignans*, and *coumestans*.

The highest concentration of isoflavones is found in soy and soy products, and they're especially rich in two types, daidzein and genistein. Research shows that they may help the body use estrogen more effectively and support heart health. They may also be associated with a lower risk of some hormone-related cancers, especially breast cancer.

Lignans are found in flaxseeds, sesame seeds, whole grains, and veggies like carrots and broccoli. They're activated in the gut by your microbes, and they help keep stronger forms of estrogen in check (think of them as a dimmer switch that helps keep estrogens in balance). They also help your body clear estrogen that's no longer needed.

Coumestans are a more potent form of phytoestrogens, found in split peas, lima beans, mung beans, alfalfa sprouts, and smaller amounts in certain cruciferous veggies like Brussels sprouts.

For more information on the benefits of phytoestrogens in perimenopause and menopause, listen to episode #47 of my podcast, *Menopause Reimagined*, with Jennifer Harrington, ND.

Tip: Flaxseeds are the number one source of lignans by far, with about 30–50 mg per tablespoon. Grind them before eating them and add them to smoothies, yogurt, old-fashioned oatmeal, or salads. To maintain freshness, store the opened bag in the freezer. *Note:* Flax oil contains little to no lignans unless it specifically says it does on the label. Rather, it contains ALA, a vegan source of omega-3s (see Chapter 8).

Rosemary

Another ingredient worth mentioning is rosemary. This fragrant herb contains phytoestrogens and is rich in antioxidants such as rosmarinic acid and carnosic acid, which help protect cells from oxidative stress. Rosemary is delicious fresh or dried and has many culinary uses. It's fantastic in scrambled eggs, on potatoes, or roasted with chicken or lamb. Try rosemary tea or rosemary-infused olive oil:

DIY Rosemary Oil
1 teaspoon dried rosemary
½ cup olive oil

Using a mortar and pestle, coffee grinder, or blender, grind the dried rosemary until it's almost a powder. Place the rosemary into a small jar and add the olive oil. Allow it to sit for at least one day or overnight for the flavors to infuse before using. Keep refrigerated.

Bonus: You can also use it in your hair. It has been shown to help with growth, circulation, shedding, and thinning. Be sure to do a patch test to make sure it doesn't irritate your skin.

What About Soy?

"Is it safe to eat soy and soy-based foods when I'm in perimenopause or menopause?"

Soybeans and soy food products have been at the center of controversy for years due to their high concentration of isoflavones, especially genistein and daidzein, which can have mild estrogenic properties.

The concern originated from animal studies that linked high doses of isoflavones to a disruption in hormones and a higher risk of certain hormone-dependent cancers like breast and uterine. However, more recent human studies have shown that when eaten in typical food amounts, soy doesn't really raise circulating estrogen levels or thicken the uterine lining, and it may be beneficial for women in perimenopause and menopause, when eaten in moderation.

A 2024 study looked at the results from forty trials with over three thousand participants and found that eating soy foods for about three months had no effect on key estrogen markers in postmenopausal women.[*]

Another possible concern with soy is its effect on the thyroid. There are mixed results when it comes to studies on whether a high intake of soy can disrupt thyroid function, particularly in people who have a thyroid condition or who are deficient in iodine. The Mayo Clinic recommends waiting at least an hour (and some experts recommend up to three hours) after taking your thyroid medication to eat soy-containing foods or beverages, as they can interfere with its absorption.

Consume soy in its whole or minimally processed state two to three times a week. Fermented soy foods like tempeh, miso, and natto can be easier to digest and absorb because their isoflavones

---

[*] It's important to note that the study was funded by the United Soybean Board (U.S. Department of Agriculture) and the Canadian Institutes of Health Research.

have been partially broken down by beneficial microbes during the fermentation process. Choose organic soy whenever possible, as anywhere from 80–94 percent of soy crops in North America are genetically engineered, or GMO.

Be mindful of how many ultra-processed soy products you eat, like soy milk, TVP (texturized vegetable protein), soy-based cheese alternatives, nondairy soy creamers, soybean oil, soy protein isolate (found in some shakes, bars, and meal replacement shakes), and soy-based meat alternatives often found in plant-based "burgers," "hot dogs," or other foods that look and taste like meat. The reason being that they're highly processed so they don't have the same nutrient profile as whole soy foods.

Progesterone-Supporting Foods

Progesterone helps to balance estrogen, supports sleep and mood, and can help reduce symptoms like anxiety, insomnia, and heavy periods.

The following nutrients, and the foods they're found in, can help support your body's ability to produce progesterone. According to Dr. Carrie Jones, if you're in the early stages of perimenopause, these are especially beneficial during the luteal phase, or the second half of your cycle, after you've ovulated, because progesterone is only made after ovulation. In later perimenopause, you may not ovulate as often or ovulation may stop altogether. While these nutrients can still support your hormones overall, they can't stimulate progesterone production when you aren't ovulating (and in perimenopause it can be hard to know when it's happening). If you're in menopause, you can eat them any time of the month:

- **Zinc:** Supports the function of the ovaries and plays a role in the production of progesterone. Zinc also helps progesterone work properly in the body so it can do its job. Foods rich in zinc can help support healthy estrogen and progesterone levels, and it plays a role in fertility.

  Tip: Zinc in animal foods is absorbed better than in plant-based foods. Eat zinc-rich foods with vitamin C–rich foods or protein to enhance its absorption.

PROGESTERONE-SUPPORTIVE FOODS

SEEDS

- Pumpkin seeds
- Sesame seeds
- Sunflower seeds
- Flaxseeds

NUTS

- Almonds
- Cashews
- Brazil nuts
- Walnuts
- Hazelnuts
- Pistachios

LEGUMES

- Chickpeas
- Lentils
- Black beans
- Kidney beans
- Pinto beans
- Peas

WHOLE GRAINS

- Oats
- Brown rice
- Quinoa
- Whole wheat
- Barley

VEGETABLES

- Leafy greens (spinach, kale, collard greens)
- Cruciferous vegetables (broccoli, cauliflower, cabbage, Brussels sprouts)
- Sweet potatoes

FRUITS

- Strawberries
- Berries (blueberries, raspberries)
- Bananas
- Avocado

ANIMAL PROTEINS

- Poultry (chicken, turkey)
- Eggs
- Grass-fed beef, lean beef, pork

- Shellfish (oysters, crab, lobster)
- Fish (salmon, mackerel, tuna, sardines, shrimp)

HEALTHY FATS AND OILS

- Olive oil
- Fatty fish (salmon, mackerel, sardines)

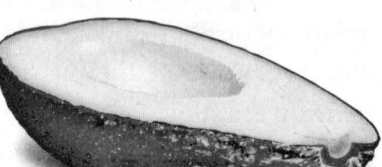

- **Vitamin C:** Helps to protect progesterone from oxidative stress (which can lower it).

- Other nutrients that may help support overall hormone health include magnesium, healthy fats, cholesterol-rich foods (as they help to make hormones), and cruciferous veggies.

Did you know? High cortisol levels from ongoing stress can interfere with your body's normal production of progesterone. This is another important reason to manage stress levels now that you're in perimenopause and menopause. Refer to Chapter 6 for tips.

Did you know? Exercise is an effective way to boost testosterone, especially resistance training. High-intensity interval training (HIIT) and lifting weights can temporarily raise testosterone levels for up to an hour after a workout. Regular exercise helps to regulate cortisol levels, which supports testosterone production.

Testosterone-Supporting Foods

Testosterone is important in perimenopause and menopause because it supports libido, mood, energy, motivation, stamina, muscle mass and strength, and bone health.

Nutrients that help support testosterone levels include:

- **Zinc:** Helps your body support the production of testosterone, and a deficiency has been linked to lower testosterone levels. A 2021 study on postmenopausal women showed that women with low zinc levels who supplemented with it saw a significant increase in their testosterone levels compared to the control group. The study concluded that those who supplemented with this mineral saw improvements when it came to libido, arousal, orgasm, vaginal dryness, and pain during intercourse.

- **Boron:** Has been shown to increase testosterone and estradiol (a type of estrogen) levels in some women with low levels.

TESTOSTERONE-SUPPORTIVE FOODS

SEAFOOD

- Oysters (very high in zinc)
- Fatty fish (salmon, mackerel, sardines, tuna)
- Shellfish (crab, lobster)
- Sea fish (general)

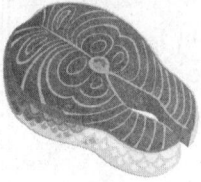

MEAT AND EGGS

- Eggs (especially yolks)
- Lean beef and red meat

NUTS AND SEEDS

- Brazil nuts (selenium)
- Almonds
- Walnuts
- Pumpkin seeds (zinc)
- Sunflower seeds

VEGETABLES

- Cruciferous vegetables (broccoli, cabbage, cauliflower, Brussels sprouts)
- Onions
- Garlic

FRUITS

- Pomegranates

WHOLE GRAINS

- Oats
- Fortified cereals
- Whole grains (general)

HEALTHY FATS AND OILS

- Extra-virgin olive oil
- Coconut
- Avocado oil
- Fish oil

OTHER PLANT FOODS

- Dark chocolate and cocoa products (cacao nibs, cocoa powder)
- Honey (boron)
- Ginger (root and tea)
- Parsley
- Fenugreek
- Maca root

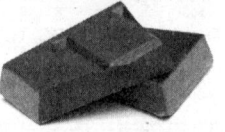

BEVERAGES

- Pomegranate juice

- **Magnesium:** Helps to support healthy testosterone levels indirectly by improving sleep and helping us cope better with stress, as chronically high cortisol can lower it.

- And other nutrients like vitamin D, cholesterol-rich foods (egg yolks, shellfish, full-fat dairy, organ and red meats), protein-rich foods (chicken and turkey with the skin, fish and shellfish, Greek yogurt, cottage cheese), quality fats, cruciferous veggies, antioxidants, and polyphenol-rich foods help your body maintain healthy testosterone levels.

Lifestyle Tip: Here's yet another reason to manage stress. As we discussed in Chapter 6, our adrenals make DHEA, which is a precursor for testosterone. When blood sugar levels and stress (cortisol) are high, they can impact our adrenal glands, potentially lowering the production of DHEA and testosterone.

For a more complete list of phytoestrogen, progesterone, and testosterone-supporting foods, visit www.nourishingmenopause book.com and click on the Resources tab.

Here are some simple guidelines to keep in mind as you plan your meals:

- **Macros:** According to Lisa Tsakos, a nutritionist with over twenty-five years of experience, cofounder of the Health Coach Collaborative, and weight-loss specialist, the ideal balance of carbs, protein, and fat varies depending on several factors, including your body, lifestyle, activity level, and personal preferences. That said, she believes a *general* guideline for most women in perimenopause or menopause is around 20–30 percent of calories from protein, 40–50 percent from carbohydrates, and 20–30 percent from fat. I recommend figuring out your macros by downloading a tracking app such as MyFitnessPal, Cronometer, Lose It!, Carb Manager, Lifesum, or Macros+.

- **Weight loss:** If your goal is to lose weight, Lisa recommends strictly avoiding any simple carbs and added sugars (like desserts) after 5 p.m. and gently lowering your current calorie intake based on your macro calculator or tracking app's recommendations. If you want to gain weight, add calories to your current daily intake.

- **Adjust portion sizes:** A portion size is the actual amount of food that's on your plate. Studies show that people tend to eat more when the portion size is larger. Portion sizes have increased over the last thirty years, and so has the average size of a dinner plate. While my preference is to focus on the quality of the foods you eat, some people find monitoring their portions helpful. To help, you can use visual cues and your hands. Here's how:

PROTEIN	CARBOHYDRATES	FATS
Palm Size	Fist Size	Thumb Size
Beef	Beans	Avocado
Chicken	Bread	Butter
Cottage cheese	Chickpeas	Cheese
Eggs	Couscous	Chocolate
Fish	Fruit	Full-fat dairy products
Pork	Lentils	Nuts
Salmon	Noodles	Oils
Tofu	Pasta	Seeds
Turkey	Potatoes	
	Quinoa	
	Rice	

- **Front-load your meals:** Research shows that eating more earlier in the day and less later on may be better for your health than eating most of your food at night. You may find that eating more substantial meals earlier in the day can be beneficial for cognition, blood sugar balance, weight management, energy levels, and overall metabolic health. After all, we need the nourishment from foods to give us energy, help us focus better, lift our mood, and protect our immune system during the day when many of us are more active.

- **Finish dinner early:** Aim to finish your last meal by 6 p.m. or 7 p.m. and try to avoid eating anything after 8 p.m. to give your body a chance to completely digest your food. Allow at least three hours between your last meal and your planned bedtime. (Drinking water or herbal tea after 8 p.m. is fine). I personally find when I finish dinner and stop eating by 7 or 7:30 p.m., my blood sugar is more stable overnight and is lower the next morning.

- **Follow the 80/20 rule:** Eat whole, unprocessed foods at least 80 percent of the time. Adapt according to your needs and goals.

- **Limit ultra-processed foods, including ultra-processed sugar:** They likely contain refined sugars, high sodium, and very few nutrients. Instead, opt for whole foods, including low-glycemic fruits, and switch to sweeteners like monk fruit, stevia, and allulose. Use in moderation.

- **Choose organic foods whenever possible:** This helps to avoid certain pesticides that can be harmful to your nervous system. You can search for the types of pesticides and their effects on human health on the U.S. Environmental Protection Agency's (EPA's) website.

- **Limit alcohol:** I know this is a hard one. But Dr. Daniel Amen, a psychiatrist who did brain SPECT scans on more than 225,000 human brains, believes that alcohol is poison to the brain. He states that even moderate drinking can age the brain faster and affect cognition, mood, and decision-making.

- **Limit caffeine:** Listen to your body and see how you feel. Don't drink it too close to bed if it keeps you awake, and avoid drinking it on an empty stomach.

Many of these guidelines are in line with the Mediterranean diet, one of the most studied and popular diets in the world, which emphasizes whole foods and provides a healthy amount of fiber, antioxidants, and other nutrients. It's also anti-inflammatory, a big plus for perimenopausal and menopausal women. Research from 2024 on menopausal women showed that it was associated with weight loss, better blood sugar control, and lower blood pressure, triglycerides, total cholesterol, and LDL levels. The Mediterranean diet has also been shown to help with lowering risk for developing type 2 diabetes.

Sample Meal Plans

Now that you've figured out your daily targets, you're ready to apply the B.A.L.A.N.C.E. principles. Choose one of the menu-planning guides below to help you get started.

Try planning your menu according to these standard guidelines:

MEALS	GUIDELINE	EXAMPLES
Drink a glass of room-temperature water with the juice of half a freshly squeezed lemon upon waking or before eating or drinking anything else. Wait at least 15 minutes before eating.		
BREAKFAST	Include a minimum of 25–30 grams protein (or what your macro calculator specified), some antioxidant-rich carbohydrates (like low-glycemic fruit), fiber, and some healthy fats	Smoothie: 1 scoop protein powder, ½ cup fruit (fresh or frozen berries), 1 scoop fiber, milk/non-dairy milk, water
MID-MORNING SNACK (IF NEEDED)	*Note: Limit snacking to improve insulin sensitivity.* Carbohydrate/protein snack. Always combine carbs with some protein to stabilize blood sugar levels	1 piece low-glycemic fruit and a handful of nuts or 1 tablespoon of nut butter or cottage cheese
LUNCH	Whenever possible, make this your largest meal of the day. Include 25–30 grams of protein, some complex carbs, and at least 1 vegetable	Chicken breast, sweet potato, stir-fried cruciferous vegetables with kimchi on the side
MID-AFTERNOON SNACK (IF NEEDED)	*Note: Limit snacking to improve insulin sensitivity.* Include at least 5 grams of protein. Always combine carbs with some protein to stabilize blood sugar levels	4 tablespoons hummus, veggie sticks (carrots, celery, green beans)

MEALS	GUIDELINE	EXAMPLES
DINNER	Include 25–30 grams of protein, fill half your plate with vegetables, and have a small amount of starch (or if you're trying to lose weight, avoid starchy foods or sweets after 5 p.m.)	3–4 oz animal protein, ⅓ cup of lentils, sweet potato, or quinoa, large green salad with colorful veggies, lightly steamed vegetables, and sauerkraut on the side

Plant-Based Sample Menu

This is a sample menu plan tailored for an active woman in midlife who prefers a plant-based diet. Adapt the portion sizes accordingly.

If you need help figuring it all out, I recommend working with a knowledgeable professional such as a nutritionist, registered dietitian, sports nutritionist, or menopause specialist who can guide you based on your needs.

Tip: To increase the protein content of your plant-based meals, top them and your snacks with hemp seeds, nutritional yeast, pumpkin seeds, chopped nuts, sesame seeds, or a spoonful of nut butter. Toss roasted chickpeas, edamame, tofu, tempeh, or lentils into salads, soups, or grain bowls, and choose higher protein pasta or grains like lentil or chickpea pasta and quinoa. You can also use higher protein plant milks, such as pea, minimally or unprocessed organic soy, or hemp, in smoothies, oatmeal, or coffee.

	BREAKFAST	LUNCH	DINNER	SNACK
DAY 1	Scrambled tofu with spinach or arugula, diced veggies, seasoned with turmeric, crushed garlic, and nutritional yeast. Top with kimchi. 1 slice avocado toast on sprouted whole-grain bread	Lentil Salad: Mixed greens topped with cooked lentils, diced cucumber, cherry tomatoes, avocado slices, and lemon-tahini dressing	Chickpea Curry: chickpeas, coconut milk, tomatoes, and spices, served over quinoa or brown rice	Guacamole and raw veggie sticks (green beans, red peppers, carrots) OR Sliced sour apple with sunflower or almond butter, sprinkled with cinnamon
DAY 2	Smoothie: Blend together almond milk, 1 scoop of plant-based protein powder, frozen berries, spinach, and almond butter	Salad: Quinoa mixed with black beans, corn, diced bell peppers, red onion, cilantro, and a lime vinaigrette dressing	Vegan eggplant lasagna, large kale or arugula salad	A handful of mixed raw nuts (almonds, walnuts, and cashews) OR Dry roasted chickpeas
DAY 3	Oatmeal power bowl made with 1 scoop plant-based protein powder, chia seeds, almond butter, and high-protein plant-based milk	Chickpea power bowl with mixed vegetables and brown rice and sprinkled with pumpkin and sunflower seeds	Portobello mushroom steaks with lentil mash and sautéed greens sprinkled with 3 tablespoons hemp hearts	Hummus and veggie sticks

12.

Perimenopause, Menopause, and Mental Health

It's interesting how the physical symptoms of menopause are better known than the mental and emotional ones, even though both types of symptoms are widespread. As we saw in Chapter 2, mental and emotional symptoms can represent up to 90 percent of the top ten most common symptoms.

In my research and social media communities, women have openly shared that they don't know who they are anymore, they don't recognize themselves, and they feel like something or someone has taken over their bodies. Perimenopausal years are tough, especially emotionally if you don't know or understand what's happening to your body. And even if you do, experiencing emotional upheaval on a daily basis is draining, exhausting, and often traumatic.

I had a conversation with someone at the gym who's in perimenopause who told me she's a shell of the person she used to be. We were both in tears because I understood exactly how she was feeling.

But I want you to know this: It does get better for many women once they go into menopause. It did for me. And while you may still have symptoms, you'll begin to feel more like yourself again.

Stories like the woman at my gym and my research inspired me to dedicate an entire chapter to addressing our mental and emotional symptoms with self-love and self-care practices. To write it, I collaborated with my mom, Myra Giberovitch, MSW, to draw on her research and expertise as a licensed social worker with more than thirty-five years of clinical experience under her belt. She's a trauma recovery specialist, and if you follow me on social media, you may already be familiar with her direct, no-nonsense, yet compassionate approach to self-love, self-care, and spiritual growth. I've included some strategies in this chapter that can help support your mental health. However, you should always seek the assistance of a qualified professional for your specific needs, particularly if you're experiencing anxiety, depression, or another condition. If you're having suicidal thoughts, please seek professional help right away. There are many hotlines you can call.

Self-Reflection

As we move through life, we go through different stages, from infancy to old age. And each stage brings its own unique experiences, lessons, and skills that help us to develop into mature, responsible adults.

One of these stages is called "middle adulthood," and it occurs between the ages of forty and sixty-four, which often coincides with when we enter into perimenopause and menopause. This is the stage when many of us are busy with family responsibilities, career demands, aging, and achieving or maintaining financial security.

It's also a period when we may question *who* we are and *where* we're going, and we may struggle with our identity.

This reflection can make us think about our lives and reconsider what's truly important and what might need to change, from relationships to accomplishments to career and personal growth goals.

Some people see this time as a chance to reinvent themselves. Others may struggle with regrets about things they could have done differently and find themselves at a crossroads trying to figure out what's next.

Action Plan

If this is something you identify with, here are some things you can do to help you through the process:

Take an inventory of self: By the time you turn forty, you've achieved so much in your life, and it's easy to forget just how awesome you are. Take an "Inventory of Self": Once a year, or whenever you feel like it, write down things you've accomplished, big and small. Try it now. Think of five things you've accomplished this year, week, or even today. It could be getting out of bed when you didn't feel like it, facing a fear, getting through your to-do list, standing up for yourself, setting boundaries, or getting a promotion or an award. Do it as often as you'd like or need. The key is to take the time to honor yourself for something you're proud of. If you find it's a hard exercise to do on your own, ask a friend, colleague, or family member to help. Other ways to take an inventory of self are to write down five things you're really good at, or have someone else share five things they love about you. Keep your list(s) accessible so you can read them whenever you need a gentle reminder of how incredible you are. I came up with this term because I find it helps to put things into perspective, and it may even help guide you in a direction you didn't expect.

Let go of what no longer serves you: Another thing you can do is to let go of parts of yourself that no longer feel right or no longer serve you. For example, you might be dealing with unresolved issues from past or current struggles, such as:

- Coming to terms with dreams or goals you haven't achieved;

- Examining your relationships;

- Evaluating the people you rely on for support;

- Caring for children and other family members;

- Dealing with being the "sandwich generation" between young families and aging parents;

- Feeling a sense of loss or sadness when your kids move out (empty nest syndrome);

- Coping with financial issues;

- Balancing your personal life with your career;

- Rethinking your career (e.g., job satisfaction, career changes, or job loss);

- Experiencing health challenges and/or dealing with any of the 103+ symptoms of perimenopause and menopause;

- Adjusting to life as you age; and

- Coping with past trauma.

The first step is to become aware of what your unresolved issues or current struggles are and name them. The second step is to process them by confiding in a friend or family member, journaling, or seeking professional help.

How Can You (Re)Connect with Who You Truly Are?

Our childhood experiences, life events, and the pressure to meet others' expectations shape who we are. Whether you had a great or difficult upbringing, your sense of self can weaken over time, and as we saw from my research, 43 percent of women struggle with low self-esteem now that they're in perimenopause and menopause.

Myra recommends that as you step into this next chapter of your life, one goal is to try and let go of any self-doubt or fear that holds you back from living the life you envision for yourself. To do that, you first need to understand where these feelings are coming from: Are they pressure from others, or pressure from yourself? Once you understand the origins of these feelings, you can then begin to connect with who you really are. In her words: "It's important to be yourself. This means letting go of the pressure to fit in and celebrating what makes you unique. How you see yourself, and how much you appreciate and love yourself, matters. Learning to be kind to yourself helps you grow and feel fulfilled. And it means accepting yourself, flaws and all, and treating yourself with compassion and respect. Only then can you let go of self-doubt and live in a way that feels authentic."

While this process can take time, here are some tips to help guide you.

Practice self-awareness: Spend time alone, free from distractions and demands. Start by reflecting on your thoughts, feelings, and behaviors. Identify any old programs, negative thought patterns, self-sabotage, and limiting conscious and unconscious beliefs that may be holding you back. Expect negative thoughts to pop up. They're normal and natural. The goal, however, is not to give them so much power. When a negative thought comes up, notice it. Acknowledge it and remember that thoughts aren't commands. Then visualize a large red X to cancel it and replace it with a positive one. For example, instead of "I can't do this," try "I'm doing the best I can."

Ask yourself some pointed questions about your present life and answer them honestly.

- Are there any unresolved issues that may be preventing you from moving forward?

- Are you living the life you imagined for yourself, trying to live up to other people's expectations, or settling?

- Are you *truly* happy?

- What do you wish for yourself?

Some tools to help you become more self-aware include therapy, journaling, spending time in nature, reading, taking a course, listening to podcasts, and incorporating mindfulness into your daily routine.

Commit to your growth: Personal growth takes time, effort, and patience. Be kind to yourself, even when it's hard.

Take responsibility: At the end of the day, you're in control of your choices and actions. Notice what *is* and *isn't* working and do your best to make the appropriate changes. Focus on what you *can* control and take steps toward building the life you want. Outside pressures and limitations are real and oftentimes unavoidable, so do what you can within your means or circumstances.

Seek support: It's okay to ask for help from a friend, family member, mentor, life coach, teacher, spiritual leader, another woman in perimenopause/menopause, or a therapist/other licensed provider. Having someone to speak to for encouragement and support can make a big difference.

Let go of excuses: Do you find yourself making excuses for why you can't move forward? Have you ever said: "I'm too old," "I'm afraid," "I don't deserve to be happy," "It's too hard to start over," or "My family wouldn't approve"? These kinds of beliefs can keep us feeling stuck and powerless. If excuses have become a habit, try challenging them. Let go of limiting beliefs that may be holding you back. Taking action, even in small steps, can help you move forward and reach your full potential.

Here are some tips on how to empower yourself. As Myra puts it, the voice of power says:

- I am facing my fears, mustering my courage, and doing it anyway.
- I am creating my reality, one experience at a time.
- I am responsible for myself.
- I am releasing my scarcity consciousness.
- I am willing to have it all.

Loving Yourself

Can you look into the mirror and comfortably say "I love you"? Does it come easily, or does it feel awkward? When we love and accept ourselves unconditionally, we're in a better position to set boundaries, follow our passions, and make self-care a priority. Self-love also influences how we relate to others, as it sets the foundation for healthy, balanced, and nurturing relationships. Even if looking yourself in the eyes seems unnatural or uncomfortable, keep on doing it until you believe it. Basically, fake it until you make it!

How Do You Show Yourself Love?

As women, many of us naturally know how to nurture and care for others. Estrogen makes us more caring, protective, empathetic, maternal, attached, and socially connected. It's one reason we value relationships. It can act like a Pollyanna filter that makes us more focused on keeping the peace, even when it means putting other people's needs before our own. While this can be a great trait, it often results in putting ourselves last.

Many women also suffer from the "disease to please." In her book *The Disease to Please: Curing the People-Pleasing Syndrome*, Dr. Harriet B. Braiker describes it as a compulsive behavior where individuals feel driven to seek others' approval, often at the expense of their own happiness.

Once we go into menopause and our estrogen levels drop, for many of us, that Pollyanna filter disappears. Poof! We're no longer that people-pleaser we once were. To put it another way, we don't give any more f*cks or we have no f*cks left to give. We're also better able to put down boundaries, say no, assert ourselves, recognize our strengths, and embrace our superpowers. This change can be upsetting for people around us, especially if they're benefiting from our people-pleasing behavior, and it could potentially strain relationships.

One of my good friends was nonconfrontational her whole life. She'd keep things to herself, and she'd never speak up. But once she went into menopause, it was as if she became a whole new person. Now she doesn't hold back what she's thinking, and she's not afraid to speak her mind. Sometimes we have a good laugh about it, especially when she does or says something that is so out of her old character.

So how can we go from wanting to please others to loving our-selves?

Start by building your self-esteem, the mental and emotional perceptions you have of yourself, by changing your mindset to believing in yourself.

When you truly believe in yourself, you value, accept, respect, and love yourself and don't allow others to treat you disrespectfully. You naturally set higher standards for how you're treated. The better you feel about yourself, the more you feel you deserve to be treated with dignity and respect.

Myra did an amazing video for my social media pages about self-esteem. She explained how it's either high, low, or somewhere in between. With healthy self-esteem, we're in touch with our needs and ensure they're met. We know when to ask for help, are com-fortable setting boundaries, take pride in our accomplishments, live a healthy lifestyle, and generally feel good about ourselves. With low self-esteem, we neglect our needs, look to others for validation, and put ourselves down. We look for outside approval and suffer from the disease to please. The better we feel about ourselves and the higher our self-esteem, the more we can tolerate criticism and people's disappointments in us. We no longer need to do things to please others because we want them to like us or seek their approval.

You also need to pay attention to your self-talk. As I mentioned earlier, the words you use to speak to yourself matter. Are you put-ting yourself down with comments such as "I'm so stupid," "I'm lazy," and "I never get anything right"? Think of the power those words hold. Instead, rephrase them to "I am smart," "I can handle this," and "I am doing my best."

What's your body language like? Do you stand with your shoul-ders hunched over, or tall with them pulled back? Do you walk with confidence, or are you afraid to take up too much space? Your body language says a lot about how you feel about yourself. Create a power pose that exudes confidence and strength. For example, stand with your legs apart and your hands on your hips and walk with your head held up high. Practice it at home in front of a mirror to help you feel more confident about yourself. Take up as much space as you'd like. For more information on this topic, I recommend watching Amy Cuddy's TED Talk "Your Body Language May Shape Who You Are." It's excellent.

According to Dr. Kristin Neff, PhD, *practicing self-compassion* and treating ourselves as kindly as we treat our friends can reduce stress and potentially lower cortisol levels. It may also increase oxytocin, the body's love and feel-good hormone. Self-compassion is strongly linked to having better mental health. It can help lower stress, anxiety, depression, and perfectionism and boost happiness, motivation, and overall satisfaction with life. By being kind to ourselves, we can make better choices, resulting in improved health and happiness.

Another important aspect of building self-esteem is *looking at your relationships and how they affect you.* Do you surround yourself with people who drain your energy? Do others speak to you with respect? Do you find your relationship with your significant other is changing?

The better you feel about yourself, the more you surround yourself with people who treat you with kindness and respect. When you feel worthy and deserving of this type of treatment, you won't tolerate anything less.

Partner Relationships in Perimenopause and Menopause

My husband and I have had our share of challenges over the years, but things got much more difficult in my late thirties. What made it even harder was the fact that I didn't know I was in perimenopause at the time. We made it through, but it wasn't easy. Looking back on those rockier years, one thing that I believe helped our relationship was his sense of humor. He'd often try to make me laugh, even when I was upset. Communication also worked well once I understood *why* I was losing my sh*t all the time. When I read my husband this paragraph, he said, "All true." While humor worked for us, my husband suggests finding a communication method that works best for you and your partner to help defuse stressful situations.

I've spoken to many women over the years who are unhappy and unfulfilled in their relationships with their male partners. The divorce rate for women over fifty is on the rise. Research by AARP shows that women in their forties, fifties, and sixties initiate more than 60 percent of divorces. In fact, the divorce rate for people over fifty has become so common that it has its own term: Gray Divorce.

But *why* is it so common now?

The mix of physical, mental, and emotional changes that come with perimenopause and menopause can be hard for many women to navigate.

It can also be challenging for our partners, who are often on the receiving end of our mood and behavior changes, and they don't understand why.

Let's take a closer look at some of the reasons relationships can become strained during this time:

Physical changes: The many physical changes that menopause brings can affect intimate relationships. Two 2018 studies found that menopause-related symptoms like decreased libido/sex drive, vaginal dryness, and pain during intercourse can contribute to challenges in intimate relationships and marriages. And our own Morphus libido/sex drive* research published December 2025 in the journal *Menopause* showed that 91 percent of women in perimenopause and menopause had a noticeable decrease in libido or sexual desire, and 66 percent had a harder time reaching orgasm.

Physical symptoms can affect our self-esteem, causing us to shut down, avoid hanging out with others, shy away from intimacy, or struggle to keep close relationships. Changes like weight gain and hair loss or thinning can make us feel insecure and self-conscious. Over time, this emotional isolation can push others further away, making it harder to reconnect.

---

* "Women's Sexual Health: Understanding Libido Changes During Perimenopause and Menopause."

Mental and emotional changes: Emotional ups and downs like mood swings, irritability, rage, increased stress and anxiety, a lack of patience, and depression can have a major impact on partnerships. Changes in estrogen and progesterone can affect brain chemicals like serotonin and dopamine, which help to regulate mood. The combination of both physical and emotional symptoms makes it hard to manage daily life, let alone relationships. Estrogen helps regulate oxytocin, the "love hormone" that's responsible for helping us bond, trust, and feel emotionally connected to others. When oxytocin levels drop, women may feel more distant from the people they love most. Women in our research and online community describe it as feeling "numb" or "dead inside." Add in stress, exhaustion, overwhelm, unresolved past traumas, and changing nutritional needs, and it's understandable that women in this phase of life can have very little energy left to give anyone else. All these emotional changes can make it harder to talk openly about your feelings, which can create tension with your partner. But understanding why it's happening and being open about how you're feeling and what you're going through is the first step toward working through them together.

Existing marital stress: Research shows that the quality of your marriage can have a big impact on both your mental and physical health. Women in rocky relationships are more likely to have higher rates of depression and health issues like metabolic syndrome when there's ongoing conflict. Studies also show that marital stress can worsen health outcomes for women between the ages of thirty and sixty-five who have coronary heart disease (CHD). In addition, issues that have been dormant for many years may surface now. When couples don't communicate well or start growing apart, it can cause more tension and arguments if it's not addressed. Talking openly and making time for each other can help keep the relationship strong, especially when you don't feel like it.

Also, hormonal changes, like mood swings, less interest in sex, and lower self-confidence can affect the dynamic of a marriage. At the same time, this phase of life often brings a clearer picture of what we want and don't want in a relationship.

If you're feeling unhappy or unfulfilled in your marriage, consider having an open and honest conversation with your partner. Talking to a therapist or someone you trust can help you get through this challenging time.

Lack of understanding: When one partner feels misunderstood, or unheard, it can lead to frustration and loneliness. Many women going through this stage of life feel like their partners don't understand what they're experiencing or have empathy for their symptoms, especially if their partner is younger or a different gender. That's why having honest, heart-to-heart conversations and really listening can help both partners understand each other better. Myra calls this "active listening."

I had an open conversation with Jesse Robertson, a male content creator, who has been very outspoken about perimenopause and menopause now that his wife is going through it. His goal is to educate men about this phase of life so they can show up for their partners. He shared: "I know there are so many more husbands who would want to support their wives through menopause if they only understood what she was going through. If they just understood how difficult it can be both physically and mentally, they could not only strengthen their relationship, but they could literally save their marriage." And according to Bryce Wylde, a functional medicine clinician and founder of Husband™, "men in midlife often undergo their own set of hormonal, metabolic, and neurological changes sometimes called andropause. These shifts can affect sleep, stress, mood, energy, and recovery, all of which directly influence the emotional and physical environment women are navigating. When men understand what women are experiencing, and take steps to support their own midlife well-being, both partners benefit." You can listen to both discussions on my podcast, *Menopause Reimagined*, episodes #168 and #162, respectively.

Suppressed anger: Women who put the needs of others first may hide their feelings, especially anger, in order to keep the peace in their relationships. But as they start focusing on their own needs and their sense of self improves, their suppressed feelings can come out as sudden bursts of anger or rage. See if you can figure out what the true feelings are behind the anger, like frustration, irritation, disappointment, fatigue, stress, or sadness, and talk about them before they build up. Checking in with yourself about your feelings and expressing your needs to your partner on a regular basis can make the relationship more supportive and emotionally stable.

Changing interests: In a monogamous relationship, both partners work together toward a shared goal, but each person is also responsible for their own growth. Sometimes, regardless of how they try, a relationship can't be fixed, and it's healthier for both partners to go their separate ways. Some women choose to explore new connections that bring them joy and fulfillment, such as open relationships, polyamory, or same-sex partnerships.

Empty nest syndrome: When children move out, many couples find they no longer share the same interests, and they can drift apart. Myra recommends finding new common interests or rediscovering the parts of the relationship that initially brought you together. It can be as simple as scheduling a regular date night, going on walks, reading books together, exercising as a couple, and any other activity that helps to bring you together. Another option is to go for couples counseling or therapy.

Action Steps to Improve Relationships

If you want to improve the quality or your relationship(s), here are some action steps you can take:

Develop a vocabulary for open communication: It's important to have the words to be able to express yourself and explain the difficulties you're having, including the symptoms you're experiencing. However, it can be tough to do when you don't even realize you're in perimenopause. Regardless of whether you know what stage you're in, one communication tip Myra recommends is to speak from the "I," let your partner know *how* you're feeling, and express your needs. Here's an outline of a script you can follow.

Fill in the blanks:

"I feel [insert how you feel]

because [insert the reason].

As a result [insert your actions based on your feelings]."

Then express your need or want [let them know how they can support you].

It can look something like this:

"I feel *sad, irritated, angry, moody, etc.*

because *I'm having night sweats and not sleeping well.*

As a result, *I'm exhausted, get irritated easily and have no patience.*"

Then express your need or want: "*I would love for you to listen and really hear me. That would make me feel cared for by you; I would appreciate it if you could help me around the house more without me having to ask every time, etc.*"

Take a time-out: When angry feelings come up and you feel emotionally and physically overwhelmed, tell your partner you need some time to yourself. If possible, calm yourself down by taking a walk, doing deep breathing, or counting to ten. Come back when you're ready to talk. If you're not ready to continue the conversation, say so. You may need more alone time to process your thoughts and feelings so you can figure out where your anger is coming from. It's important to feel your emotions and use healthy ways to manage your anger so you can communicate better with your partner.

Take accountability: If you have regular angry outbursts, think about taking responsibility for your actions. I understand that the idea of saying sorry might trigger you or make you feel uncomfortable, especially if you don't believe you did anything wrong. That's a valid feeling. Apologizing, when appropriate, can be a powerful tool. It's not necessarily about admitting you did something wrong. It's about taking responsibility for your actions and acknowledging how they may have affected someone you love. Taking responsibility helps to calm the situation and show you care about the other person's feelings. Your actions show them that the relationship is important to you. It also shows emotional maturity, self-awareness, and that you choose to value the relationship over your personal pride. Most important, it makes it easier to talk openly, understand each other better, and grow together, helping to make your relationship stronger over time. However, there are also times when you may be in an unhealthy relationship where your partner isn't kind to you, doesn't treat you with respect, or may be abusive, so you lash out, which is understandable. If this is the case, Myra recommends exploring other options like getting outside help from a counselor or therapist or leaving the relationship.

Self-Care: Making Time for You

Whenever possible, schedule time, without interruptions, to give yourself permission to rejuvenate and recharge. This sends the message to yourself and others that you're deserving of it. If you have young kids, it can be hard to find the time, so do what you can, even if it's only five minutes.

- Start your day with a ritual or practice to anchor you and protect you against stress: listen to calming music, go for a walk, journal, express gratitude, exercise, meditate, pray, etc.

- Do something special for yourself on a regular basis. If you have a hard time carving out personal time, reach out to a friend or family member who can help (e.g., by babysitting so you can take a short walk).

- Be gentle with yourself. Treat yourself the way you'd treat a good friend, with kindness and respect.

- Tune in to your needs. Ask yourself what you're prepared to say yes or no to. As I mentioned in Chapter 6, "no" is a complete sentence. No explanation is needed.

- Create a space that nourishes and replenishes you, a place you can call your own. Surround yourself with objects and mementos that hold special meaning. It could be a sunlit nook, a table with fresh flowers or keepsakes, artwork or pictures that you love looking at, sitting in nature, or a personal altar with gemstones or objects you connect with.

- Inject "glimmers" into your everyday life, a term introduced by trauma specialist Deb Dana to describe micro-moments of joy, safety, and connection. Find what makes you happy, safe, and connected, and savor those moments.

- Repeat mantras/affirmations to yourself daily. These are positive statements we say to ourselves to reframe our negative self-talk and limiting beliefs to more compassionate ones. You can say them out loud, post them somewhere you'll see them often, or write them in your journal.

  Here are some examples:

  » I believe in myself.

  » I can handle this! I've got this.

  » I am resilient.

  » I treat myself with kindness and compassion by having patience for my process.

  » I am doing my best and now I can rest.

  » I face my fear by finding my courage and doing it anyway.

  » My body is strong and healthy.

  » I take care of myself and do what nourishes me.

When it comes down to it, we all want similar things: We want to be happy and feel loved. We want to live a life with meaning and purpose and feel valued for who we are. We want to be seen and heard and to know that our voices and lives matter, that we matter. These are things we have in common as perimenopausal and menopausal women and as human beings.

And it all starts with how we decide to care for ourselves. Myra often reminds me that self-love and self-care are not selfish acts. Rather, they're the foundation for how we show up every day. In her words: "When we nourish ourselves physically, mentally, and emotionally, we honor our needs, speak our truth, and live authentically in our power."

What are three things you do, or want to do, to nourish your self-care and self-love? Write them below:

- _____
  _____

- _____
  _____

- _____
  _____

13

Exercise During Perimenopause and Menopause

"Eat less, exercise more."
  "Cardio is the best way to lose weight."
  "Lifting heavy will make you bulky."
  "No pain, no gain!"

As Gen Xers and older millennials, we grew up bombarded by mixed messages about fitness and body image. We were told to eat less and move more, count calories, weigh our food, avoid eating fat because it makes us fat, and that no pain meant no gain. We were taught that lifting weights made women bulky and that cardio was queen, and we needed to do endless amounts if we wanted to stay in shape and be thin.

In my teens and early twenties, I spent hours at the gym on the StairMaster and treadmill and in aerobic classes trying to "burn off" the calories I ate that day, and I avoided the weight room altogether because I didn't want to look like the Hulk.

Think about how many times you told yourself over the years that you *needed* to go to the gym, or for a run, or to lose five or ten pounds so you could fit into your [insert event] dress. Too many to count, right? We've all been there. Those beliefs ran deep, and many of us, including me, carried them into midlife without realizing our bodies have changed (or are changing).

In my late forties, before I knew what perimenopause was, I thought my body was failing me because I was doing what I always did when it came to nutrition and exercise, but it wasn't working anymore and I didn't understand why.

Here's the thing: Your body has different needs now. Working out the way you did in your twenties and thirties doesn't necessarily serve you anymore, and in some cases can backfire by increasing inflammation and stress. This is the time to train smarter, not harder.

Along with the other changes you're making, it's important to reevaluate how you look at and approach exercise during midlife. It's no longer just about outward appearances or fitness goals. The health benefits of exercise and movement are endless, but how does it benefit perimenopausal and menopausal women specifically? Exercise serves a deeper purpose now. It's about feeling good, becoming or staying strong, and being able to do the things you love for as long as possible. Exercise at this stage is about energy, flexibility, confidence, resilience, and independence. It's a powerful tool for maintaining muscle mass, bone density, and strength, and reducing the risk for falls and fractures. It also strengthens your immune system, supports heart health, helps you bounce back from stress or illness more easily, balances your mood and blood sugar, improves sleep, and helps to keep hormones regulated. And at any age, exercise helps to reduce stress and triggers endorphins to make us feel amazing!

Rethinking how we move fits well with how we're rethinking food, rest, mindset, and boundaries. The goal now is to feel physically and mentally strong, capable, and confident.

Exercise Is Critical During Perimenopause and Menopause

Starting at around age thirty, we typically begin to lose about 3–8 percent of our muscle mass per decade. By the time we're in our forties, we may have 10–20 percent less muscle strength than we did in our twenties and thirties. And by our fifties, our muscles become less efficient at building and repairing themselves, which can lead to smaller, weaker muscles over time. After age sixty, the loss of lean muscle speeds up if we're not doing strength training or getting enough protein.

Once we go into menopause, we're more prone to losing muscle. Losing noticeable muscle mass, along with a drop in strength or function, is called sarcopenia, and when your muscles lose strength, even if the size of your muscles doesn't change, it's called dynapenia. Both can make you weaker and make everyday movements like climbing stairs and carrying groceries more challenging. Women with sarcopenia often have weaker grip strength and lower bone density, which puts them at a higher risk for osteoporosis. They're also more likely to be insulin resistant (refer to Chapter 5 where I talked about how muscles are your body's main glucose sponge, as they soak up sugar from your bloodstream). Recent research also suggests that sarcopenia may increase the risk of dementia. The best approach for slowing down sarcopenia is resistance training combined with eating enough protein.

According to Heather Creamer, a personal trainer, cancer exercise specialist, cofounder of the Health Coach Collaborative, and executive director of the Nova Scotia Fitness Association, it's never too late to start exercising and seeing the benefits! Heather trains women in their forties, fifties, sixties, seventies, and eighties who have never lifted weights before and sees firsthand how it increases their confidence, and how that confidence translates into other areas of their lives.

Strategic Training for Changing Hormones

The American College of Sports Medicine (ACSM) recommends the following activity guidelines for all healthy adults aged nineteen to sixty-five. These guidelines are widely adopted by both the U.S. and Canadian governments, as well as many other major organizations. They recommend a *minimum* of 150 minutes (2.5 hours) of moderate-intensity cardiovascular activity (such as brisk walking, or swimming, depending on your ability), or at least 75 minutes of vigorous-intensity exercise *a week* to see benefits for your cardiovascular health, with an additional minimum two times a week of resistance training, along with balance and flexibility training. You can combine moderate and vigorous activity to reach these goals. This is especially important for women in perimenopause and menopause, because as hormones shift, balance, strength, and flexibility can change too.

Dr. Stacy Sims, an exercise physiologist and nutrition scientist known for her research on women's performance and hormone health, recommends the following for women over forty: resistance and strength training (using weights, resistance bands, or body weight) at least three times a week to maintain muscle mass and metabolic health, along with *brief* high-intensity interval training (HIIT) once or twice a week to support cardiovascular health and metabolism.

Dr. Sims advises against relying too heavily on moderate-intensity cardio like long jogging sessions or frequent spin classes, because doing *too* much of this type of exercise can raise stress hormones, like cortisol, and over time may not provide the same hormonal or muscle-building benefits. Lower-intensity exercises or movements, like walking, hiking, and swimming, are great for active recovery days or in between harder workouts.

Practically speaking, the most important thing you can do is move your body. Most of us don't move enough. Research shows that more than 50 percent of adults in North America don't meet the recommended aerobic activity guidelines, and about 75 percent fall short of the combined aerobic and strength training recommendations from the ACSM. So start where you are and do what you can, when you can. Every bit of movement counts, and it adds up.

According to Melissa Hyde, a personal trainer with thirty-nine years of experience, a women's health and fitness expert and co-founder of the Loving Her Project, strength training is nonnegotiable for women in perimenopause and menopause for all the reasons I've already mentioned. And resistance training helps to build and protect your muscle mass and bone density. Melissa recommends keeping strength workouts to a maximum of four times a week to avoid overtraining. By strength training, Melissa means lifting heavy, whatever that means for you. In her words: "The definition

Did you know? Emerging research from 2025 found that if you're on a GLP-1 medication, you may lose a considerable amount of lean body mass (which includes muscle), along with fat. Since women between the ages of fifty and sixty-four are more likely to use GLP-1 medications, strength training and getting enough protein are crucial for preserving muscle. Check out my interview with Ashley Koff, a registered dietitian (RD), where we talked about GLP-1 agonist medications (episode #177 on my podcast, *Menopause Reimagined*).

of heavy is different for each of us, and it's not about competing with anyone else, it's about challenging yourself." Choose a weight that feels hard but doable for eight to ten repetitions (the last few should feel more challenging than the first few), and gradually increase the weight or number of reps over time. For most women, lifting heavier won't lead to bulky muscles but rather strength, shape, and definition. This involves doing upper- and lower-body exercises using dumbbells, barbells, weight machines, resistance bands, kettlebells, and even your own body weight. Melissa and I discussed this in more detail on episode #116 of my podcast, *Menopause Reimagined*.

There's a lot of fitness advice out there, but the most important advice I can offer is to listen to your body. If you feel good after a workout, that's a good sign that the exercise is right for you at that time. If it drains your energy, then try something else.

An important concept when it comes to strength training and building muscle, especially for this time in our lives, is a principle called progressive overload (PO). PO is when you slowly increase the intensity or strength of your workouts by doing more repetitions or sets, or by using heavier weights. It's how your body responds and gets stronger over time. If you repeat the exact same exercises at the same weights without changing things up, your body adapts, and you may experience a plateau. For beginners,

Heather recommends increasing the weight by no more than 2–5 percent over the course of a week to reduce the risk of injury or stress on the joints. For example, if you're doing bicep curls with five-pound dumbbells, begin with one to two sets of eight to twelve reps, and make sure you're also focusing on using good form. As your strength and confidence grow, gradually work your way up to three sets. You know you're working with the right weight for your body when the last few reps in the set feel more challenging than the first few, and you can only do a few more while still maintaining proper technique. Once you get to a point where all the reps feel equally easy, it's time to increase the weight to six pounds. At this point you can begin with three sets of eight to twelve reps. Repeat the process when the new weight is no longer challenging. You can also increase the intensity of your workout by gradually adjusting the number of reps or sets, slowing down the tempo of the lift, or adding lengthened partials (which means doing a few extra reps at the hardest part of an exercise when your muscle is fully lengthened. For example, during a bicep curl, when your arm is extended, bring the weights halfway up, then lower them back down. Working in that fully lengthened part of the movement helps with muscle strength and growth).

The key to reducing your risk of injury is to ensure proper form and make small progressive changes over time.

How to Exercise During Perimenopause and Menopause

It's important to differentiate between cardiovascular activity, which strengthens heart and lung health, and weight training, which strengthens muscles and bones, and supports your ligaments, cartilage, tendons, and other structures. Ideally, you'll want to incorporate both as part of your weekly exercise activities.

Research shows that it can take about eight to twelve weeks of regular training (at least two to three times per week) for women in menopause to see an increase in strength. And it's important to allow your muscles to recover in between workouts by alternating muscle groups or taking days off so they can grow, repair, and strengthen. I talk more about recovery later in this chapter.

Accumulating activity in short spurts throughout the day can still provide significant metabolic, cardiovascular, and mental health benefits. This type of approach may make it easier to stay consistent and reach your total weekly activity goals, especially if you're just starting with an exercise routine. It all adds up!

Below, you'll find Heather's recommendations for weekly cardiovascular and resistance training goals for women in both perimenopause and menopause.

During Perimenopause

This is a critical time to work on our cardiovascular health and build bone and muscle strength to help prevent loss as we go into menopause.

A good formula to follow is cardiovascular + resistance + flexibility + balance training.

Cardiovascular

Aim for an *accumulated minimum* of 150 minutes of moderate to vigorous cardiovascular activities each week. This can be broken into small increments of more intense exercise (like HIIT) or can include a long walk, and anything in between.

Depending on your goals, how hard you work during a workout matters. To find the right intensity for *your* workouts, you can use your heart rate as a gauge. First, figure out your maximum heart rate, which is the highest number of beats per minute (BPM) your heart should reach during exercise. The formula is 220 minus your age. Then multiply that number by the percentage of effort you want to work at (I'll explain this in a minute). You can track your heart rate with a wearable device, or you can tune in to your own body using the perceived rate of exertion (RPE) scale. This concept is based on how hard your workout *feels*, for example, how heavy your breathing is, how tired your muscles feel, and your overall effort or strain.

- **Moderate intensity:** Many of us in perimenopause (and menopause) will work out at this intensity, which is also known as the heart-healthy or fat-burning zone. Moderate intensity is working out at 50–70 percent of your max heart rate. For example, if you're fifty years old, your max heart rate would be 220 minus 50 = 170 bpm. So, multiply 170 by 50 percent and 70 percent and you get a range of 85–119 bpm. How do you know if you're working at a moderate-intensity pace? Do the "talk test." You should be able to hold a conversation but not be able to sing.

- **High intensity:** This is more suitable for those who have been training for a while or if you're an athlete, as you'll be working at an intensity level of 80–95 percent of your max heart rate (MHR). It'll be challenging to hold a conversation at this intensity since you'll be breathless and working near your physical limit.

There are many ways to sneak in cardiovascular exercises. Find an activity you enjoy doing, like going to the gym for aerobic classes or using their machines before or after a strength-training workout, roller skating, biking, rock climbing, pickleball, skiing, swimming, gardening, active housework (like vacuuming or mopping), or taking a brisk walk after a meal.

Resistance Training

Include at least two full-body, weight-bearing sessions a week and work your way up to three or four, working all major muscle groups. Challenge yourself to lift heavier weights than you normally would (this applies to whatever activity level you're starting at), always prioritizing safety and technique. Use the progressive overload principle to gradually increase the intensity and weight over time, reducing the risk of injury while maximizing results.

Before starting any resistance-training exercises, it's important to warm up your muscles first to increase circulation, improve joint mobility, and lower the risk of injury. A five to ten minute warm-up that includes light cardio, mobility drills, dynamic stretching, or bodyweight movements helps prepare your body for safe and effective training.

When it comes to (resistance) training, Stacy Sims recommends

Research shows that strength training is linked to lower rates of cardiovascular disease and death from all causes.

using compound movements such as squats, lunges, deadlifts, hip thrusts, or bent-over rows, which work several muscle groups at once. These exercises save time and build strength for everyday functions like lifting, pushing, pulling, and twisting. They also help to lower the chances of injury by improving coordination and balance.

If you're working out four or more times a week, you can do split workouts, for example, upper-body and lower-body exercises on separate days.

Flexibility

Lower estrogen levels in perimenopause and menopause can reduce collagen production and decrease elasticity and hydration in connective tissues such as tendons and ligaments. This can lead to increased stiffness, less flexibility, and a higher risk of injuries from strain or overuse. Incorporate stretching and mobility exercises several times a week to maintain range of motion and support recovery. Since muscles need to be warmed up before stretching, a great time to do it is after a workout or activity to help improve flexibility and mobility.

Tip: Hold each stretch for at least fifteen to thirty seconds to give the muscle time to relax. Do each stretch two to three times. If you're stretching regularly, you'll increase your flexibility over time. Yoga and Pilates are also great for this.

Balance

Balance training is especially important at this stage because hormonal fluctuations can affect stability and coordination, and can increase the risk of falls and injury. Our small stabilizing muscles such as the obliques, hip flexors, and rotator cuffs, which are crucial for posture and joint stability, can lose strength and responsiveness earlier than larger muscles because they're often underused. Balance training can help to counter that loss. It also helps to retrain your nervous system by improving communication between your brain, sensory organs (like the inner ears and eyes), and muscles, helping you stay steady and lowering the risk of falls. Aim for at least ten to fifteen minutes of balance-focused training a couple of times a week. Try yoga, tai chi, bird-dog holds, planks, heel-to-toe walking, standing three-way kicks, and stability ball work. Slowly increase the challenge by combining balance exercises with mental exercises like counting backward while standing on one leg.

During Menopause

In Chapter 8, I discussed how we're most susceptible to being diagnosed with osteoporosis, and one in three women over the age of fifty will experience a fracture because of it in her lifetime. This is another reason that weight-bearing exercises and resistance train-

---

Fact: Falls are a leading cause of injury-related deaths and the most common cause of injury-related hospitalizations in adults aged sixty-five and older. Women are more prone to falling as they age because of lower muscle mass and strength, hormonal changes, and the fact that we're more often prescribed antidepressants and sedatives, which can affect balance and coordination. Other medications, including muscle relaxants, blood pressure, and sleep aids, may also affect balance and coordination, so balance and strength-focused exercise becomes even more important in menopause. Low bone density and osteoporosis can make fall-related injuries more serious. A simple way to test your balance is to stand on one foot for ten seconds without putting your other foot down or holding on to something for support. If you're unable to do it, you may be at an increased risk of falling. In addition to balance training, you can also look into fall prevention programs, where they teach you how to fall properly to minimize injury.

ing are so critical in this time of life. So, if you haven't been exercising regularly up to this point, it's a great time to start.

If you're just beginning, keep in mind that the recommendations or guidelines mentioned earlier are something to work toward. Start slowly, and build on it. It can be overwhelming to jump right into a weekly schedule, so do what you can. It takes an average of about sixty-six days to build a habit, so consistency is key. Every bit of movement counts.

The formula in menopause is the same as perimenopause: cardiovascular + resistance + flexibility + balance training. However, at this stage, prioritizing resistance, flexibility, and balance training, as well as recovery, is even *more* important to help strengthen bones and muscles, and prevent falls and fractures.

Weight training is queen. For many of us now, our mindset shifts to being more health aware and focused on how we feel and move in our bodies, so looking for exercises that translate to our everyday life becomes important. For example, squats help us get on and off the toilet, bicep curls help us lift and carry what we need in our daily lives, and working our core muscles (abs and back) improves posture and helps with everyday movements.

When it comes to strengthening muscles, focus on your chest, shoulders, arms, legs, back, and core (muscles that work together to stabilize your spine, pelvis, and torso). And don't skip leg day! Research shows that the stronger our legs are (especially our quadriceps), the healthier our brains tend to age, and the lower our risk may be for developing dementia later in life. In addition, leg strength is also associated with better cognitive performance. Basically, overall muscle strength is a good indicator of brain health and function.

The same goes for grip strength. Studies show that menopausal women with stronger grip strength have higher bone mineral density and greater muscle strength. Having a weaker grip strength is associated with an increased risk of developing osteoporosis. A stronger grip is also associated with a lower risk of cardiovascular disease, type 2 diabetes, and early death. You can measure your grip strength with a handgrip dynamometer, a small device that records your strength when you squeeze it. Track your scores and compare them over time. The average strength for women over fifty typically falls between 50–60 pounds (or 23–27 kg), which is considered normal for this age group.

Exercise Tips in Perimenopause and Menopause

Here are some tips to keep in mind:

Mobility (the range of motion around a single joint): This relates to how well we're able to move through everyday tasks. For example, how well can you get on and off a chair? Or up and down off the floor? Can you walk up and down the stairs easily? Pick something up off the floor? Or move quickly to grab or catch something? All the exercises I talked about already will help with mobility. This is one of my favorite things to do because it helps with range of motion, flexibility, circulation, reducing stiffness, and stress relief. And the more you do it, the greater results you'll see. Try using resistance bands, massage balls, and foam rollers, as well as cat-cow stretches, shoulder rolls, hip circles, arm extensions, and child's pose. Somatic movement, tai chi, and other stability-building exercises like single-leg stands are also great because they improve stability, coordination, and mind-body connection. Pain is often related to not moving properly or at all, which can lead to compensations in other areas. Doing regular mobility exercises can help undo many of those patterns and reduce many of the aches and pains we associate with aging.

Note: Mobility matters just as much while strength training. For example, when doing chest presses, can you lower the bar all the way to your chest before pressing it back up? The director of my gym always emphasizes proper form and range of motion to make every rep count.

Have proper form. Fundamental mechanics are really important to avoid injuring yourself. If you're unsure how to do a specific exercise properly, ask a fitness professional to show you. At my gym, the instructor will often correct my form or adjust how much weight I'm lifting during class, which I appreciate because I want to make sure I'm doing it right. You can ask someone to show you, watch a video, follow fitness experts who understand perimenopausal and menopausal physiology, or hire a personal trainer who can tailor workouts to your body. There are also many group fitness classes (online and in person) you can join.

Try resistance bands. These are great for any level of fitness to help build strength, flexibility, balance, and mobility. They're gentle on joints, and you can use them anywhere (they're compact, versatile, and great for travel!). They're also a good option if you're less mobile, as you can adapt your workouts to accommodate your specific situation. My dad can't walk very well due to knee problems, so he uses them consistently to strengthen his upper and lower body while he's sitting and watching TV.

Incorporate plyometric work (quick explosive movements to improve strength and coordination and the brain-muscle connection). This type of training helps strengthen your muscles, joints, and tendons, improves coordination and athleticism, and can help stimulate or maintain bone density. When it comes to everyday movements, this helps you move quickly, for example, if you have to get out of the way of something or someone. Try hopping, skipping, jumping, medicine ball slams, jumping jacks, and burpees. Move in different directions including forward, backward, and laterally. Again, always move at a pace that feels comfortable for you.

Keep in mind that once you're in menopause, you're more prone to pelvic floor issues because lower levels of estrogen can affect connective tissue and pelvic floor support. If you're concerned or have a preexisting pelvic floor condition, exercise with intention to protect that area. For example, choose low-impact movements like gentle hopping, mini jumps, skipping with soft landings, or modified versions like step-ups or step-down hops, marching jacks (high knees while lifting your arms overhead), or step jacks (where you're alternating your side steps while lifting your arms). If you have leaking, heaviness, pain, or discomfort, it's important to talk to a pelvic floor specialist who can provide insight into your specific needs.

Brief sessions: If you don't have the time for one longer workout, consider breaking it up into three shorter sessions throughout the day. Several studies suggest that walking for about ten minutes three times a day at a moderate pace is just as, or more effective, at lowering post-meal blood sugar and insulin levels, and improving overall cardiometabolic markers compared to one longer session. It may also be easier to fit into your schedule.

A study on (post)menopausal women who trained for two sessions a week over a period of ten weeks found that they got stronger in both upper- and lower-body strength. However, if your goal is to gain muscle mass, or lose fat, researchers suggest training more often than twice a week, lifting heavier weights, and doing more than six to eight challenging sets per muscle group per week. This increased level of training is more likely to make a difference when it comes to losing weight and building muscle.

Walking: Walking has a ton of mental and physical health benefits, including heart health, mood, energy, stress relief, sleep, weight, and blood sugar management. A 2023 meta-analysis of nearly 227,000 adults (aged eighteen and up) published in the *European Journal of Preventive Cardiology* found that the risk of dying from heart issues started to drop at a relatively low number of steps, around 2,300 a day, and taking around 3,800 to 4,000 steps a day was enough to start significantly lowering the risk of dying from any cause. Each extra 1,000 steps was linked to about a 15 percent lower risk of death from any cause, and every extra 500 steps to about a 7 percent lower risk of dying from cardiovascular disease. The benefits continued to increase with more steps. And observational research published in 2025 in *The Lancet Public Health* found that walking around 7,000 steps a day (as opposed to 2,000) was linked to significantly lower risks of dying from any cause (47%), dementia (38%), and falls (28%).

Walk after you eat: When it comes to managing blood sugar, going for a short ten- to fifteen-minute walk after eating a meal, especially dinner, can significantly help lower post-meal (postprandial) blood sugar levels. Any form of exercise after eating can help prevent your blood sugar from spiking as high as it would if you ate and then stayed sitting (refer back to Chapters 5 and 11). Going for a walk or doing light activity after eating can help lower blood sugar for up to three hours and a single, longer session of exercise (like a brisk walk or workout) can help improve insulin sensitivity for up to twenty-four hours. There's also peer-reviewed research from 2022 that shows that doing soleus push-ups (a standing or seated exercise that activates the deep muscle in the calf) can lower post-meal blood sugar levels by about 52 percent and reduce insulin levels by around 60 percent over a three-hour period.

Fitness or exercise "snacks": Did you know that sitting for long periods of time can raise blood sugar, triglycerides, and inflammation in your body? What's the solution? Short bursts of movement. Melissa Hyde recommends incorporating fitness snacks into your day by getting up and moving every hour on the hour. These can be push-ups on the counter during your break, squats while brushing your teeth, calf raises while watching TV, or wall sits while you're on a call. Set an alarm to remind you to get up and move. I first heard of fitness snacks from Lisa Borden, founder of The Wellness Intelligence Collective (TWIC). She recommends "stacking your snacks" by doing several small fitness snacks a day. We went into detail about what that could look like on episode #121 of my podcast, *Menopause Reimagined*.

NEAT: According to board-certified naturopathic endocrinologist and nutrition scientist Dr. Jolene Brighten, while structured exercise is valuable, the real key to longevity and hormone health is how often we move throughout the day. This is a concept referred to as NEAT, which stands for "non-exercise activity thermogenesis." She explains that "integrating natural movement, like walking instead of driving short distances, carrying groceries, dancing while cooking, or taking the stairs, helps regulate blood sugar, improve insulin sensitivity, and balance cortisol rhythms." Studies consistently show that moving your body regularly throughout the day, even at an easy pace, supports better metabolic and hormonal health than spending most of the day sitting and squeezing in short, intense workouts.

WHAT ABOUT WEIGHTED VESTS?

Weighted vests have become very popular on social media. According to Selene Yeager, NASM-certified personal trainer and GGS menopause coaching specialist, "If wearing a weight vest motivates you to move more, then that's terrific, and if it adds a little bit more of a challenge than your usual exercise routine, that's great too. There have been a handful of small studies suggesting potential bone health benefits when used as part of an exercise program, but you shouldn't count on a weighted vest to build or protect your bones. If you're wearing it to build muscle strength, just lifting weights is a better strategy. If you're looking for weight-loss bene-fits, the vest needs to be pretty heavy to have a measurable impact on calorie burn, which can put undue stress on your lower back and joints. You may be able to get a bit of a car-diovascular boost adding a weighted vest to your workouts, just keep your expectations in check. And if you decide to wear one, focus on keeping your posture, core, and pelvic floor muscles strong to avoid injury."

Exercise timing: If you find exercising later in the day interferes with your sleep, try moving your workouts to earlier in the day when your cortisol is naturally highest. Save gentle exercises like stretch-ing, yoga, or walking for the evening to unwind and help prepare your body for bed.

Go slow: It's never too late to move! Start slow and build your strength and stamina over time. If you have a health condition or if you're in pain, look for a professional who specializes in this area, like a physiotherapist, personal trainer, exercise physiologist, occupa-tional therapist, rehabilitation specialist, or sports medicine doctor. If you're newer to exercise, Melissa Hyde wants you to know there's no need to "make up for lost time." In fact, that mindset can lead to burnout or injury. Instead, do what you can and gradually increase the intensity and difficulty of your workouts over time.

Why We Need to Rest in Between Workouts

Rest is just as important as the workout itself. It's important to give your body time to recover between sessions now that you're in perimenopause and especially menopause. Here's why: Lower levels of estrogen and progesterone can slow down how quickly your body recovers after exercise and contribute to greater muscle loss over time. Chronically high cortisol from ongoing stress can make your body more sensitive to those changes, which can interfere with repairing and rebuilding muscle. When cortisol stays high for too long, your body may spend more time in breakdown mode than growth mode. Too much of any intense exercise, done too often or for too long, along with poor sleep, high stress, or not eating enough nutrient-dense foods (including protein), makes it harder to build and maintain muscle at this stage of life.

Rest gives your body the chance to lower cortisol and inflammation, and it reenergizes you so your muscles can grow stronger. It also allows your hormones and nervous system to reset. It does this by shifting your body into parasympathetic mode, helping the body rest, digest, repair, and regulate your hormones. It also helps prevent injury and burnout from overtraining.

Overtraining can look different for us now than it used to. In addition to, or instead of, sore muscles, it might show up as irritability, fatigue, weight gain or trouble losing weight, or sleep issues. That's your body telling you it needs less intensity and more time for recovery.

During a weight-training session, longer rest periods between sets are also important now as they can help muscles recover and perform better during workouts. When you're working in the eight- to twelve-rep range per set, allow two to five minutes between sets (instead of thirty to ninety seconds, which is still recommended for younger people). If you still feel fatigued, wait a little longer. Research from 2022 on older women who rested for three minutes in between sets showed that they had more endurance during their workouts than those who only rested for one minute. Hopefully, we'll see more research on resting intervals specifically for women in perimenopause and menopause in the coming years.

Since being in perimenopause and menopause can impact your energy levels and affect how quickly you recover after exercise, it's important to adjust your workouts and rest times to what works best for you.

Recovery Tips

This is something I've been experimenting with recently as I've been feeling the aftereffects of my workouts, especially on leg day.

- **Magnesium oil:** Rub magnesium oil into your muscles after showering and reapply it a few times a day to relieve soreness. The oil penetrates your skin and muscles and helps to relieve the pain.

- **Epsom salt baths:** Soaking in a warm bath with Epsom salts, also known as magnesium sulfate, or magnesium chloride flakes can help soothe and relax sore muscles. Add two cups and soak for twenty minutes.

- **Bodywork:** My favorite therapies for helping my muscles recover and improving circulation are massage and stretching. I find them especially helpful if I have an injury.

- **Protein:** Have protein in your meal or snack within a couple of hours of working out to help with muscle repair and strength (refer back to Chapter 11 for how much).

- **Stay hydrated:** Drink before and after you exercise, as staying hydrated helps you feel more energized and can help prevent injury. Drink electrolytes to replace what you lose during workouts (I shared some beverage options in Chapter 11).

- **Keep moving:** Even on rest days, gentle movement can improve circulation and reduce stiffness.

- **Eat anti-inflammatory foods:** Here's another great reason to add omega-3s, leafy greens, and berries to your diet. Anti-inflammatory foods help to lower inflammation caused by exercise and help your muscles repair and grow.

- **Consider creatine:** Creatine is made in your body and stored mainly in your muscles, with smaller amounts in the brain. It's one of the most-studied nutrients, with thirty-plus years of research to back it up. Women naturally tend to have slightly less creatine stored in their bodies than men, and it's becoming very popular among perimenopausal and menopausal women. Creatine helps your body make energy and may support your brain, mood, and heart. When it comes to exercise, it can help build and maintain muscle mass, increase strength, especially in older adults, support faster recovery, and lessen post-workout soreness.

  You can find creatine in animal-based foods like meat and fish (herring and salmon), and you can take it as a supplement. When taken as a supplement, the recommended form is creatine monohydrate, and the typical dose is 3–5 grams a day. You can take it any time of day.

  Note: Once you start taking creatine, you might feel bloated or notice some weight gain, since it draws water into your muscle cells. This is usually temporary and tends to go away after a few weeks. Be sure to stay hydrated and find the dose that works best for you.

Exercise and Mental Health

Another major benefit of exercise in perimenopause and menopause is how it helps your body manage and cope with stress. Since we're more stressed now, it's a welcome distraction, giving us a break from daily stressors.

Exercise is amazing for our mood and mental health because it increases "feel good chemicals" in our brain and nervous system like serotonin, dopamine, and endorphins. It also helps to regulate cortisol, which as you know can run high during this time in our lives.

Exercise has been shown to improve symptoms of depression in menopausal women.

A 2024 meta-analysis found that mind-body exercises like yoga, tai chi, Pilates, and qigong improved bone mineral density, sleep quality, anxiety, depression, and fatigue in perimenopausal and (post)menopausal women. Exercising outdoors, often called "nature therapy," can improve mood, reduce blood pressure, and lower cortisol levels. Avoid heavily polluted areas.

Since many of us are dealing with anxiety, mood fluctuations, and a lack of sleep at this time, staying active can help regulate many of our symptoms.

Exercise and Vasomotor Symptoms

Research from 2022 shows that exercise might reduce the severity of hot flashes and night sweats for some women, but not necessarily their frequency. Other research suggests that regular moderate-intensity exercises like pickleball, brisk walking, light cycling, swimming at a steady pace, dancing, and gardening or yard work that gets your heart rate up may also ease symptoms.

If You Can't Exercise Regularly

If you're unable to exercise, for whatever reason, consult with a fitness specialist who can work with you and tailor a program for your particular needs.

Balancing Stress and Exercise in Midlife

According to Melissa Hyde, "Midlife is a time when our body is asking to be cared for differently. But before we even talk about exercise intensity, we need to address something crucial: how much stress you're under and how well you're recovering from it. Intense workouts can set you back because your body is already working hard just to keep up, and adding physical stress only drains it further."

Melissa's point is important and backed by research. As we saw in

Chapter 6, when we go into perimenopause and menopause and our estrogen and progesterone levels drop, our adrenal glands step in by making small amounts of hormones, mainly androgens like DHEA and androstenedione. The adrenal glands also produce cortisol, and chronic stress can change how much of these adrenal hormones are produced, often increasing cortisol and decreasing DHEA, which can leave us feeling fatigued or overwhelmed. It can also increase inflammation and make it harder to build muscle or recover properly from workouts. Research also shows that ongoing high cortisol and low DHEA are linked to more menopause symptoms, including hot flashes, sleep issues, mood changes, increased sensitivity or lower tolerance to pain, and other inflammatory conditions.

That's why when you're already under a lot of stress, whether from lack of sleep, emotional stress, or overtraining, Melissa recommends focusing on more gentle movements like yoga, Pilates, stretching, walking outdoors, mobility work, and breath work until you're feeling stronger. It's also important to prioritize sleep (Chapter 7), eat protein with every meal (Chapter 11), and be mindful of how much alcohol and caffeine you're consuming. These steps help support your stress system (including your adrenal glands) and calm your body so you can resume your regular training at a later date.

Pre- and Post-Exercise Nutrition

As I talked about in Chapters 8 and 11, protein is the foundation for building and maintaining muscle, and women who eat enough protein maintain more muscle and strength as they age.

Having protein after a workout helps your muscles recover and grow stronger. Eating protein with carbs around the time of your workouts helps with recovery: Carbs give your muscles energy, and protein helps to repair them. Having carbs before you exercise can give you extra energy and help your muscles stay strong.

Having antioxidant-rich foods, such as colorful veggies; low-glycemic fruits like berries; herbs, spices, nuts, and seeds; and omega-3 fatty acids from salmon, sardines, hemp seeds, chia, and walnuts may help support recovery and lower inflammation.

Research also shows that eating omega-3 rich foods combined with resistance training can significantly increase muscle strength (but not muscle size). Together, these nutrients can help reduce inflammation and improve metabolic health during perimenopause and menopause.

From a nutrient standpoint, a 2024 analysis found that getting enough of two types of B vitamins, B1 (thiamine) and B2 (riboflavin), was associated with a 22 percent and 16 percent lower risk of developing early-onset sarcopenia, respectively. Include foods rich in both these B vitamins on a regular basis. Legumes, nutritional yeast, whole grains, and nuts and seeds are good sources of B1, and sources of B2 include dairy products, eggs, spinach, kale, and broccoli.

In summary, the advantages of exercise go beyond weight and appearance. Shifting the focus from losing pounds to gaining strength, energy, and confidence improves our self-esteem, something many of us find diminishes during this time (low self-esteem is on the 103+ list of symptoms). I've personally felt the incredible benefits of exercise! To give you one example, I'm proud of how I'm now able to lift my carry-on suitcase in one fell swoop over my head and into the overhead bin when I'm traveling by plane. As simple as that sounds, it wasn't something I could do when I was younger, and it makes me very happy!

Doing activities you enjoy that get your body moving and build strength can help you stay strong, mobile, and resilient for years to come.

Not the Final Chapter: Where Do We Go from Here?

As I write this final chapter, I'm excited for your next one.

You've spent years pouring energy into everyone around you. Now, this is your time to prioritize your health and focus on what *you* want moving forward.

I also hope this book helps you feel seen, supported, and validated. I hope it gives you the insight and direction to move into this next chapter with confidence and curiosity.

Grab a pen or pencil and write down three new mindset or lifestyle strategies that you'd like to implement immediately after reading this book.

1. _____

   _____

2. _____

   _____

3. _____

   _____

I recently heard Dr. Jessica Shepherd, MD, MBA, FAGOG, speak about the importance of building your healthcare team. She shared that no single person can meet all of your mental, physical, and emotional needs during this phase of life, so assemble a team that you trust and who will support you holistically. This team should also include your biggest cheerleaders, the people you can lean on when you need someone to talk to or to confide in.

Lisa Brookman, MSW, PSW, cofounder of West Island Therapy and Wellness Centre, recommends surrounding yourself with people, including professionals, who get it. People who truly understand women's health and more specifically perimenopause and menopause, who listen, and who make space for your experiences. If a professional is dismissive, that's a red flag. Your relationship with healthcare providers should be grounded in trust, respect, and genuine understanding. As a psychotherapist, she urges us to truly love ourselves because when we do, we become whole, stronger, and more grounded. And we show up in ways that change our relationships, health, and happiness.

As you strengthen your support network, I also want to acknowledge our partners. In 2025, my company Morphus and I published research on men's perspective of menopause* in the journal *Menopause*, and what we discovered is that many of them want to help but don't know how. As discussed in Chapter 12, talk to your partner. Share how you're feeling and what you need so they can support you better.

We can't do this alone. Although each one of us is unique, we're connected through our shared experiences. Some days will be easier than others; that's normal, but it's important to always be gentle with yourself and give yourself grace throughout this process.

Because the majority of us will spend anywhere from a third to half of our lives in menopause, this book can serve as a guide for your nutrition, lifestyle, mindset, and supplement choices. Keep asking questions. Information is constantly evolving, so seek answers from multiple experts and sources you trust. If you'd like to connect with others who are also going through perimenopause and menopause, check out in-person and online communities who talk about it openly. I'd love you to join our private Morphus Facebook community at www.facebook.com/groups/wearemorphus.

---

* "Understanding Men's Perspectives of Perimenopause and Menopause" with Marcella Hill and Danielle Meitiv.

I'd like to hear your story. Send me a note at book@wearemor
phus.com.

For additional resources on the topics covered in this book,
please visit www.nourishingmenopausebook.com and click on the
Resources tab.

As I mentioned in Chapter 2, our research is ongoing, and your
lived experience matters. By completing our surveys at www.weare
morphus.com and clicking on the Research tab, you help make this
work possible.

While this may be the last chapter of this book, it's not the final
chapter of your story. I'd like to leave you with a quote I wrote that
captures our shared experiences and what is still being written:

> *"Women in menopause are like butterflies. First, they*
> *undergo metamorphosis, then they take flight to become*
> *their true, authentic, and free selves."*

Your wings are ready. How will you take flight as you live this
new chapter of your life as your true, authentic self?

With love and gratitude,

Andrea ♥

ACKNOWLEDGMENTS

This book has truly been a team effort. When you have over twenty-six years of experience, information, and research stored in your brain, it doesn't make for an easy edit. Before my publisher received the final copy of my manuscript, many of the chapters ran over a hundred pages, some even close to 150. I'm not exaggerating! I owe Brittany Lavery, Amanda Lewis, and my amazing colleague Lisa Trepanier-Tsakos all the kudos in the world for helping me shape this book into something I'm super proud of.

To my incredible editor, Brittany Lavery, thank you for believing in me, and in this book, from day one. Your curiosity and drive to understand perimenopause and menopause gives me hope for your generation and those that follow. Your guidance, patience, understanding, and contributions were exactly what the book (and I) needed, and you were a pleasure to work with! I'm grateful for you and your team at Simon & Schuster Canada, including the marketing and publicity departments, the wonderful production team, and particularly Muna Hussein, whose heroic efforts ensured this book reached production on time.

Amanda Lewis, while it was no easy feat, you were able to comb through the chapters and find the heart of the message. You're a true magician and I can't thank you enough for your help with this book.

To the production team at Simon & Schuster, I'm deeply grateful to all of you who helped bring this project to life: Rachael DeShano, Kayley Hoffmann, and Kaitlyn Lonnee. I'm particularly grateful to Sabrina Futia in editorial for her help with the references.

To Alana Kluver, thank you from the bottom of my heart for your time, devotion, and attention to detail in helping me with the edits. I'm thrilled you got to read this book as a Gen Zer who will now know what to expect when you enter into perimenopause and menopause, and how to navigate it.

To my agent, Stacey Glick, thank you for saying yes to me and for believing in me and the topic from day one. You matched me with the perfect publishing team and for that I'll always be grateful!

Samantha Harris, thank you for introducing me to Stacey after that long and passionate conversation we had at Expo West. We could have gone on for hours! Your connection opened the door to everything that followed.

To my colleague Lisa Tsakos. This marks our fourth book together, and I couldn't imagine doing it without you. I'm so blessed to have someone with your experience by my side. How fitting is it that we both went through menopause at the same time? I knew back in 1999, in our twenties, when you taught me Fundamentals of Nutrition at the Canadian School of Natural Nutrition (CSNN) that we'd be partners in some capacity; it just so happened to be as authors of health and wellness books. Thank you for pouring your heart and soul into this book and for being an invaluable sounding board. I'm so proud of what we've accomplished, and I cherish our friendship.

Deborah Mitchell, you were there from the very beginning when writing this book was just an idea and vision I had. You helped me lay the foundation and envision what this book could become. I couldn't have started this project without you, and I'm grateful for the fifteen years we worked together. Your loyalty and dedication meant so much to me and I'm so thankful we met all those years ago in New Mexico at that press conference.

To Randy Boyer, my business partner of twenty-six years. Writing this book in the third act of our lives feels like a full-circle moment. Helping women feel educated and empowered as they go into perimenopause and menopause is our mission at Morphus, and I'm excited to continue our legacy of helping others. Thank you for your support and understanding over the past three years while I worked on the proposal and then the book itself. Your loyalty, patience, and most of all friendship over the past three decades means the world to me. I couldn't have done this book without your unwavering support.

Lisa Collins, my left-hand, get-it-done, techy gal. Thank you for managing the details, reviewing chapters, and coordinating the graphics. You're a rock star and I'm grateful for you and having you as an integral part of our team at Morphus.

To my mom, Myra. It was an honor to collaborate with you on Chapter 12. As a master of social work and therapist for over thirty-five years, your insights, empathy, compassion, understanding, and tips will help women for generations to come. Thank you for being my sounding board and for reviewing my chapters several times over. You're my best friend and I love you!

To my colleagues and friends Bonnie Wisener, Lorene Sauro, Heather Creamer, Melissa Hyde, Amanda Thebe, and Lori Schacter, thank you for your generosity in reviewing specific chapters. Your input was so appreciated, and I have a tremendous amount of respect for all of you.

A big thank-you to Lise Walton, Lisa Tsakos, Crystal Krandel, Alana Kluver, and Sylvianne Borenstein for contributing delicious, nourishing recipes.

To all the doctors, healthcare practitioners, and experts who provided quotes, endorsements, and insight, thank you for lending your voices to this important conversation and for shaping it with incredible expertise.

To my dear friend Scott Lazerson. Thank you for your unwavering support, enthusiasm and most of all friendship of 20 years. I adore you and Heidi, and I'm grateful for all that you do.

To the woman who first opened my eyes to menopause long before I experienced it, Lorna Vanderhaeghe. I had no idea what a wild and transformative ride was ahead, but working for you and speaking on this topic years before I went through it laid the foundation for what was to come.

Dr. James Simon, MD, and Dr. Carrie Jones, ND, I'm so grateful for both of your support. Having you in my corner for my research means the world to me. Thank you for writing the forewords and for believing in me, my work, and this book.

To my kids, thank you for your patience, humor, and understanding. I wrote this book for you, because I want you to know that perimenopause and menopause are a natural phase of life that every woman who's blessed to live long enough will go through. I want you to feel informed, prepared, and confident when you eventually go through it, or when you support a partner who does. Thank you for putting up with me and my constant writing. I love you and you make me so proud. I'm honored to be your mom.

To my incredible husband, Rich. There aren't enough words to express my gratitude. You're a freakin' superstar. You've been so supportive and patient with me over the last two years. Thank you for picking up the slack at home, for making me dinners, and for taking over driving duty. I couldn't have done this without your unwavering support and help. Thank you from the bottom of my heart for always being in my corner and giving me the confidence and inspiration to accomplish great things. You're my rock, my biggest cheerleader, and I'm so grateful to call you my husband and partner. I love you.

To our Morphus online and social media community, I'm so grateful for each and every one of you. For your support, for filling out our research surveys, for being part of a bigger mission to help women navigate this time in their lives. Your comments, input, and responses to our surveys are helping women globally.

And finally, to you—the reader. Thank you for choosing to read this book, for wanting to understand your body, and for taking ownership of your health and symptoms. Together, we're breaking the silence around perimenopause and menopause and redefining what it means to thrive at every age. You're part of a movement that's changing the conversation, and I'm honored you're here with me.

Recipes

SPICES

Homemade Everything Spice

By Crystal Krandel

This is my favorite go-to spice blend. You can add it to pretty much everything! You can buy the ingredients at a bulk store and mix them together. It's perfect for topping homemade bagels or breads, adding to roasted vegetables and eggs, or seasoning meats. If you're looking to lower your salt intake, you can leave it out.

2 tablespoons poppy seeds
2 tablespoons sesame seeds (white or black, or a mix)
2 tablespoons dried minced garlic
2 tablespoons dried minced onion
2 tablespoons Himalayan pink or black salt

Combine all the ingredients in a small bowl.

Mix well until everything is evenly distributed.

Transfer to an airtight container for storage.

Storage: Store in an airtight container in a cool, dry place away from direct sunlight. The spice blend will stay fresh for up to 6 months.

Serving size: 1 teaspoon
Protein: ~0.3 g
Carbs: ~1.1 g
Fat: ~0.5 g
Sodium: 367 mg (with added salt)
Sodium: ~20 mg (without added salt)

DIPS, DRESSINGS, AND SAUCES

Artichokes and Dip Dressing

By Sylvianne Borenstein

Artichokes contain antioxidants, prebiotic soluble fiber, and nutrients, including vitamin C, vitamin K, folate, phosphorus, potassium, and magnesium, that help support bone and liver health and can help lower oxidative stress. Avocado and olive oil have healthy monounsaturated fats, and shallots belong to the allium family of foods, compounds that help protect cells from damage caused by free radicals. In addition to using it as an artichoke dip, you'll have some left over to dress salads or drizzle over proteins like fish or chicken.

6 artichokes

DRESSING
1 heaping tablespoon of Dijon mustard
3 tablespoons extra-virgin olive or avocado oil
1 tablespoon red wine vinegar
4 shallots, chopped
2 pinches salt

Use kitchen scissors to trim the artichoke leaves and cut the tops and bottoms off each artichoke.

Wash the artichokes well, especially between the leaves, to remove dirt.

You can either boil or steam the artichokes in salted water until they are soft (Sylvianne prefers boiling them). Once soft, the leaves come off easily with a fork.

Drain the water and soak the artichokes in cold water to serve them warm but not burning hot.

Whisk together the dressing ingredients and serve on the side in a small bowl for dipping.

Note: If using olive oil, remove the dip from the fridge 20 minutes before using it to allow it to become room temperature.

Serving size: 2 tablespoons of dressing
Protein: ~1.8 g
Carbs: ~6.6 g
Fat: ~2.8 g

Cauliflower Sauce

This simple-to-make creamy cauliflower sauce is a lower-carb twist on a classic comfort food. The combination of ingredients provides nutrients including protein, calcium, magnesium, and vitamin K. Nutritional yeast contains B vitamins, which are important for mood and brain health. It's a tasty and versatile way to incorporate more vegetables into your diet. Pour it over pasta, drizzle it on veggies, or use it as a white pizza sauce.

1 cauliflower, steamed and cooled
1 cup cottage cheese
1 clove garlic, grated
1 teaspoon salt
3 teaspoons black pepper
¼ cup nutritional yeast

Add all ingredients to a blender (or food processor) and blend for 30 seconds.

Scrape down the sides and blend again until the sauce is smooth. If the sauce is too thick, add a little water or milk and blend again.

Note: You can also use this sauce as a dip. Add chili powder or cayenne pepper (to your taste).

Serving size: ¼ cup
Protein: ~4 g
Carbs: ~5 g
Fat: ~1 g

Black Bean, Olive Oil, Feta, and Mint Dip

By Lisa Tsakos

This dip is great for snacking and entertaining. It's high in protein and has a refreshing flavor profile from the mint.

1 can (15 oz) black beans, drained and rinsed
2 tablespoons extra-virgin olive oil
1 small garlic clove, minced (optional)
¼ cup crumbled feta cheese (or your preferred cheese)
¼ cup fresh mint leaves, finely chopped, plus a few whole leaves
1 tablespoon fresh lime juice (optional)
Sea salt (or Himalayan salt) and pepper, to taste
A pinch of chili flakes (optional for some heat)

In a food processor, combine the black beans, olive oil, and minced garlic (if using). Blend until smooth. If the mixture is too thick, you can add a little water or more olive oil until the desired consistency is reached.

Transfer the mixture to a bowl. Stir in the crumbled cheese and chopped fresh mint.

Add the lime juice (if using), salt, pepper, and chili flakes (if using). Adjust the seasoning to your taste.

Garnish with a few whole mint leaves or an extra drizzle of olive oil on top, if desired.

Serve the dip with crackers, pita chips, or fresh veggies.

Serving size: 1 tablespoon
Protein: ~1.1 g
Carbs: ~2.2 g
Fat: ~1.5 g

SOUPS AND SALADS

Superhero Soup

This delicious soup is loaded with anti-inflammatory veggies and spices that help lower inflammation. If your hot flashes are intense, this soup tastes great at any temperature.

1 large white onion, diced
1 large carrot, diced
2 stalks celery, diced
3 to 4 cloves garlic, diced
1 tablespoon extra-virgin olive oil
1 medium sweet potato, peeled and diced

A pinch of cayenne pepper
1 teaspoon salt
1 teaspoon pepper
1 head of broccoli, cut into pieces
4 to 6 cups vegetable or chicken stock

In a large pot over medium heat, sauté the onion, carrot, celery, and garlic in olive oil until it gets a bit golden, about 1-2 minutes.

Add the sweet potato and all the spices. Cook for 3-4 minutes.

Add the broccoli and cook for another 1-2 minutes.

Add 4-6 cups of vegetable/chicken stock (enough to cover the vegetables fully).

Cover the pot and bring it to a gentle boil. Lower the temperature and simmer for 30 minutes or until the vegetables are tender.

Use an immersion blender or a regular blender to blend the soup into a creamy, delicious texture. (Before using an immersion blender, allow the soup to cool slightly to prevent it from burning you if it splatters).

Tip: Swap chicken stock for chicken bone broth to increase the protein.

Serving size: 1 cup
Protein: ~3 g
Carbs: ~12 g
Fat: ~2 g

Squash, Pomegranate, and Quinoa Salad

By Alana Kluver

This bright, colorful salad feels like summer and will leave you feeling fresh and naturally energized. The squash and quinoa combo keeps you satisfied while delivering a burst of antioxidant-rich flavor.

1 medium butternut squash
Extra-virgin olive oil
Salt and pepper
½ cup uncooked quinoa (I use mixed quinoa, but any variety works)
1 pomegranate
½ cup pumpkin seeds
1 large handful of baby spinach
½ cup crumbled feta cheese (or vegan alternative)

DRESSING
1 tablespoon whole-grain mustard
1 teaspoon low-sugar liquid sweetener (my favorite is yacon syrup)
2 tablespoons balsamic vinegar
2 tablespoons extra-virgin olive oil
Salt and pepper, to taste

Remove both the outer skin and seeds from the butternut squash, and chop into roughly 1-inch cubes. Drizzle with a small amount of olive oil, lightly season with salt and pepper, and roast in the oven at 400°F (204°C) for 40–50 minutes (or until it's soft enough to pierce with a fork). Once cooked, remove and allow to cool slightly.

At the same time, cook the quinoa on the stovetop according to package instructions (which should be approximately 10–15 minutes of simmering and 5–10 minutes of resting).

Deseed the pomegranate, ensuring that all the white pith is removed.

Make the salad by combining the roasted squash, cooked quinoa, pomegranate seeds, pumpkin seeds, baby spinach, and feta cheese.

(Continues)

Whisk together the dressing ingredients and pour over salad. Toss to combine, and enjoy!

Tip: This salad can be served as a side dish or adapted to create a delicious, filling meal (that happens to be great for meal prep!). To make this a well-rounded meal, add your favorite protein either on top or tossed in (my personal go-to is grilled chicken).

Serving size: 1 cup
Protein: ~11 g (not counting optional added protein)
Carbs: ~30 g (this will vary depending on your choice of sweetener)
Fat: ~19 g

Green Apple, Cabbage, and Cucumber Slaw

By Alana Kluver

Crisp, fresh, and naturally sweet, this green slaw adds a refreshing twist to any meal and takes only minutes to throw together.

½ green cabbage
2 Persian cucumbers
1 green apple

DRESSING
2 tablespoons rice wine vinegar
2 tablespoons soy sauce (look for brands with no added MSG)
2 tablespoons sesame oil
2 tablespoons low-sugar sweetener (like stevia, monk fruit, or allulose)

To prep your salad ingredients, finely shred the green cabbage, chop the cucumbers (either in rounds or half moons), and julienne the green apple (make sure to keep the green skin for extra fiber!).

Whisk together the dressing ingredients and adjust to your taste preference (e.g., if you prefer a sweeter slaw dressing, add more of your sweetener, or if you prefer a tangier slaw dressing with a bit more zip to it, add more rice wine vinegar).

Toss all the salad ingredients together with the dressing, and enjoy!

Serving size: 1 cup
Protein: ~1 g
Carbs: ~11 g (this will vary depending on your choice of sweetener)
Fat: ~7 g

SIDE DISHES

Easy Roasted Cauliflower Bites

Goodbye greasy chicken wings, hello tasty cauliflower bites. These healthy cruci-ferous bites help support your hormones. Serve hot as a side dish or snack.

1 large head of cauliflower, cut into bite-sized florets
2 tablespoons extra-virgin olive oil
1 teaspoon ground turmeric
½ teaspoon garlic powder or 1 clove garlic, minced (optional)
Salt and pepper, to taste
Fresh lemon wedges, for serving (optional)

Preheat oven to 425°F (220°C). (You can also roast the cauliflower in an air fryer.)

In a large bowl, toss the cauliflower florets with the olive oil, making sure they're evenly coated.

Sprinkle the turmeric, garlic powder (or minced garlic), salt, and pepper over the cauliflower. Toss again to ensure the spices are evenly distributed.

Spread the seasoned cauliflower florets on a baking sheet in a single layer. Roast for 25–30 minutes, or until the cauliflower is golden brown and crispy on the edges, tossing halfway through.

Remove from the oven and squeeze fresh lemon juice over the roasted cauliflower, if desired.

Serving size: 1 cup
Protein: ~4 g
Carbs: ~12 g
Fat: ~7 g

MEAL IDEAS

Easy Spinach Wraps

This high-protein, high-fiber combo forms a wrap that can be used with nitrate-free sliced meats, avocado, and hummus to make a delicious meal any time of the day. Spinach contains fiber, magnesium, and iron (refer to Chapter 8 for why these minerals are important), and each egg contains 5–6 grams of protein.

Extra-virgin olive oil
1½ to 2 cups of baby spinach
2 large eggs

Place the spinach and eggs in a high-speed blender and puree into a smooth liquid.

Warm a lightly oiled large frying pan over medium-high heat, and pour ¼ to ½ cup spinach-and-egg liquid into the pan.

Spread it around the pan to form a thin layer.

Cook for about 4–5 minutes until the wrap is partially cooked.

Flip and cook the other side for about 1–2 minutes.

Repeat with remaining mixture.

Put it onto a plate and enjoy it with nitrate-free sliced meats, avocado, and hummus, or your favorite wrap fixings.

Serving size: 1 egg wrap (macros not included for fixings)
Protein: ~14 g
Carbs: ~3 g
Fat: ~10 g

Sardine Patties

Sardines are a delicious way to incorporate omega-3- and protein-rich fish into your diet. These turn out crispy on the outside and moist on the inside. Plus, sardines are an excellent source of calcium, and they provide a depth of flavor when mixed with all the other ingredients. They are quick to make and perfect for meal prep. Leave a few in the fridge to grab for a quick lunch with a salad.

2 cans of sardines, drained
2 teaspoons extra-virgin olive, avocado, or coconut oil
1 small onion, diced
1 stalk celery, diced
1 small carrot, grated

A pinch of sea or Himalayan salt
1 teaspoon black pepper
1 teaspoon grated ginger
1 egg
2 tablespoons all-purpose, almond, or gluten-free flour

Place the drained sardines in a medium bowl.

Warm a frying pan over medium-high heat. When warm, add the oil, onion, and celery, and sauté until the onion is translucent and celery is softened.

Add the carrot, salt, pepper, and ginger, and sauté for an additional 2 minutes.

Add the mixture to the sardines, along with the egg and flour. Mix well.

In the same frying pan, add a little more oil. Scoop ¼ of the sardine mixture into the pan and flatten.

Cook on one side for 3–4 minutes until golden brown; flip and cook the other side for 1–2 minutes.

Repeat with the remaining mixture.

NOTES

- *Add chili flakes for a little extra zing. Chili flakes can help rev up your metabolism too.*
- *Wrap in lettuce leaves instead or add to spinach wraps (see the previous recipe).*

Serving size: 1 patty
Protein: ~8 g
Carbs: ~5 g
Fat: ~6 g

Lentil Curry with Poached Egg

This dish can be eaten for breakfast, lunch, or dinner (fresh and as leftovers).

1 tablespoon extra-virgin
   olive oil
1 small onion, finely diced
2 cloves garlic, grated
1 inch ginger, grated
2 teaspoons fish sauce
1 tablespoon tamari
1 tablespoon mild green curry
1 Thai chili, finely chopped

1 cup chopped broccoli, chopped
   into small florets
1 tomato, chopped
1 cup chicken or vegetable stock
2 cups green lentils, cooked
½ cup coconut milk
2 to 4 eggs
1 tablespoon finely chopped
   chives

In a large frying pan, heat the olive oil over medium-high heat, then add onion and sauté until translucent. Add the garlic, ginger, fish sauce, tamari, green curry, and chili; sauté for 5 minutes.

Add the broccoli, tomato, stock, and lentils, then reduce the heat to medium low and let simmer for approximately 20 minutes or until thickened.

Add the coconut milk and warm through.

Meanwhile, in a small saucepan, bring water to a gentle boil. Crack 1 egg into a small bowl. With a spoon, stir the water to create a vortex, gently place the egg in the water, and cook for 2–3 minutes or until desired doneness. Repeat with the rest of the eggs (alternately, you can use fried eggs).

Serve the curry in a bowl topped with an egg and some chives.

Note: For the lentils, you can buy them cooked in a can or cook them according to the directions on the package.

Tip: Boost the protein in your ground meat dishes by mixing in at least half a cup of cooked lentils, beluga lentils, or canned black beans. This sneaky heart-healthy swap also adds fiber and doesn't sacrifice flavor or texture!

Serving size: 1 cup curry with 1 poached egg
Protein: ~20 g
Carbs: ~12 g
Fat: ~33 g

Greek-Style Chicken Thighs

These chicken thighs are tangy and moist and loaded with anti-inflammatory herbs that contain antioxidants.

½ cup Greek yogurt
2 teaspoons dried oregano
2 teaspoons dried basil
2 cloves garlic, grated
Zest and juice of 1 lemon
1 teaspoon salt
1 teaspoon ground pepper
1 teaspoon chili flakes (optional)
8 to 10 skinless, boneless chicken thighs

In a large mixing bowl, combine the yogurt, oregano, basil, garlic, lemon zest and juice, salt, pepper, and chili flakes, if using.

Reserve half of the marinade in a separate bowl for later.

Place the thighs in the remaining marinade.

Marinate in the fridge for at least 1 hour, but overnight is best.

Preheat oven to 375°F (190°C).

Place the chicken in a single layer on a baking pan. Bake the chicken for 25–30 minutes until it is cooked through.

Serve with rice or roasted potatoes. It also tastes great in a lettuce wrap.

Drizzle the reserved sauce on top.

Serving size: 1 chicken thigh
Protein: ~21 g
Carbs: ~1 g
Fat: ~11 g

Roasted Tomato and Onion with Shrimp Pasta

This is a quick, easy-to-clean-up meal. Eat the leftovers with lettuce and extra vegetables for lunch the next day.

8 Roma tomatoes, quartered
2 onions, quartered
3 cloves garlic
4 tablespoons extra-virgin olive oil
2 teaspoons salt
2 teaspoons pepper
4 teaspoons dried basil
4 teaspoons dried oregano

2 teaspoons dried chili flakes
1 lb peeled shrimp, thawed and
   drained
High-fiber pasta, or spaghetti
   squash or spiralized zucchini
   for grain-free options
1 tablespoon chopped fresh basil
Grated parmesan, to taste

Preheat the oven to 400°F (204°C).

On a rimmed sheet pan, layer the tomatoes, onions, and garlic. Drizzle with 3 tablespoons olive oil, 1 teaspoon salt, 1 teaspoon pepper, 2 teaspoons dried basil, 2 teaspoons oregano, and 1 teaspoon chili flakes. Mix until tomatoes and onions are well coated. Roast in the oven for 20–30 minutes. The tomatoes and onions should be charred slightly and most of the liquid should be gone.

Meanwhile, place the shrimp in a small bowl and drizzle with the remainder of the olive oil, salt, pepper, dried basil, oregano, and chili flakes (if using). Set aside.

For the last 10 minutes, add the shrimp to the sheet pan and cook through.

While the shrimp is cooking, boil the water for the pasta and cook to al dente.

Once the pasta is cooked, drain and return to the pot. Carefully add the tomato mixture to the pot with the juices, then top with the fresh basil. Mix and serve with a side salad for a quick, easy weeknight meal. Top with grated parmesan, if desired.

If using spaghetti squash or zucchini, place in a large bowl and add the shrimp and tomatoes to warm through.

Serving size: 1 cup (before adding the pasta or noodles)
Protein: ~17 g
Carbs: ~12 g per cup
Fat: ~9 g

Lasagna Rolls

This twist on the classic Italian dish combines cabbage rolls and lasagna. The rolls take some time to make, but it's worth it, and they freeze very well. Make them on the weekend for a ready-to-cook weekday meal. Add 20 minutes to the cooking time if you're preparing them from frozen.

1 head savoy cabbage
1 cup cottage cheese
2 teaspoons dried oregano
2 teaspoons dried basil
1 egg
1 tablespoon extra-virgin olive oil
1 lb ground beef or ground chicken
1 leek, sliced thinly
1 clove garlic, grated
1 teaspoon salt
2 teaspoons black pepper
2 cups pasta sauce

Cut out the core of the cabbage and carefully peel apart the leaves.

Bring a large pot of water to a boil. Place the cabbage leaves in the pot for 3–4 minutes (this may need to be done in batches if the cabbage was large).

Place the cooked leaves in a colander and drain well.

In a large bowl, mix together the cottage cheese, oregano, basil, and egg. Set aside.

In a large frying pan, heat the olive oil over medium-high heat and sauté the beef or chicken, breaking it up as you cook it.

Add the leek and garlic to the beef or chicken, and sauté until translucent. Add the salt and pepper and mix again. Then set the mixture aside to cool slightly before assembling the rolls.

In a large baking dish, spread ¼ cup of the pasta sauce.

In each cabbage leaf, put ½ cup of the cottage cheese mixture and ¼ cup beef or chicken.

Roll each leaf and place the seam down in the baking dish.

Continue until the baking dish is full and all the mixture is gone.

Top with the remaining pasta sauce.

Cover with foil and place in a 375°F (190°C) oven for 30-40 minutes.

With 15 minutes left, remove the foil to brown the tops.

Note: Top with dollops of goat cheese in the last 15 minutes.

Serving size: 1 roll (approx. 3 inches long and 2 inches wide)
Protein: ~14 g
Carbs: ~10 g
Fat: ~10 g

Easy Chickpea and Spinach Curry

2 tablespoons extra-virgin olive oil
1 onion, diced
2 garlic cloves, minced
1 tablespoon fresh ginger, minced
1 tablespoon curry powder
1 teaspoon cumin
1 teaspoon turmeric powder
½ teaspoon chili powder
1 can (28 fluid ounces) diced tomatoes
1 can (19 fluid ounces) chickpeas, drained and rinsed
2 cups fresh spinach
Sea salt or Himalayan salt, to taste

Heat the olive oil in a pan over medium heat. Add the onion, garlic, and ginger, and sauté until softened.

Stir in the curry powder, cumin, turmeric, and chili powder, and cook for another minute.

Add the diced tomatoes and cook for 5 minutes, allowing the flavors to meld.

Add the chickpeas and spinach and simmer for 10 minutes, until the spinach wilts and the curry thickens.

Serve over brown rice or quinoa. Add salt to taste.

Serving size: 1 cup curry
Protein: ~4 to 6 g
Carbs: ~25 to 35 g
Fat: ~9 to 13 g

DESSERT

Banana-Coconut-Oatmeal Chocolate Chip Cookies

By Lisa Tsakos

Cookies with benefits. These provide protein from coconut flour, fiber from the oats, potassium from the bananas, and magnesium from the chocolate chips, although they are optional.

DRY INGREDIENTS

1 cup gluten-free rolled oats (old-fashioned, not instant)
½ cup almond flour
¼ cup coconut flour
½ teaspoon baking soda
½ teaspoon cinnamon
¼ teaspoon sea salt
1 tablespoon ground flaxseed (optional, but recommended for binding)

WET INGREDIENTS

2 very ripe bananas
¼ cup Medjool dates (about 3 to 4 dates, soaked and mashed)
½ cup coconut oil or grass-fed butter, melted and cooled
1 egg
1 teaspoon pure vanilla extract

EXTRAS

½ cup dark chocolate chips
        (I like to chop up an extra-dark chocolate bar and
        mix in some raw cacao nibs)
¼ cup shredded unsweetened coconut
¼ cup dried goji berries or dried cranberries

OPTIONAL

¼ cup chopped walnuts or pecans

(Continues)

Preheat oven to 350°F (177°C) and line a baking sheet with parchment paper.

In a large bowl, mix all the dry ingredients.

In a separate bowl, mash the bananas thoroughly. Mix in the dates, coconut oil, egg, and vanilla.

Stir the wet ingredients into the dry ingredients until combined.

Let the dough rest for 5–7 minutes so the coconut flour absorbs moisture.

Fold in the chocolate and any other extras.

Drop 1-tablespoon mounds of the cookie dough onto the baking sheet.

Bake for 11–13 minutes, until bottoms of cookies are golden.

Cool the cookies on the pan for 5 minutes before transferring.

Note: On average, coconut flour has about 4–6 grams of protein per ¼ cup (30 g) serving, depending on the brand.

Makes about 20 cookies

Serving size: 1 cookie
Protein: ~3.5 g
Carbs: ~13 g (Fiber: ~3 g)
Fat: ~8 g

INDEX

Note: Page numbers followed by *t* indicate tables